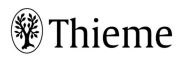

Critical Care Radiology

Cornelia Schaefer-Prokop, MD

Associate Professor of Radiology
Medical School Hanover, Germany

Radiology Department
Meander Medical Center
Amersfoort
Academic Medical Center (AMC)
Amsterdam
The Netherlands

With contributions by

M. Cejna, E. Eisenhuber-Stadler, M. Fuchsjaeger, G. Heinz-Peer, M. Hoermann, L. Kramer, S. Kreuzer, C. Loewe, S. Metz-Schimmerl, I. Noebauer-Huhmann, B. Partik, P. Pokieser, M. Prokop, T. Sautner, C. Schaefer-Prokop, W. Schima, E. Schober, A. Smets, A. Stadler, M. Uffmann, M. Walz, P. Wunderbaldinger

561 illustrations

Thieme
Stuttgart · New York

Library of Congress Cataloging-in-Publication Data
is available from the publisher.

This book is an authorized translation of
the German edition published and copyrighted 2009 by
Georg Thieme Verlag, Stuttgart,
Germany. Title of the German edition:
Radiologische Diagnostik in der Intensivmedizin.

Translator: Terry C. Telger, Fort Worth, Texas, USA

Illustrator: Helmut Holtermann, Dannenberg, Germany

© 2011 Georg Thieme Verlag,
Rüdigerstrasse 14, 70469 Stuttgart, Germany
http://www.thieme.de
Thieme New York, 333 Seventh Avenue,
New York, NY 10001, USA
http://www.thieme.com

Cover design: Thieme Publishing Group
Typesetting by: Druckhaus Götz GmbH,
Ludwigsburg, Germany
Printed in China by Everbest Printing Ltd,

ISBN 978-3-13-150051-9   1 2 3 4 5 6

This book is dedicated to my children

Preface

Perhaps more than in any other setting, the interpretation of radiological images in postoperative and intensive care patients requires an interdisciplinary exchange of information, and cooperation between the radiologist and the clinical team. The low specificity of many findings—especially in bedside chest radiographs and postoperative abdominal studies—does not diminish the value of intensive care radiology. Regular and active interdisciplinary information sharing will contribute greatly to accurate image interpretation and resulting management decisions. This book places special emphasis, therefore, on the differential diagnosis of morphologic findings and their interpretation within the clinical context, and on accurately discriminating between normal and abnormal findings.

The quality of radiographic images has improved dramatically in recent years as a result of digital technology. Computed tomography (CT) has assumed an expanding role owing to its rapid availability, short examination times, new indications, and its unrivaled diagnostic accuracy and efficiency. This efficiency results not only from short scan times, but also from the ability to image the body in arbitrary planes of section.

Consistent with my own interests, the reader will notice a particular emphasis on illustrative radiographic and CT images. I am indebted to all my friends and colleagues who contributed to this book, whether in the form of manuscripts or images. I thank the staff at Thieme Medical Publishers—especially Dr. S. Steindl and Dr. C. Urbanowicz—for their patience and help in bringing this project to completion. I am grateful to Prof. U. Moedder for his personal support. I thank my husband, and especially my children, for their support, their patience, and their understanding for the many hours of hard work.

I hope that this book will help radiologists, residents in radiology, and even clinicians to interpret the often difficult and nonspecific findings in children and adults, and that it will help to advance interdisciplinary cooperation in the diagnostic imaging of intensive care unit patients.

Cornelia Schaefer-Prokop

Contributors

Editor

Cornelia Schaefer-Prokop, MD
   Associate Professor of Radiology
   Medical School Hanover, Germany

   Radiology Department
   Meander Medical Center
   Amersfoort
   Academic Medical Center (AMC)
   Amsterdam
   The Netherlands

Contributing Authors

Manfred Cejna, MD
   Associate Pofessor of Radiology
   Chairman, Department of Radiology
   University Teaching Hospital LKH Feldkirch
   Feldkirch, Austria

Edith Eisenhuber-Stadler, MD
   Department of Radiology and Diagnostic Imaging
   Göttlicher Heiland Hospital and Herz-Jesu-Hospital
   Vienna, Austria

Michael Fuchsjaeger, MD
   Associate Professor of Radiology
   Department of Diagnostic Radiology
   Medical University of Vienna
   Vienna, Austria

Gertraud Heinz-Peer, MD
   Associate Professor of Radiology
   Department of Diagnostic Radiology
   Medical University of Vienna
   Vienna, Austria

Marcus Hoermann, MD
   Associate Professor of Radiology
   Department of Diagnostic Radiology
   Medical University of Vienna
   Vienna, Austria

Ludwig Kramer, MD
   Associate Professor of Internal Medicine
   Medical Clinic I
   Hietzing Hospital
   Vienna, Austria

Soeren H. Kreuzer, MD
   Assistant Professor of Radiology
   Department of Diagnostic Radiology
   Medical University of Vienna
   Vienna, Austria

Christian Loewe, MD
   Associate Professor of Radiology
   Department of Diagnostic Radiology
   Division of Cardiovascular and Interventional
   Radiology
   Medical University of Vienna
   Vienna, Austria

Sylvia Metz-Schimmerl, MD
   Assistant Professor
   Department of Diagnostic Radiology
   Medical University of Vienna
   Vienna, Austria

Iris-M. Noebauer-Huhmann, MD
   Assistant Professor of Radiology
   Department of Diagnostic Radiology
   Division of Osteology and Neuroradiology
   Medical University of Vienna
   Vienna, Austria

Bernhard Partik, MD
   Brigittenau Diagnostic Center
   Vienna, Austria

Peter Pokieser, MD
   Associate Professor of Radiology
   Chairman, Medical Media Services
   Vienna, Austria

Mathias Prokop, MD
   Professor of Radiology
   Chairman, Department of Radiology
   Radboud University Nijmegen Medical Center
   Nijmegen, Netherlands

Thomas Sautner, MD
   Associate Professor of Surgery
   Chairman, Department of Surgery
   St. Elisabeth Hospital
   Vienna, Austria

Wolfgang Schima, MD, MSc
   Associate Professor of Radiology
   Chairman, Department of Radiology
   Göttlicher Heiland Hospital and Herz-Jesu-Hospital
   Vienna, Austria

Ewald Schober, MD
   Department of Diagnostic Radiology
   Social Medical Center Baumgartner Höhe
   Otto Wagner Hospital
   Vienna, Austria

Anne Smets, MD
   Pediatric Radiologist
   Department of Radiology
   Academic Medical Center (AMC)
   Amsterdam, Netherlands

Alfred Stadler, MD
   Department of Radiology and Nuclear Medicine
   Hospital Hietzig
   Vienna, Austria

Martin Uffmann, MD
   Associate Professor of Radiology
   Chairman, Department of Diagnostic Radiology
   Landesklinikum Neunkirchen
   Neunkirchen, Austria

Michael Walz, MD
   Hessen Center for Quality Assurance in Radiology
   Life Science GmbH
   Eschborn, Germany

Patrick Wunderbaldinger, MD
   Favoriten Diagnostic Center
   Vienna, Austria

Abbreviations

ALI	acute lung injury		HPS	hypertrophic pyloric stenosis
AP	anteroposterior		HRCT	high-resolution computed tomography
ARDS	adult (acute) respiratory distress syndrome		IAPB	intra-aortic balloon pump
ATS	American Thoracic Society		ICD	implantable cardioverter defibrillator
AV	arteriovenous		ICRP	International Commission on Radiological
BAL	bronchoalveolar lavage			Protection
BPD	bronchopulmonary dysplasia		ICU	intensive care unit
BPF	bronchopleural fistula		IPPB	intermittent positive pressure breathing
CAP	community-acquired pneumonia		IRDS	infantile respiratory distress syndrome
CAPD	chronic abdominal peritoneal dialysis		IVP	intravenous pyelogram
CCAM	congenital cystic adenomatoid malformation		LDH	lactate dehydrogenase
CDH	congenital diaphragmatic hernia		LIS	Lung Injury Score
CK	creatine kinase		MAS	meconium aspiration syndrome
CLL	chronic lymphoblastoid (lymphocytic)		MCL	midclavicular line
	leukemia		MPR	multiplanar reformation
CMV	cytomegalovirus		MRI	magnetic resonance imaging
COP	cryptogenic organizing pneumonia		MRSA	methicillin-resistant *Staphylococcus aureus*
COPD	chronic obstructive pulmonary disease		NEC	necrotizing enterocolitis
CPAP	continuous positive airway pressure		NOMI	nonocclusive mesenteric ischemia
CPIS	Clinical Pulmonary Infection Score		NSIP	nonspecific interstitial pneumonia
CR	computed radiography		PA	posteroanterior
CT	computed tomography		PBB	protected brush bronchoscopy
CTDI	computed tomography dose index		PCN	percutaneous nephrostomy
CVC	central venous catheter		PCP	pneumocystis pneumonia
DAD	diffuse alveolar lavage		PD	pancreaticoduodenectomy
DAP	dose–area product		PE	pulmonary embolism
DLP	dose–length product		PEEP	positive end-expiratory pressure
DR	digital radiography		PEG	percutaneous endoscopic gastronomy
DSA	digital subtraction angiography		PG	prostaglandin
EBV	Epstein–Barr virus		PIE	pulmonary interstitial emphysema
ECG	electrocardiography		RAO	right anterior oblique
ECMO	extracorporeal membrane oxygenation		RSV	repiratory syncytial virus
EPF	esophagopleural fistula		SDD	surfactant deficiency disease
ETT	endotracheal tube		SLE	systemic lupus erythmatosus
FFD	film–focus distance		TTN	transient tachypnea of the newborn
FRC	functional residual capacity		TUR	transurethral resection
GI	gastrointestinal		UAC	umbilical artery catheter
GvHD	graft-versus-host disease		UVC	umbilical vein catheter
HFV	high-frequency ventilation		VAP	ventilator-associated pneumonia
HIV	human immunodeficiency virus		VILI	ventilator-induced lung injury
HMD	hyaline membrane disease		VZV	varicella-zoster virus

Contents

1   Basic Principles: Radiologic Techniques and Radiation Safety ... 1

Radiologic Techniques in the Intensive Care Unit ..   1
C. Schaefer-Prokop

Radiation Exposure and Radiation Safety   3
A. Stadler

**Communication, Reporting of Findings,
and Teleradiology**   7
M. Walz and C. Schaefer-Prokop

2   Thoracic Imaging of the Intensive Care Patient ... 9

Technique of Portable Chest Radiography   9
C. Schaefer-Prokop

Communication between Radiologists and Clinicians   13
C. Schaefer-Prokop

Catheters and Monitoring Devices   14
E. Eisenhuber-Stadler and P. Wunderbaldinger

**Pulmonary Hemodynamics and Edema in ICU
Patients**   29
S. Metz-Schimmerl and C. Schaefer-Prokop

Adult Respiratory Distress Syndrome   37
I. Noebauer-Huhmann, L. Kramer, and C. Schaefer-Prokop

Pneumonia   49
C. Schaefer-Prokop and E. Eisenhuber-Stadler
Aspiration and Aspiration Pneumonia   56
Pneumonia during Mechanical Ventilation   61

ARDS and Pneumonia   63
Septic Pneumonia   63
Pneumonia in Immunodeficient or Immuno-
suppressed Patients   64
Complications of Pneumonia   67

Atelectasis   70
E. Eisenhuber-Stadler

Pneumothorax   74
E. Eisenhuber-Stadler and S. Metz-Schimmerl
Tension Pneumothorax   78

Pleural Effusion   80
C. Schaefer-Prokop

Acute Pulmonary Embolism   86
S. Metz-Schimmerl and C. Schaefer-Prokop

3   Imaging of Intensive Care Patients after Thoracic Surgery ... 93
M. Fuchsjaeger and C. Schaefer-Prokop

Pneumonectomy   93

Lobectomy   101

Segmental Lung Resection   102

Sleeve Resection   103

Lung Transplantation   103

Cardiovascular Surgery   106

Heart Transplantation   109

Esophageal Surgery   110

4 Acute Abdomen in Intensive Care Patients ... 113

Acute Pancreatitis 113
M. Uffmann

Acute Cholecystitis and Cholangitis 120
M. Uffmann

Acute (Pyelo)nephritis (Urosepsis) 123
G. Heinz-Peer

Acute Renal Failure 127
G. Heinz-Peer

Acute Gastrointestinal Bleeding 129
C. Loewe, E. Schober, and M. Ceijna

Inflammatory Bowel Diseases 135
E. Schober and C. Schaefer-Prokop

Infectious Enterocolitis 135
Pseudomembranous Enterocolitis 136
Graft-versus-Host Disease of the Bowel 136
Toxic Megacolon 136
Diverticulitis 137

Acute Intestinal Ischemia 140
W. Schima and M. Prokop

5 Imaging of Intensive Care Patients after Abdominal Surgery ... 147

Abdominal Drainage 147
B. Partik and P. Pokieser

Types of Abdominal Drains and their Applications . 147
Feeding Tubes 148
Biliary Drainage 148
Urinary Tract Drainage 149

Normal Postoperative Findings 150
S. Kreuzer and C. Schaefer-Prokop

Postoperative (Physiologic) Fluid Collections 150
Postoperative (Physiologic) Intestinal Atony 150
Postoperative Pneumoperitoneum 150

Postoperative Complications 151
C. Schaefer-Prokop, S. Kreuzer, T. Sautner, and W. Schima
Postoperative Bleeding 153
Postoperative Sepsis and Focus Identification 154

Peritonitis 156
Abscess 158
Postoperative Bowel Obstruction 163

Complications of Specific Operations 169
C. Schaefer-Prokop, S. Kreuzer, and T. Sautner

After Esophageal Surgery 169
After Pancreatic Surgery (Whipple Operation) 171
After Biliary Tract Surgery 173
After Cholecystectomy 173
After Colorectal Surgery 174
After (Partial) Nephrectomy 176
After Renal Transplantation 176
After Liver Transplantation 178
After Surgery or Stenting of an Aortic Aneurysm .. 179

6 Thoracic Imaging of the Pediatric Intensive Care Patient ... 183
A. Smets and C. Schaefer-Prokop

Normal Thoracic Findings in Newborns 183
During Mechanical Ventilation 185

Catheter Position: Normal Findings and Malposition 185

Transient Tachypnea of the Newborn (Wet Lung) .. 187

Infantile Respiratory Distress Syndrome 188

Meconium Aspiration Syndrome 190

Neonatal Pneumonia 190

Complications during or after Mechanical Ventilation 191
Pulmonary Interstitial Emphysema 191
Pneumomediastinum 191
Pneumothorax 192
Postextubation Atelectasis 193

Hemorrhage 193
Bronchopulmonary Dysplasia 193

Congenital Lung Diseases with Respiratory Failure at Birth 194
Tracheoesophageal Fistulas 194
Congenital Lobar Emphysema 195
Congenital Cystic Adenomatoid Malformation 196
Congenital Diaphragmatic Hernia (Bochdalek Hernia) 196
Congenital Lymphangiectasia and Chylothorax 197

Acute Obstruction of the Upper Airways 197
Acute Retropharyngeal Abscess 197
Foreign Body Aspiration 198
Acute Epiglottitis, Croup, Exudative Tracheitis, and Tonsillitis 200

Asthma 200

(Viral) Bronchiolitis 201

Pneumonia 203

7 Acute Abdomen in the Pediatric Intensive Care Patient ... 207

M. Hoermann

Meconium Ileus 208

Necrotizing Enterocolitis 209

Malrotation and Volvulus 211

Gastrointestinal Atresia and Stenosis 213

Congenital Megacolon (Hirschsprung Disease) 214
Clinical Aspects 214

Hypertrophic Pyloric Stenosis 215

Intussusception 215

Appendix ... 219

Further Reading 219

Index 231

Basic Principles: Radiologic Techniques and Radiation Safety

Radiologic Techniques in the Intensive Care Unit 1
Radiation Exposure and Radiation Safety 3
Communication, Reporting of Findings,
and Teleradiology 7

Radiologic Techniques in the Intensive Care Unit

C. Schaefer-Prokop

Radiologic examinations in the intensive care unit (ICU) are most commonly performed at the bedside. They consist mainly of portable chest radiographs, followed by ultrasound scans. Projection radiographs of the skeleton are only rarely obtained. Much as in other clinical settings, computed tomography (CT) has assumed an expanding role in the ICU. CT scans are obtained at an increasingly early stage for addressing diagnostic problems of the chest and abdomen. This relates to the generally higher diagnostic efficiency of CT over other modalities, the capabilities of modern scanners in the detection of vascular pathology (pulmonary embolism, intestinal ischemia), and the use of CT for image-guided interventions (e. g., abscess drainage).

The following typical problems are encountered in the diagnostic imaging of ICU patients:

- Patients have limited ability to cooperate with the examiner.
- Imaging conditions are more difficult than in the radiology department (chest imaged in a supine or sitting position, limited access for ultrasound scans, etc.).
- Radiographic interpretation is often hampered by superimposed foreign materials (dressings, metal implants, catheters, tubes, wires).
- Radiographic equipment is frequently limited (portable radiography machine), and images are obtained without automatic exposure control.
- If the patient is taken to the radiology department (e. g., for CT, MRI, DSA), the gain in diagnostic information must be weighed against the increased risk of transporting the patient.

Radiographic Equipment

The following basic radiological equipment should be available in the ICU:

- a portable radiography machine
- storage phosphor cassettes, or cassette-based direct detectors with a 35 × 43 cm format—may be used as a grid-film cassette or with a Bucky device for inserting standard film cassettes
- radiation protection aprons (lead equivalency of 0.25–0.5 mm) and protective gloves
- portable radiation screens for some applications
- viewboxes or video monitors for viewing images (large enough for viewing and comparing two or three large-format films)
- ultrasound scanner with documentation system

The number of radiography machines and the scope of accessory equipment will depend on the number of ICU beds and on special hygienic requirements. Larger units and suites should be equipped with their own film processor or digital reader device. A portable fluoroscopy machine with its own table should be available in a separate examination room. Portable CT scanners have been tested under study conditions but have not come into practical use due to technical limitations.

Conventional Film–Screen Radiography

⬚ Digital radiography has almost completely replaced conventional film–screen radiography in ICUs.

Conventional film–screen radiography has been replaced by digital radiography in almost all ICUs and is mentioned here only for completeness. A conventional cassette contains the x-ray film and a pair of intensifying screens placed at the front and back of the cassette. These film–screen combinations are characterized by their spatial resolution and dose requirement, which determine the speed rating of the system (50, 100, 200, 400, 800, or 1600). Faster systems require a lower radiation dose but also sacrifice some degree of spatial resolution. Film–screen combinations with a speed rating of 400 ("400 systems") are used for radiographs in ICU patients and for most applications in emergency medicine, while 100 or 200 systems are used only in the evaluation of limb injuries (traumatology). Imaging with a scatter-reduction grid provides higher image quality than filming without a grid. While the use of a grid requires a higher exposure level (dose is generally increased by a "grid factor" of 2–3), this can be partially offset by using a higher tube voltage (120 kV instead of 80 kV for chest films).

Digital Radiography

⬚ Computed radiography is the standard in ICUs and emergency rooms; digital radiography machines have also become available in recent years.

Digital radiography has become the mainstay for image acquisition and documentation in ICUs and emergency rooms owing to its technical advantages.

The advantages of digital technology relate to organizational aspects (digital data format with capabilities for data transfer and image distribution to multiple users) and its lack of sensitivity to underpenetration and poor contrast due to exposure errors. These advantages are based on the digital data format, image processing including automated signal normalization, and the greater dynamic range of digital detectors compared with x-ray film.

Computed radiography (CR), or storage phosphor radiography, is the current standard in intensive care radiology. Mobile flat-panel or direct radiography (DR) systems have recently become available in the 35 × 43 cm format. The advantage of DR is the greater dose efficiency of the system, which permits ca. 50% dose reduction during the examination.

Computed radiography. CR (**Fig. 1.1a**) is comparable in its handling to a daylight system. It is a cassette-based system that requires a special reader device. The detector consists of a photostimulable storage phosphor plate housed in an aluminum cassette. After the plate has been exposed, the cassette is placed into the reader. The radiographic image can either be printed on film (hard copy) or displayed on a video monitor (soft copy).

— **Practical Recommendation** —————————

Computed radiography basically uses the same technical factors (kV, grid, mAs) as film–screen radiography. Dose reduction to below 400 speed is not recommended, even when modern imaging plates are used. Neither should the dose be increased, as this does not add to diagnostic information, at least under study conditions.

Direct detector units. Direct detector units (**Fig. 1.1b**) consist of the imaging cassette, which contains the detector and is hardwired to the readout unit by an electric cable. This means that the technician must take the readout unit to the patient's bedside along with the rest of the system, which will naturally affect workflow and organizational details. The advantage of DR over CR is its higher dose efficiency, which allows for a significant dose reduction (30–50%, depending on the patient's condition). Another advantage is the direct availability of the image on the readout unit, which provides immediate feedback on imaging parameters.

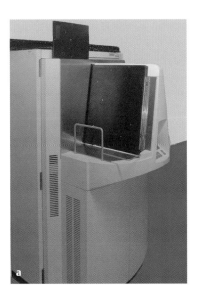 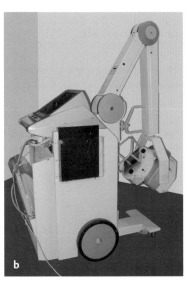

Fig. 1.1 a, b **Equipment for digital radiography.**
a Computed radiography.
b Flat-panel system for direct radiography.

Radiation Exposure and Radiation Safety

A. Stadler

Issues of medical radiation safety are rarely a priority concern in emergency and ICU patients, even though the patients may be exposed to considerable dose levels. One problem is that trauma patients in particular must often undergo comprehensive imaging protocols that involve high individual doses during the acute phase of treatment. Another problem is that even low individual doses per examination may well produce a significant cumulative exposure when continued over a period of weeks.

Radiation Exposure to Patients and Staff

The supine anteroposterior (AP) chest radiograph is the most common imaging examination in the ICU, especially in patients on long-term ventilation. More than 100 radiographs may be taken during a prolonged stay in the ICU. While various dose values have been reported in the literature, the effective dose in all cases was less than 0.2 mSv per radiograph. CT examinations expose patients to significantly higher effective dose values than chest radiographs (**Table 1.1**). The values listed in the table are only approximations, however, as the effective dose depends strongly on equipment and examination parameters.

Assessment of Patient Risk

A portable chest radiograph generally exposes the patient to more radiation than a film taken on a wall-mounted cassette holder, depending on the selected parameters (**Table 1.2**). This is due mainly to the shorter film–focus distance (FFD) at the bedside and the use of an AP rather than posteroanterior (PA) projection (increasing the effective dose to females by a factor of 1.9, to males by a factor of 1.6). The dose increase associated with the use of a scatter-reduction grid (grid cassettes) can be partially offset by a higher kilovoltage setting.

The risk coefficients defined by the ICRP (International Commission on Radiological Protection) in 1991 are useful for estimating the bioeffects of radiation. The likelihood that a 30-year-old individual will develop a radiation-induced malignancy is estimated at 5% per sievert (4.5%/Sv for solid cancers, 0.5%/Sv for leukemia; ICRP 60; see also **Table 1.5**). The latent period for developing leukemia is ca. 15 years compared with 40 years for other malignant diseases. This latent period is a particular concern in older individuals. Based on the above percentages, an ICU patient who receives 100 chest radiographs (total dose of 0.02 Sv based on single doses of 20 µSv) will have an additional 0.1% risk for developing a malignant disease (**Table 1.3**). Since approximately one in four people

will develop a malignancy during their lifetime, the chest radiographs in the above example will increase the risk from 25% to 25.1%.

Thus, even in a setting of long-term intensive care involving multiple radiographic examinations, the patient will not face a significant additional cancer risk, especially when we consider the severity of the condition for which the patient is receiving intensive care.

Radiation Exposure during Pregnancy

Acute illness or injury in a pregnant woman, while rare, is a challenging management problem. One aspect of the problem concerns the use of roentgen rays and the resulting radiation exposure to the embryo or fetus. Antenatal

> ▸ Even numerous radiographic examinations do not pose a significant additional cancer risk in ICU patients.

> ▸ A portable chest radiograph exposes the patient to more radiation than a film taken on a wall-mounted cassette holder.

Table 1.1 Typical effective doses from various radiographic examinations

Type of examination	Typical effective dose
PA chest radiograph	0.025 mSv
AP chest radiograph	0.06 mSv
AP abdominal radiograph	1 mSv
Cranial CT	2.3 mSv
Thoracic CT	8 mSv
Abdominal/pelvic CT	10 mSv

Table 1.2 Radiation exposure from a portable chest radiograph compared with a radiograph taken on a wall-mounted cassette (modified from Luska)

	Upright chest radiograph (wall-mounted cassette)	Portable chest radiograph (Mobilett)	Relative dose increase
Projection	PA	AP	1.6–1.9
kV	125	80	1.4
FFD	2 m	1 m	1.2
Grid	12:40	Without a grid / grid cassette	0.2–0.8
Effective dose	25 µSv	20–60 µSv	0.8–2.4

FFD, film–focus distance.

Table 1.3 Examples of total effective dose and risk assessment in several radiologic examinations

Radiologic examinations	Total dose	Risk of a malignant disease
20 Chest radiographs	4 mSv	0.02%
5 Abdominal radiographs	5 mSv	0.025%
3 Cranial CTs	6.9 mSv	0.0345%
5 Thoracic CTs	40 mSv	0.2%
5 Abdominal CTs	50 mSv	0.25%

exposure to ionizing radiation can potentially lead to two types of pathology: malignancies and malformations.

Malignancies. As in adults, radiation exposure of the fetus increases the risk of malignant disease. For example, antenatal exposure to 10 mGy leads theoretically to a 3.5-fold increase in cancer risk. This means that the natural risk of 0.07 % would be increased to 0.25 %.

Malformations. It is generally agreed that antenatal radiation exposure must exceed a threshold value to induce malformations. Exposure below the threshold is not considered harmful, while exposure above the threshold within a certain time window (2nd to 15th week of gestation) may cause a developmental abnormality. The exact threshold is difficult to define, but a value of 100 mGy is generally assumed. Because the fetal dose from a single examination tends to be well below 50 mGy, even high-dose examinations should not cause fetal harm. As an example, one of the most common emergency examinations in pregnant patients, the CT detection of pulmonary embolism, will deliver a fetal dose less than 0.2 mGy. This dose is several orders of magnitude below the threshold value.

> The threshold uterine dose in pregnant patients is generally considered to be 100 mGy. Exposures below that level do not pose a risk to the fetus.

Management after radiation exposure. In pregnant women who have undergone a radiographic examination, it is often appropriate to ask whether pregnancy termination is necessary or should at least be considered, especially in cases where the pregnancy is not detected until after the examination. A three-stage concept should be used for assessing the level of exposure and deciding on further management:

1. Tables are used initially to make a gross estimate of the radiation dose to the uterus. If the gross estimate is less than 20 mSv, the physician indicates this in the patient's record and notes also that there is no radiologic indication for terminating the pregnancy.
2. If the gross estimate exceeds 20 mSv, the dose should be estimated more precisely by taking into account the imaging technical parameters, equipment data, and patient data. If the revised estimate is less than 100 mSv, this is noted in the patient's record. The patient is informed of the result, and again the physician does not recommend pregnancy termination.
3. If the estimate exceeds 100 mSv, the dose is calculated as accurately as possible based on all available information. If this confirms that the exposure exceeded 100 mSv, the physician consults with the patient and weighs the risk of continuing the pregnancy against the patient's desire to have a child. Given the risks involved, the physician would support a desire to terminate the pregnancy. If the calculated exposure exceeds 200 mSv, the physician will usually recommend termination.

> Low-dose examinations of pregnant patients may be performed without concern, whereas high-dose examinations should be subject to rigorous selection criteria.

Table 1.4 High-dose and low-dose categories of emergency radiographic examinations

Low-dose examinations	High-dose examinations
Radiography of the limbs	Pelvic radiography
Chest radiography	Abdominal radiography
Thoracic CT	Abdominal CT
Cranial CT	Abdominal fluoroscopy

Again, it should be emphasized that below a uterine threshold dose of 100 mSv, the expectant mother may be assured that all emergency (noninterventional) radiologic examinations are safe. In all cases the imaging parameters should be documented in full detail. Ideally, patients should be given a dosimeter, especially in combined or interventional procedures, so that an accurate retrospective determination of uterine dose can be made with the help of a medical physicist.

There is no evidence that the use of nonionic contrast media poses a hazard to the fetus or embryo.

High-dose and low-dose examinations. Emergency radiologic examinations can be conveniently divided into high-dose and low-dose examinations (**Table 1.4**). Low-dose examinations may be performed without concern, whereas high-dose examinations should be based on rigorous patient selection criteria and should be weighed against alternative modalities (ultrasonography, MRI).

— **Practical Recommendation** —————————

In summary, there is no need to alter management protocols for radiation safety reasons in the acute care of pregnant patients when careful selection criteria are applied. There are isolated instances where repeated high-dose examinations during long-term care and interventional procedures may pose a potential risk to the fetus, in which case management should be discussed in consultation with the clinician, radiologist, and possibly a medical physicist.

Radiation Exposure in Children

Children should be considered separately in the evaluation of radiation-induced risks. On the one hand, children are more radiosensitive than adults. For any given dose, the risk of developing a radiation-induced malignancy is several times higher in a newborn than in an adult (**Table 1.5**). Another consideration is that for any given examination such as cranial CT, the effective dose to a pediatric patient will be several times higher than the dose to an adult. As an example, the statistical risk of abdominal CT in a 1-year-old child is of the order of one induced cancer per 1000 examinations—a risk that is by no means negligible.

CT scans are most likely to cause significant radiation exposure in emergency radiology, especially during abdominal examinations. By comparison, the exposure from

Table 1.5 Calculated radiation-associated risk of dying from cancer (ICRP 60)

Age	Risk (deaths/mSv)
Newborn (4 weeks)	18/100 000
Small child (2 years)	13/100 000
Child (7 years)	10/100 000
Adolescent (14 years)	7.5/100 000
Adult (30 years)	6/100 000
Adult (60 years)	2.5/100 000
Adult (80 years)	1.5/100 000
Average	5/100 000

Table 1.6 Recommended reduction of mAs in pediatric cranial CT examinations as a function of age

Age	% of adult mAs dose
<6 months	25
6 months to 3 years	40
3–6 years	65
>6 years	100

Table 1.7 Recommended reduction of mAs in pediatric abdominal and thoracic CT examinations as a function of body weight

Body weight (kg)	% of adult mAs dose	
	Abdomen	Chest
<15	15	15
15–24	25	25
25–34	40	35
35–44	60	50
45–54	80	75
<54	100	100

conventional radiographs is several orders of magnitude less. This emphasizes the importance of modifying the scan protocols in CT for dose optimization.

The original dose can be reduced by almost half by decreasing the tube voltage to 80–100 kV. The smaller diameter of pediatric patients compared with adults allows for a significant reduction of the mAs while maintaining an acceptable signal-to-noise ratio (**Tables 1.6, 1.7**). Equipment manufacturers have offered increasingly optimized protocols in recent years. Regardless of this, it is absolutely essential to select patients carefully and to use alternative modalities (ultrasonography, MRI) whenever possible, especially in the pediatric age group.

Principles of Dose Reduction to Staff

The best way to avoid radiation exposure to staff is by following the *distance squared law*. For example, the radiation dose from laterally directed scattered radiation may equal 2 μGy at a distance of 1 m from the source,

but falls to 0.5 μGy at a distance of 2 m. Thus, doubling the distance reduces the radiation dose by 75%.

The effect of *lead aprons* can be assessed in terms of their lead equivalency, which is indicated on the apron. An apron with a lead equivalency of 0.1 mm will reduce the radiation dose by half, while a value of 0.4 mm will reduce the dose by 90%.

Further dose reduction can be achieved by using *lead screens* in conjunction with the portable radiography machine.

— Practical Recommendation —

CT is associated with a characteristic spatial distribution of scattered radiation. Radiation exposure can be greatly reduced by standing in the *radiation shadow* cast at a *lateral oblique angle* to the gantry. This is particularly advised in cases where patients require ventilation or close surveillance, and for persons who must be present in the scanning room during interventional procedures.

Assessment of Risk to Staff

Various studies performed in ICUs and emergency rooms have consistently shown that even without a lead apron, staff exposure is reduced to a negligible level by keeping a minimum distance of ca. 1.5 m from the radiation source. When this rule is followed in the ICU, there is no need to interrupt nursing actions or medical procedures when a patient is admitted to the adjacent bay. At a distance of 3 m, the scattered radiation from a bedside chest radiograph is no greater than one hour's exposure to natural environmental background radiation.

Regarding protection from scattered radiation when patients are admitted to the same room, regulations state that only cross-table projections require the use of a portable lead screen (while also maintaining a minimum distance of 1.5 m from the source tube).

Typical extrapolated values for nursing staff are less than 0.1 mSv/year. This is less than 10% of the permissible dose, which is 1 mSv/year for the general population, and less than 5% of the natural background radiation dose of 2.4 mSv/year. Studies performed in neonatal ICUs have indicated even lower levels of radiation exposure to nursing staff, other patients, and visitors.

Dose Reduction in Computed Tomography

The volume CT dose index ($CTDI_{vol}$) is the most important radiation dose measure used in designing protocols for CT examinations. The $CTDI_{vol}$ indicates the average *local* dose within the scanned volume and is directly displayed on most modern scanners. It permits an immediate assessment of the relative dose delivered by the selected scanning protocol. The effect of technical factors such as

Emergency abdominal CT examinations deliver the highest radiation dose to children, making it necessary to apply rigorous criteria in patient selection.

Staff members can avoid significant x-ray exposure by keeping a distance of at least 1.5 m from the radiation source.

pitch, mAs, kV, filtering, etc. is already included in the index. The dose-length product (DLP) also takes into account the scan length. This means that standard CT scanning protocols can be modified for dose optimization by documenting the dose indices displayed on the scanner and evaluating the diagnostic accuracy that is obtained. The approximate effective patient dose can be estimated by using "conversion factors" that additionally take into account the anatomical region that is scanned.

The following parameters are essential in achieving the desired dose reduction in CT:

- number of passes (biphasic studies, delayed scans)
- scan length (preferably limited to the region of interest)
- Patient dose is directly proportional to mAs. But as the mAs is decreased, image noise increases correspondingly. Often the mAs can be significantly reduced in thin patients and children compared with standard protocols.
- The CTDI depends on the tube current. Reducing the voltage from 120 to 80 kV decreases the CTDI by a factor of 2.2. It is advisable to use a high kilovoltage, however, when scanning regions of high radiographic density in obese patients.
- Greater slice thicknesses result in less image noise and allow for a reduction in mAs.
- Imaging with soft kernels will also reduce image noise, allowing for lower mAs values.
- Wherever possible, the gonads and breasts should be outside the scanned region. This can often be achieved with careful positioning technique. The gonads should be protected with a leaded rubber apron or gonad shield. It is good practice in children to protect the unscanned body region (even outside the gonads) with leaded rubber shields.

Dose Reduction in Digital Radiography

Computed radiography. Digital radiographic techniques are widely used in modern ICUs. The detector used in computed radiography (CR) is a storage phosphor plate housed in a rigid cassette. The dose efficiency of these detectors has been continuously improved in recent years. The latest generation of imaging plates (Fuji ST-Vn or comparable plates from other manufacturers) requires the dose for a conventional 400-speed film and provides an image quality that is superior in many respects to conventional radiographs.

While dose reduction in CR does not underexpose the image owing to automatic contrast and density control, it does lead to increased image noise and thus poorer structural contrast, especially in high-absorption regions like the mediastinum. Increasing the dose reduces image noise but does not improve the delineation of structures (under standardized study conditions) and does not add diagnostic information. Consequently, there is no rationale for using increased dose levels in CR.

The imaging dose cannot be visually assessed on the basis of film blackening as it can in conventional radiography, but image noise in CR provides feedback that is useful for dose evaluation.

Manufacturers also offer various types of data that serve as "dose indicators" (S values in Fuji-based systems, LgM values in Agfa systems, EI values in Kodak systems). These values may be based on the histogram of image pixel values (S value), they may indicate the dose-area product (Philips), or they may indicate deviations from the average imaging dose for that body region (Agfa). Their purpose is to permit a relative dose assessment while preventing the dose level from creeping upward or downward. This is a particular hazard with bedside radiographs in the ICU, which are taken without automatic exposure control.

— Practical Recommendation

The S numbers in Fuji based CR systems may deviate over time by as much as 30–50%. These deviations result from histogram changes and do not indicate a true, significant change in the imaging dose. Variations of the mean initial value that are greater than 50% should be investigated by a technician.

Direct detector systems. Flat-panel direct detector systems give a direct readout of the dose-area product in mGy (patient entrance dose). These systems have recently come onto the market, and portable models are also available. Recent publications and our own experience indicate an option for 30–50% dose reduction compared with a 400 system, without causing a significant loss of image quality. Images acquired at conventional dose levels yield better quality in the high-absorption region of the mediastinum.

A general dose reduction (<400 speed) is not recommended for CR. Increasing the dose does not add diagnostic information and should be avoided.

Communication, Reporting of Findings, and Teleradiology

*M. Walz and
C. Schaefer-Prokop*

Ordering Examinations and Reporting Findings

Type of order. The orders for radiology services fall into two main categories: routine and emergency.

- Routine services can be smoothly integrated into the workflow of the ICU and require a one-time coordination of the departments involved. Persons should be available in the ICU to assist with setting up the equipment or taking the radiographs; other staff members may exit the area to avoid exposure.
- Emergency orders should be performed immediately and rely on the prompt availability of necessary staff and equipment, usually furnished by the radiology department.

Content. A written or electronic request for radiology services should include all patient data, the desired examination, the radiology history, and the clinical problem with up-to-date clinical information. In women of childbearing age, the order should note an existing or possible pregnancy or confirm that pregnancy has been excluded. This information forms the basis for a clinically meaningful radiology report while providing a justified indication for the examination itself. From an organizational standpoint, it is also important to designate a physician responsible for x-ray use—someone who is present on site, available at short notice, and authorized to give instructions to the radiologic technologist. A different physician may exercise this role on different days of the week or at different times of day (e.g., a radiology department physician during routine work hours, an ICU physician at night and on weekends). If the physician making the justified indication is in the radiology department, he or she must be able to rely on the clinical information that has been provided, and so a legally valid order signed by a physician is recommended.

Clinical information. The following clinical information is relevant to the interpretation of radiologic findings:

- patient's history and condition (level of consciousness, mechanical ventilation)
- nature, course, and dates of previous operations, trauma, hemorrhage, aspirations, mass transfusions, shock, or adverse drug reactions
- nature, course, and dates of previous endoscopies, biopsies, or catheterizations of hollow organs, body cavities, vessels, or parenchymal organs
- acute or preexisting impairment of cardiac, renal or cerebral function
- current values for blood-gas analysis, blood pressure, and ventilation
- previous radiographs, including radiographs taken elsewhere

Reporting of findings. The protocols for interpreting images and reporting the findings are different for routine orders and emergency orders. While joint conferences in the ICU have proven best for routine services, emergency orders require direct reporting of findings because the results may have immediate therapeutic implications. Depending on circumstances, the findings may be reported by telephone, by direct conversation, in written form, or as a voice recording if an electronic dictation system is available. Other, digital options are the use of text blocks or a speech recognition system for the rapid creation of digitized text.

Conferences. Regular joint conferences are held to review relevant historical and clinical data, discuss current findings, and consider possible further diagnostic and therapeutic actions. Interdisciplinary clinical/radiologic/pathologic conferences for retrospective case analysis and the discussion of errors are a useful tool for quality assurance and improvement.

Information sharing. The frequent low specificity of morphologic findings in the chest underscores the importance of interdisciplinary cooperation in the care of ICU patients, as the interpretation of radiologic findings is greatly influenced by an awareness of clinical parameters such as fluid balance, ventilation therapy, and inflammatory markers.

The necessary flow of information between the clinician and radiologist is most effectively maintained by conducting regular joint rounds, but should also function when needed in response to acute problem cases. Clinical information plays a crucial role in intensive-care radiography, because image analysis must take into account not only the multitude of primary pathologic processes, but also any previous therapeutic and/or diagnostic measures, which may influence the detectability of findings and will definitely affect their interpretation.

> A system must be in place for the immediate implementation of emergency radiology orders in the ICU.

> A radiology report has high "evidential value" only when validated by a handwritten or digital signature.

▬ *Summary* ▬

Radiologic examinations in the intensive care unit (ICU) are most commonly performed at the bedside and consist mainly of portable chest radiographs followed by ultrasonography. **Digital radiography** has almost completely replaced conventional film–screen radiography in this setting. Computed radiography has become the standard in ICUs and emergency rooms, and digital radiography machines have also become available in recent years.

Portable chest radiographs are associated with higher **radiation exposure** than films taken on a wall-mounted cassette holder, but even numerous examinations in ICU patients will not significantly increase their cancer risk.

Pregnant patients can safely undergo low-dose examinations in an emergency, whereas high-dose examinations should be subject to rigorous selection criteria.

Staff members in the ICU can avoid significant x-ray exposure by keeping a distance of at least 1.5 m from the radiation source.

A system must be in place in ICU for the **immediate implementation** of emergency radiologic orders. The radiologist must be provided with clinical information that is relevant to interpreting the radiologic findings. Emergency orders require the **direct reporting of findings** because the results may have immediate therapeutic implications. **Hospital information systems** can expedite and facilitate workflow by providing an efficient framework for distributing images and radiology reports.

Thoracic Imaging of the Intensive Care Patient

Technique of Portable Chest Radiography   9
Communication between Radiologists and Clinicians .   13
Catheters and Monitoring Devices   14
Pulmonary Hemodynamics and Edema in ICU Patients   29
Adult Respiratory Distress Syndrome   37

Pneumonia   49
Atelectasis   70
Pneumothorax   74
Pleural Effusion   80
Acute Pulmonary Embolism   86

Approximately 30% of all chest radiographs are taken at the bedside. The American Thoracic Society (ATS) still recommends that daily routine chest radiographs be obtained for:

- patients on mechanical ventilation
- patients with acute cardiopulmonary problems

Immediate chest radiographs are recommended:

- after the insertion or replacement of most medical devices (endotracheal tubes, catheters, drains, etc.)

A clinical indication for chest radiographs exists in:

- patients under cardiac surveillance

However, the old policy of "routine daily radiographs" in the intensive care unit (ICU) is no longer followed today, owing to greater awareness of the radiation risks and mounting pressures to curtail costs.

Published reports on the frequency of "unexpected" findings on routine chest radiographs range from less than 1% to more than 40%. A study of 525 routine portable chest radiographs taken in a surgical ICU yielded significant cardiopulmonary findings in less than 1% of the patients. In a medical ICU, on the other hand, 45% of 500 routine chest radiographs were abnormal while more than 40% yielded unexpected findings, and ca. 40% of the radiographs had a direct influence on patient management.

Recently, a paradigm shift has been observed on the work floor, away from routine daily radiographs to imaging based on clinical indication and for control after interventions. It appears that a differential strategy is called for, depending on whether the setting is a predominantly medical ICU (older, multimorbid patients) or a surgical ICU. While routine chest radiography has indeed been proven inadequate, clinical experience has also taught that the time interval between bedside chest radiographs should not be stretched over several days. Interpreting pulmonary opacifications in an ICU patient frequently involves consideration of the aspect "alterations over time," and this information might be lost if control radiographs were spread over too-long a period.

C. Schaefer-Prokop

Daily routine portable chest radiographs are no longer standard in the ICU, owing to concerns about radiation safety and cost.

Technique of Portable Chest Radiography

Technical Factors

In the absence of automatic exposure control, the exposure (dose) must be estimated by the technologist. The principal variables are:

- kV and mAs
- film–focus distance
- patient size
- grid factor (if a grid is used)

Changing the tube voltage or kilovoltage (in kV) significantly affects image contrast. No single guideline is given in the literature, with values ranging from 70 to 125 kV. When the kilovoltage is reduced by 20% (e. g., from 100 to 80 kV), the milliampere-seconds (mAs) value must be approximately doubled to deliver the same dose.

Film–Focus Distance

The film–focus distance (FFD) is controlled manually. It should be remembered that even small changes in the FFD result in sizable dose changes. For example, changing an FFD of 1 m by just 10 cm will cause a 20% change in dose.

An FFD of 1 m can be used for bedside radiography in either the sitting or supine position. An FFD of 1 m allows a shorter exposure time than the FFD of 1.8 m that is typically used for upright chest radiographs. This is advantageous for dyspneic patients who are unable to perform breath-holds.

Motion artifacts are more likely to occur when exposure times exceed 10 ms. The x-ray source should *not* be closer than 1 m to the film, as this would result in undesired magnification. Also, most grids require a minimum distance of 1 m.

Scatter-Reduction Grid

Radiographs without a grid. In the majority of institutions, portable chest radiographs in ICU patients are taken without a grid.

─── **Practical Recommendation** ───

That the majority of chest radiographs are taken without a grid is due in large part to the increasing use of digital techniques and the image processing capabilities of digital radiography.

Radiographs without a grid have poorer quality in the high-absorption regions of the mediastinum and retrocardiac space, especially in heavy-set patients. This results in poorer delineation of lines and tubes. Retrocardiac and retrodiaphragmatic abnormalities, such as infiltrates and small pleural effusions, are difficult to detect. It is uncertain, however, whether the poorer imaging characteristics of gridless radiographs actually affect the management of ICU patients. The authors are unaware of any studies on this topic.

Radiographs with a grid. The use of the grid technique in chest radiography requires a higher dose than radiography without a grid (factor of 3–6 = ca. 2 exposure points). or grid encasement that can be slipped over a standard cassette. Disadvantages of these grid cassettes are the increased weight of the assembly and the need for precise centering. The advantage of a linear grid over a focused grid is that only one direction is vulnerable to off-centering (perpendicular to the grid lines); angulation of

the beam along the direction of the grid lines will not adversely affect image quality. The higher the grid ratio, the smaller the tolerance angle before a "grid effect" will occur (e.g., 0.5° with an 8 : 1 grid and 10° with a 4 : 1 grid). The tolerance angle is asymmetrical in a parallel grid, being greater on the side that is farther from the x-ray tube.

"Hole grids" are less sensitive to grid effects but are less effective in reducing scattered radiation.

─── **Practical Recommendation** ───

The kV and grid should be properly matched: the higher the kV value, the higher the necessary grid factor. A 12 : 1 grid is recommended for 125 kV, although this type of grid requires accurate centering. An 8 : 1 grid is a good tradeoff for bedside radiographs, especially when the tube voltage is lowered to ca. 90 kV. Grid factors less than 6 : 1 are considered ineffective.

Projections

Chest radiographs in ICU patients are usually obtained in the supine position. On the one hand, it is good practice to position the patient "as upright as possible" to eliminate potential sources of error in the interpretation of supine films. But it is equally true that a good supine radiograph still has greater diagnostic utility than a poor radiograph in the sitting position. Consequently, patients should be elevated to a sitting position only if their general condition will allow it.

Additional views. Some clinical questions may require the acquisition of additional radiographic views:

1. Cross-table views of the supine patient with a laterally placed cassette may be useful for the localization of pathology in the retrocardiac space and posterior mediastinum.
2. Left or right lateral decubitus views with a cross-table beam may be ordered to differentiate an effusion from pleural plaque or intrapulmonary infiltrate.
3. Tangential views in an oblique anteroposterior (AP) projection are useful for detecting an anterior pneumothorax.
4. A 60–70-kV radiograph in the supine position or with the right or left side elevated is useful for detecting rib fractures.

Indications 2 to 4 can be addressed more easily and efficiently with bedside ultrasonography in cases where an experienced sonographer is available.

When the kV is reduced by 20%, the mAs must be doubled to achieve the same exposure.

With an FFD of 1 m, changing its value by 10 cm will alter the exposure by 20%.

Chest radiographs with a grid require greater exposure than radiographs without a grid.

Causes of Poor Image Quality

Incomplete visualization of the lungs. The radiographs should completely cover the lung fields with no cut-off of the apices or costophrenic angles (**Fig. 2.1**).

Incomplete visualization of devices. All tubes and lines should be defined fully and with adequate contrast, especially in the initial radiograph. This requires complete visualization of the pulmonary apex and, if necessary, the distal cervical soft tissues for evaluating a central venous catheter. The radiograph should include the upper abdomen to define the position and tip of a nasogastric tube. It can be difficult in heavy-set patients to distinguish a tracheostomy tube from a nasogastric tube in the high-absorption region of the mediastinum and upper abdomen; this may require the special processing of digital data (window leveling, edge-enhancing filter) or even repeating the exposure at a higher dose, greater collimation, or a different patient position. Another option is to opacify the device with radiographic contrast medium.

Undesired oblique projection. The medial ends of the clavicles provide anterior landmarks for detecting an oblique projection, while the spinous process of the upper thoracic vertebrae serve as posterior landmarks. In a patient with a symmetrical physique, these landmarks should be symmetrically positioned in an unrotated frontal view. If the view is rotated, the lung that is more posterior will appear smaller and more opaque (whiter) and the mediastinum will appear widened (**Fig. 2.2**).

Undesired lordotic projection. The central ray is angled toward the patient's head in a lordotic view, causing the lung fields to appear foreshortened and projecting the diaphragm at a higher level. A lordotic projection will inevitably occur when the patient lies flat and the x-ray machine is positioned at the foot of the bed, causing relative angulation of the central ray (**Fig. 2.3**). The easiest way to correct the projection is by elevating the patient's upper body.

Inadequate depth of inspiration. If the radiograph is not taken at full inspiration, both lungs will show increased opacity making it more difficult to distinguish between atelectasis and pneumonia. The heart will be transversely oriented and appear enlarged, and there will be apparent widening of the mediastinum (**Fig. 2.4**). An adequate depth of inspiration is confirmed on supine radiographs by noting that the hemidiaphragm is well defined in the midclavicular line (MCL) at the level of the anterior fifth rib.

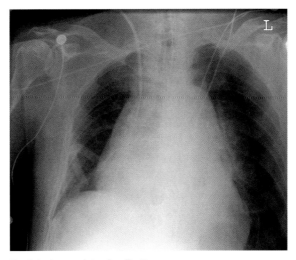

Fig. 2.1 **Incomplete visualization.**
Tension pneumothorax with incomplete visualization of the left costophrenic angle.

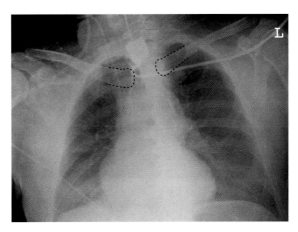

Fig. 2.2 **Oblique projection.**
This view is rotated to the right, causing an apparent widening of the mediastinum on the right side. Note the asymmetric position of the heads of the clavicles.

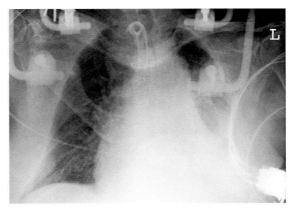

Fig. 2.3 **Lordotic view.**
The stand for the x-ray tube was placed too near the foot of the bed, causing the central ray to be angled toward the patient's head. This causes an apparent foreshortening of the lung and elevation of the diaphragm. Normally the anterior first rib is projected below the clavicle, but it appears above the clavicle in this projection.

▓ The depth of inspiration for a supine radiograph is adequate when the hemidiaphragm is displayed in the MCL at the level of the fifth anterior rib.

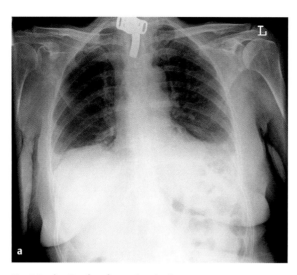

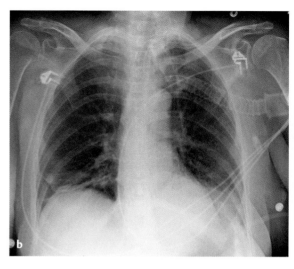

Fig. 2.4 a, b **Good and poor inspiration.**
Note the apparent change in lung density and shape of the cardiac silhouette.

a   Shallow inspiration.
b   Full inspiration.

Grid effect. If the central ray is not perpendicular to the film cassette when a grid is used (**Fig. 2.5**), a "grid effect" may result (**Fig. 2.6**). This effect causes one side of the chest to be underexposed (diffuse haziness of one hemithorax) due to the increased absorption of primary roentgen rays by the metal strips of the grid. The laterally asymmetric opacity throughout one lung should not be mistaken for a pleural effusion tracking toward the apex. A grid effect can be confirmed by noting that the extrapulmonary soft tissues on the affected side also appear hazy.

Faulty processing. Constant processing conditions should be maintained when digital technology is used. Any change in processing should be noted, and suboptimal processing (excessive edge enhancement or structural contrast) should be avoided.

Dose Control in Digital Radiography

Due to a lack of automatic dose control (automatic shut-off), *underexposure and overexposure* were the most frequent causes of poor image quality in conventional radiography; they could be recognized by the direct visual

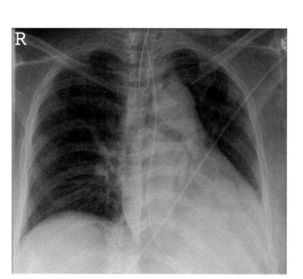

Fig. 2.5 **Scatter-reduction grid.**
Radiographs with a scatter-reduction grid require up to triple the dose (even in digital radiography) but improve penetration of the mediastinum. (This film, though taken in a heavy-set patient, shows a retrocardiac air bronchogram and clearly defines the nasogastric tube.)

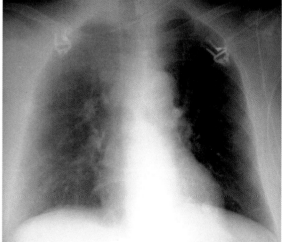

Fig. 2.6 **Grid effect.**
Off-centering of the grid has caused diffuse haziness over the right hemithorax that mimics a pleural effusion (note the extension of haziness over the extrathoracic soft tissues on the right side).

assessment of film density. This method cannot be used for dose estimation in digital radiography, because image density and dose are independent variables when digital technology is used. Nevertheless, dose control is still an essential concern in digital radiography:

- If the dose is *too low*, it will result in greater image noise and poorer image quality, especially with low-contrast structures. This could result in a loss of diagnostic information.
- If the dose is *too high*, it will not degrade image quality but may pose a radiation hazard to the patient (especially in children and other radiosensitive patients).

Dose indicators. Dose indicators are numerical values that are displayed on the film or monitor screen. They vary in their definition and calibration, depending on the manufacturer (**Table 2.1**). It should be noted that a dose indicator does not correlate with the patient entrance dose but with the dose delivered to the detector. Thus, two images from the same patient with or without pneumonia may have exactly the same patient entrance dose but different dose indicator readings. Similarly, the dose indicator will vary in different projections and body regions while the patient entrance dose remains the same. In our own analysis of follow-up chest radiographs of ICU patients, we found that the dose indicator varied over a range of approximately ± 50 % of the mean value. But despite these variations with individual absorption charac-

Table 2.1 Manufacturer-specific dose indicators in digital radiography

Dose ($K_Q/\mu Gy$)	Fuji: S value	Agfa: LgM value	Kodak: EI value
0.1	20000	1.0	0
1	800	1.4	1000
2.5	400	1.9	1400
5	200	2.3	1700
10	100	2.6	2000
Deviation*	± 50 %	± 0.3	± 150

* Denotes the range of variation in the detector dose (exposure index) as a function of patient positioning and clinical status with no associated change in the patient entrance dose (manually set exposure factor).

teristics, the dose indicator—when averaged over one group of patients and a prolonged time period (longitudinal studies)—is useful for detecting any creeping upward of the radiation dose over time. As a result, both medical and technical personnel should be familiar with the dose indicator and how it functions.

Newer systems. Newer detector systems are based on mobile flat-panel direct radiography technology. They automatically give a direct readout of the current dose–area product (DAP; patient entrance dose) and therefore allow for immediate dose control.

> Manufacturer-specific dose indicators allow for immediate dose control in digital radiography.

Communication between Radiologists and Clinicians

C. Schaefer-Prokop

Ordering Radiology Services

The orders for radiology services fall into two main categories: routine and emergency.

Routine orders. Routine services can be smoothly integrated into the workflow of the ICU and require a one-time coordination of the departments involved. Staff should be available in ICU to assist with setting up the equipment or taking the radiographs, while other staff members may vacate the room to avoid exposure.

Emergency orders. Emergency orders are performed immediately and rely on the prompt availability of necessary staff and equipment, usually furnished by the radiology department.

Clinical information. The following clinical information is relevant to the radiologic evaluation of ICU patients:
- patient history and status (level of consciousness, mechanical ventilation)

- nature, course, and dates of previous events (e. g., surgery, trauma, hemorrhage, aspiration, transfusions, shock, resuscitation, adverse drug reactions)
- nature, course, and dates of previous interventions (e. g., endoscopies, punctures, intubations, catheterizations)
- acute or preexisting impairment of cardiac, renal, or cerebral function
- recent changes in blood-gas analysis, temperature, blood pressure, or ventilation (indicating numerical values as needed)

— **Practical Recommendation** —

The hard copy (film) or soft copy (monitor image) should display information on the date and time of the image, technical factors such as kV and mAs or DAP, and number of follow-ups. It would also be desirable to include information (not generally provided) on patient position, mechanical ventilation (PEEP, FIO$_2$), and fluid balance.

Reporting of Findings

Routine orders. Daily joint conferences should be held with ICU physicians for reporting the findings of radiology services. The purpose of these interdisciplinary conferences is to review relevant clinical data, discuss current findings, and consider possible further diagnostic and therapeutic actions.

The frequent low specificity of morphologic findings in the chest underscores the importance of this interdisciplinary teamwork in the care of ICU patients, as the interpretation of radiologic findings is critically influenced by an awareness of clinical information such as fluid balance, ventilation therapy, and inflammatory markers.

Clinical information plays a vital role in intensive-care radiography, because image analysis must take into account not only the variety of primary pathologic processes, but also any previous therapeutic and/or diagnostic actions, which may affect the detectability of findings and will definitely affect their interpretation.

Emergency orders. Emergency orders require the direct reporting of findings because the results may have immediate therapeutic implications. The findings should be promptly reported by telephone, by direct conversation, in handwritten form, or as a voice recording if an electronic dictation system is available. Other digital options are the use of text blocks or speech recognition technology for the rapid creation of digital text files.

As a document with high evidential value, the radiology report is valid only when accompanied by a handwritten or digital signature. Otherwise the recognition of unsigned or verbal findings in court will depend on the degree to which their integrity or actual transmission (timing, contents) can be substantiated by proper documentation.

Catheters and Monitoring Devices

E. Eisenhuber-Stadler and P. Wunderbaldinger

One of the principal tasks of intensive care radiology is to evaluate the placement of monitoring and therapeutic devices (catheters, lines, tubes, electrodes, drains). The chest radiograph is the method of first choice for detecting device malposition and complications while also providing a document for medicolegal purposes.

The following basic rules apply in evaluating the position of tubes and lines:

- All catheters and monitoring devices introduced into the body should be radiopaque so that they will be visible on chest radiographs. If this is not the case, the catheter should be opacified with contrast medium during the initial position check.
- The insertion of any catheters, lines, tubes, electrodes, or drains should be followed by a chest radiograph to evaluate and document the position of the device and detect any complications.
- An unsuccessful percutaneous procedure should also be followed by a chest radiograph to exclude possible complications.
- Despite a correct initial placement, it is always possible for catheters, tubes, lines, electrodes, and drains to become shifted or dislodged spontaneously or as a result of position changes or spontaneous movements of the patient. This is why chest radiographs should be obtained regularly (daily if necessary) in ICU patients.
- The position of all tubes and lines should be individually checked and evaluated whenever a new chest radiograph is obtained.

Diagnostic Strategy

Radiography

Evaluating the position of tubes and lines makes it imperative to define the complete intrathoracic course of these devices. Conventional chest radiographs should employ a high kilovoltage (and a slightly higher dose if necessary) to improve mediastinal detail. In digital radiography, adjusting the contrast level (window leveling for monitor images, processing for films) is more effective than increasing the dose or adjusting the kV (**Fig. 2.7**).

Device localization. As a rule, line and tube placements in ICU patients are checked entirely on the basis of AP radiographs. This can cause problems with the accurate localization of these devices. Thus it is correct to describe the position of a catheter, for example, by stating that it is "projected onto" a certain vascular structure. If correct positioning cannot be definitively confirmed based on a single radiographic view, additional measures should be taken. These include obtaining additional views and injecting contrast medium into catheters or drains and documenting the contrast distribution.

Contrast use. The correct intravenous placement of central venous catheters is confirmed at some institutions by opacifying the catheters with contrast medium when the initial radiograph is taken. Although very small amounts of contrast medium (about 10 mL) are generally sufficient, it is still necessary to consider the relative and

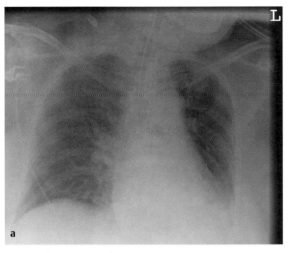
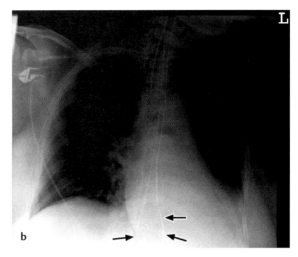

Fig. 2.7 a, b **Contrast adjustment.**
Poor visualization of tubes and lines on the monitor (a) is improved by window leveling. Note the looping of the nasogastric tube below the diaphragm (arrows in **b**).

absolute contraindications to the use of nonionic iodinated media. The examiner should check for contrast pooling or an atypical contrast distribution when evaluating the catheter position.

The current policy at most institutions—due partly to the risks of contrast use—is to withhold localization by contrast injection if the catheter is functioning normally (no resistance to blood aspiration or injection). Of course, this limits the information on catheter placement and cannot exclude potential problems such as catheter adherence.

Ultrasonography

An increasing number of reports describe the use of ultrasonography for localizing tubes and lines, especially for the detection of device-related complications. Ultrasound scanning provides a fast, sensitive, and noninvasive bedside technique for evaluating patients with a suspected myocardial perforation and hemopericardium (resulting from a catheter or pacemaker implantation). Other possible indications are evaluating the extent of a hematoma at the insertion site and, in difficult cases, accurate localization of the internal jugular vein prior to catheterization (especially in patients with low central

venous pressure). Ultrasonography is the primary modality in the ICU for detecting thrombosis of the subclavian vein or internal jugular vein in patients with a long-indwelling central venous catheter.

Fluoroscopy

Dynamic imaging modalities such as x-ray fluoroscopy provide additional information only with regard to specific clinical questions such as contrast distribution or excessive tube mobility.

Computed Tomography

CT has no role in the routine localization of catheters and monitoring devices, but it is the modality of choice in patients with equivocal findings on projection radiographs. CT can confirm the correct placement of an interlobar or pleural drain and exclude malposition outside the lung (**Fig. 2.8**). Multislice spiral CT, with its multiplanar reformatting capabilities, has further improved the accuracy of catheter localization.

The most important indication for CT is clinical suspicion of an acute complication associated with catheter

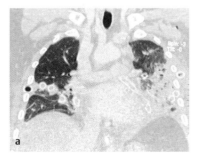
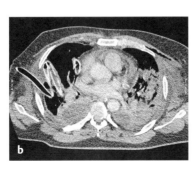

Fig. 2.8 a, b **Localization of a chest tube using CT.**
CT, with its multiplanar capabilities, is better than chest radiographs for evaluating the position of chest tubes and other devices. In this case CT shows sharp angulation and intraparenchymal placement of the tube on the right side.

▓ CT is justified by clinical suspicion of an acute complication relating to catheter insertion.

insertion. Thin slices greatly improve the accurate localization of a bleeding site related to catheter insertion.

— **Practical Recommendation** —

If ultrasonographic findings remain equivocal, CT with IV contrast administration is recommended for detecting large vein thrombosis occurring as a late complication after the insertion of a central venous catheter. It is particularly useful for defining the central extent of superior vena cava thrombosis. The contrast medium is injected into *both* arms, and imaging is initiated after an appropriate scan delay (40–60 s for the superior vena cava, 80–100 s for the inferior vena cava) to avoid an apparent filling defect caused by the mixing of opacified and nonopacified blood.

Endotracheal Tube

The chest radiograph will show malposition of the endotracheal tube (ETT) in 12–15% of intubated patients. In most cases the malposition of an orotracheal or nasotracheal tube is not detected by physical examination alone (asymmetric breath sounds or chest excursions), and so every endotracheal intubation should be followed by a chest radiograph to confirm proper placement.

▓ Every endotracheal intubation should be followed by a chest radiograph to evaluate tube position.

Since tube manipulations (e. g., retaping) or patient coughing may alter the position of the ETT, published guidelines (including recommendations from the American College of Radiology) advocate daily repetition of the chest radiograph in intubated patients. Increasingly, this practice is no longer followed in patients with stable cardiopulmonary status, although the position of the ETT should be rechecked and evaluated whenever a new chest radiograph is obtained.

Normal Position

The tip of the ETT is marked with a radiopaque strip, making it easier to locate on chest radiographs. The tip position is usually described in relation to the carina, which is at the level of the T5±1) vertebra in 95% of patients. When the head is in the neutral position, the tip of the ETT should be 5–7 cm above the carina. The tip of the tube may move considerably with flexion and extension of the neck. Because the tube is secured to the nose or mouth, only its distal end can follow movements of the head and neck, moving up to 2 cm downward with flexion and up to 2 cm upward with extension. Hence the tip of the ETT should be at least 5 cm above the carina when the head is in neutral position. If it were placed lower, a simple change in head position could cause the tip to enter one of the main bronchi. Rotation of the head may also cause the tip to move 1–2 cm. To minimize airway resistance, the lumen of the tube should occupy one-half to two-thirds of the tracheal lumen.

▓ With the head in a neutral position, the tip of the endotracheal tube should be 5–7 cm above the carina.

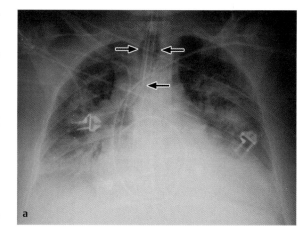

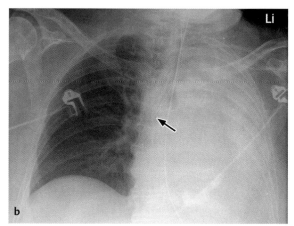

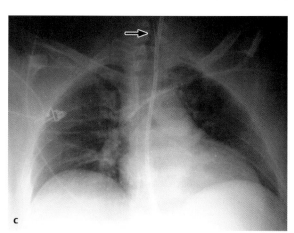

Fig. 2.9 a–c **Malposition of the endotracheal tube.**

a The endotracheal tube has been placed too low; its tip is only 1 cm above the carina. The cuff is overinflated and distends the tracheal wall. The pulmonary artery catheter and central venous catheter are normally positioned.

b The tip of the tube is in the right main bronchus (arrow), accompanied by complete atelectasis of the left lung.

c The tube has been placed too high; its tip is 8 cm from the carina, with risk of spontaneous extubation, aspiration, and injury to the larynx (vocal cords) from the cuff. The Quinton catheter and nasogastric tube are normally positioned.

Cuff. The inflated cuff of the ETT should occupy all of the tracheal lumen without distending the tracheal wall (**Fig. 2.9a**). High cuff pressures on the tracheal wall may compromise blood flow leading to ischemia of the tracheal mucosa and irreversible mucosal damage. Modern high-volume low-pressure cuffs have greatly reduced this risk by lowering the internal pressure and distributing it over a larger area. The cuff should not extend below the lower end of the tube, as a "cuff herniation" might occlude the lumen.

Malposition

In ca. 10–20% of cases, imaging localization indicates a malposition of the ETT that requires correction.

Unilateral endobronchial intubation. The most common positioning error is unilateral endobronchial intubation, usually of the right main bronchus (**Fig. 2.9b**). Unilateral intubation of the right main bronchus may lead to atelectasis of the left lung and/or right upper lobe with hyperinflation of the ventilated lung areas and risk of tension pneumothorax (ca. 15%) due to barotrauma.

Too low or too high. If the tip of the ETT is too close to the carina, it may lead to undetected unilateral endobronchial intubation or direct mechanical irritation of the mucosa. Additionally, transbronchial aspiration may cause mucosal lesions at the level of the carina. Positioning the ETT too high carries a risk of spontaneous extubation and aspiration past a leaky cuff seal within the larynx or pharynx (**Fig. 2.9c**). There is also a risk of injury to the larynx (vocal cords) from the overinflated cuff.

Esophageal intubation. Misdirected insertion of the ETT into the esophagus is recognized clinically in most cases. The ETT appears to the left of the tracheal outline on the chest radiograph, accompanied by overdistension of the esophagus and stomach and displacement of the trachea by the inflated cuff. A 25° right anterior oblique projection of the chest with the head turned to the right can clearly display the tube running posterior to the tracheal border.

Complications

Rupture of the larynx, trachea (usually the membranous part), or main bronchi (usually after a difficult intubation) is a rare but serious complication of endotracheal intubation (**Fig. 2.10**). Air escaping from the ruptured trachea or bronchus may cause a pneumomediastinum, soft-tissue emphysema, or even a pneumothorax.

— Practical Recommendation —

When a perforation occurs, CT is recommended for precise localization of the rupture site, evaluation of a possible infection in the mediastinum or neck, and for planning any surgical intervention that may be required.

A symptomatic or asymptomatic tracheal stenosis, tracheomalacia, intrathoracic vascular erosion, or tracheobronchial fistula may develop as a rare, late complication of an overinflated cuff or long-term intubation.

Tracheostomy Tube

A tracheotomy is performed in patients who require long-term ventilation or have an upper airway obstruction. When the tracheostomy tube has been inserted, a chest radiograph is obtained to assess its position and exclude complications.

Normal Position

The tracheostomy tube should run down the tracheal air column, parallel to its longitudinal axis. The tip of the tube should be located several centimeters above the carina. At least two-thirds of the straight portion of the tube should be intratracheal (**Fig. 2.11a**). The tracheostomy tube should occupy one-half to two-thirds of the tracheal lumen to minimize airway resistance.

Malposition

The tip of the tube may be pressed or jammed against the anterior or posterior tracheal wall, leading to pressure necrosis or perforation of the tracheal wall (detectable on lateral radiographs) (**Fig. 2.11b**). Very rarely, this malposition may cause pressure erosion of the left brachiocephalic artery in front of the trachea or give rise to a tracheobronchial fistula.

If the inner and outer ends of the tracheostomy tube are superimposed on the chest radiograph, occupying the same plane, the tube is not passing normally down the trachea and must be repositioned. Clinical examination is sufficient in most cases, but a lateral radiograph is helpful in rare instances.

Complications

The chest radiograph after a tracheotomy will often show mild cutaneous emphysema in the neck and a pneumomediastinum without pathologic significance. Massive subcutaneous emphysema, however, most likely indicates a tracheal perforation in the setting of the tracheotomy. A pneumothorax may result from pleural injury during the

Rupture of the larynx, trachea, or main bronchi is a rare but serious complication of endotracheal intubation.

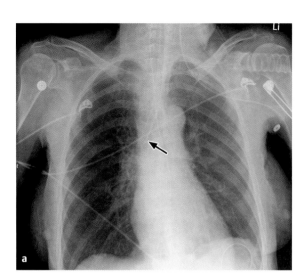
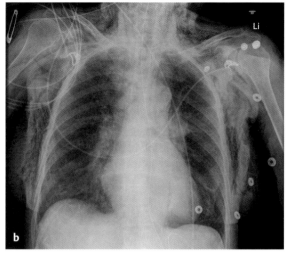

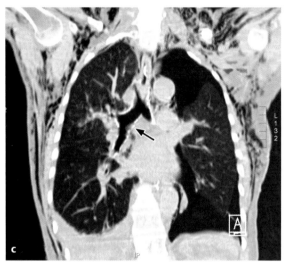

Fig. 2.10 a–d Iatrogenic tracheal rupture.

a The tip of the endotracheal tube is within the right main bronchus following a difficult intubation.

b After the tube was repositioned, the patient developed extensive mediastinal and subcutaneous emphysema.

c, d CT shows an irregular wall contour of the right main bronchus at the site of the bronchoscopically confirmed rupture (not clinically apparent until the catheter was withdrawn). There is an associated left pneumothorax.

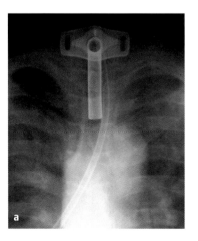
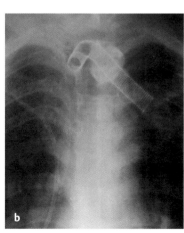

Fig. 2.11 a, b Tracheostomy tube.

a Correct position.

b The intratracheal segment of the tube is too short, causing the tip of the tube to engage against the lateral tracheal wall (risk of pressure necrosis and perforation).

tracheotomy or from a tracheal perforation. Widening of the mediastinum after a tracheotomy is suggestive of hemorrhage. Rare, late complications of tracheotomy are tracheal stenosis, tracheomalacia, intrathoracic vascular erosions, and tracheobronchial fistula.

Central Venous Catheter

Postinterventional chest radiographs demonstrate malposition of the central venous catheter (CVC) in up to 33% of patients.

The following points should be noted when evaluating the catheter position on the chest radiograph:

- The intrathoracic course of the catheter should be completely visualized from the insertion site to the catheter tip.
- Even with an unsuccessful insertion, a chest radiograph should still be obtained to rule out possible complications (hematoma at the insertion site, pneumothorax).
- Some colleagues recommend contrast instillation for the initial radiograph to check for extravascular catheterization or malposition in small vessels. In most practical situations, however, it is sufficient to assess the function of the catheter (no resistance to aspiration or infusion) and evaluate its position on plain radiographs, obtaining contrast views only in selected problem cases.

Normal Position

The catheter is usually introduced via the subclavian vein or internal jugular vein, and its tip should be visualized in the superior vena cava (**Fig. 2.12a**). In the AP chest radiograph, the catheter tip should lie close to the level of the azygos vein (between the sternal attachments of the first three ribs).

Catheters introduced via the subclavian vein and internal jugular vein should appear to cross each other on the AP radiograph. If they do not, the possibility of an extravascular or intra-arterial catheterization should be considered.

Malposition

Intracardiac malposition of the CVC in the right atrium or right ventricle may lead to valvular or endocardial lesions. Other risks are arrhythmias and myocardial perforation with hemopericardium and pericardial tamponade. *Intramural* malposition often produces no clinical manifestations but should be corrected owing to potential complications such as thrombosis or vascular erosion.

Common positioning errors. The radiographic detection of CVC malposition requires an accurate knowledge of thoracic venous anatomy (**Fig. 2.13**). The most common error with catheters placed through the subclavian vein is to advance the catheter into the ipsilateral internal jugular

If catheters introduced via the subclavian and internal jugular vein do not cross each other in the frontal radiograph, the possibility of an extravascular or intra-arterial catheterization should be considered.

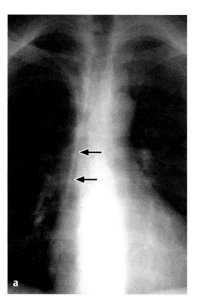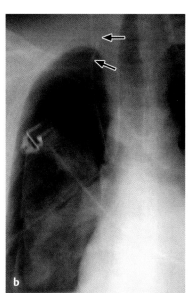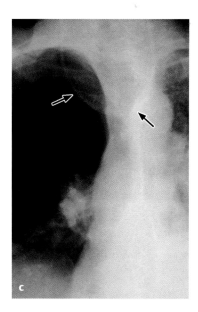

Fig. 2.12 a–c **Central venous catheter.**

a Correct position: the tip of the catheter is projected at the junction of the superior vena cava and right atrium.

b Right subclavian catheter is malpositioned in the internal jugular vein. The right jugular vein catheter occupies a normal position. A right pneumothorax is also present following chest tube insertion.

c Right jugular vein catheter is malpositioned in the contralateral internal jugular vein.

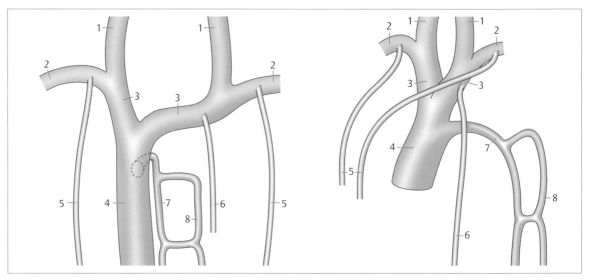

Fig. 2.13 **Diagrammatic representation (ap and lateral view) of the anatomy of the thoracic veins.**

1 Internal jugular vein	**3** Brachiocephalic vein	**5** Internal thoracic vein	**7** Azygos vein
2 Subclavian vein	**4** Superior vena cava	**6** Pericardiophrenic vein	**8** Accessory hemiazygos vein

vein (ca. 15% of cases, **Fig. 2.12b**). Another common error is to advance the catheter across the midline into the contralateral brachiocephalic vein (**Fig. 2.12c**). A catheter introduced via the internal jugular vein may erroneously enter the veins of the upper limb. These types of malposition are very easy to recognize on AP chest radiographs.

Positioning errors that are rare or difficult to detect. Catheter malposition in the azygos vein or internal thoracic vein is more difficult to detect and may require biplane radiographs or contrast opacification. Malposition of the catheter tip in the azygos vein is evidenced by a loop projecting over the termination of the azygos vein in

the superior vena cava (**Fig. 2.14a**). Malposition in the azygos vein is clearly detected in the lateral radiograph by noting posterior deviation of the catheter (**Fig. 2.14b**).

Rarely, a catheter may be positioned in the *internal thoracic vein*, recognized in the lateral radiograph by its retrosternal course (**Fig. 2.14c**). Rare sites include the pericardiophrenic vein (catheter runs along the cardiac border), left superior intercostal vein, and inferior thyroid vein.

The most common *variant of venous anatomy* is a persistent left superior vena cava, which is present in 0.3% of the normal population and in 4.3% of patients with cardiac anomalies. Typically the catheter descends through

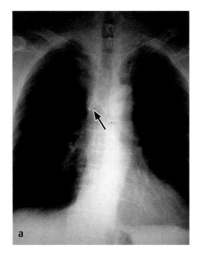
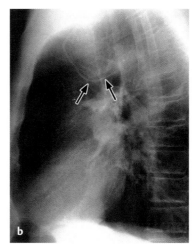
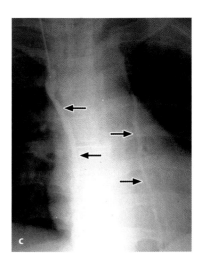

Fig. 2.14 **Central venous catheter (CVC) malpositioned in the azygos vein.**

a The tip of the CVC is in the azygos vein. Note the catheter loop projected over the proximal azygos vein.

b Lateral radiograph confirms CVC malposition in the azygos vein by the posteriorly directed catheter position.

c The internal thoracic veins on both sides have been opacified by contrast injection.

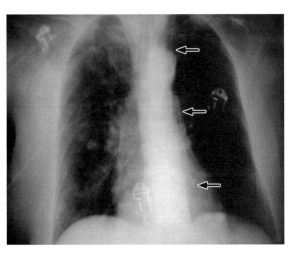

Fig. 2.15 **Persistent left superior vena cava.**
The catheter runs down the left side of the mediastinum following catheterization of the left internal jugular vein or subclavian vein.

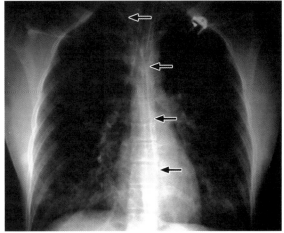

Fig. 2.16 **Intra-arterial placement of the central venous catheter.**
The catheter runs too close to the midline on the chest radiograph, having been placed inadvertently in the descending aorta.

the left side of the mediastinum following puncture of the left internal jugular vein or subclavian vein (**Fig. 2.15**).

An intra-articular CVC is recognized by its atypical course—medial to the expected location of the subclavian vein (**Fig. 2.16**).

Complications (Table 2.2)

The most frequent complication of catheter insertion is pneumothorax (6% incidence after subclavian catheterization). Pneumothorax is much less common with jugular vein catheterization but may still occur. A delayed pneumothorax should be suspected in cases where respiratory deterioration occurs hours or days after line placement.

Intracardiac placement of the catheter in the right atrium or ventricle may rarely lead to myocardial perforation with hemopericardium and pericardial tamponade.

Inadvertent *arterial catheterization* may lead to extensive soft-tissue hematomas, mediastinal hematomas, or a hemothorax. These complications are manifested on radiographs by soft-tissue opacities, mediastinal widening, and pleural effusion.

The *extravascular placement* of a CVC in the mediastinum or pleura combined with the infusion of large fluid volumes leads to an infusion mediastinum with rapidly

progressive mediastinal widening and pleural effusion (**Fig. 2.17a**).

— Practical Recommendation —

Extravascular malposition is indicated by the extravasation of contrast medium infused into the catheter. Note that with multilumen catheters, only one lumen may be extravascular.

The catheter position should be adjusted in cases where the *catheter tip rests against the right lateral wall* of the superior vena cava (**Fig. 2.17b**). This placement is most commonly seen with catheters that have been introduced via the left subclavian vein. It increases the risk of endothelial damage and vascular perforation, which typically occurs hours to days after catheter insertion (**Fig. 2.17c**).

Long-term catheterization, looping, intimal lesions, and infections promote the development of *intravenous thrombosis*. Thrombotic material is found around the CVC in up to 73% (!) of patients who have had the catheter in place for 2 weeks. Doppler ultrasound scan is the primary technique for detecting thrombosis of the subclavian vein and internal jugular vein in ICU patients. CT with IV contrast administration in both arms is recommended for assessing the extension of thrombosis toward the superior vena cava.

> A pneumothorax after subclavian catheterization is the most frequent complication of CVC.

Table 2.2 Complications of central venous catheterization

Complication	Typical radiographic signs	Comments
Hematoma at the insertion site	Soft-tissue opacity	Caution: A hematoma may form even after an unsuccessful puncture
Pneumothorax	Expanded pleural space, pleural line, loss of pulmonary vascular markings	Pneumothorax often has an anterior or subpulmonary location in supine patients
Mediastinal hematoma, hemothorax	Rapidly progressive mediastinal widening, pleural effusion	Seen with extravascular or arterial malposition

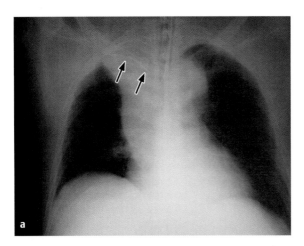

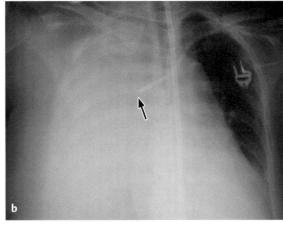

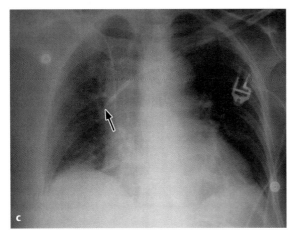

Fig. 2.17 a–c **Extravasation due to perforation.**

a The tip of the left subclavian catheter should be repositioned, as it rests against the right lateral wall of the superior vena cava.

b Two days later the tip has perforated the superior vena cava, causing complete opacity of the right hemithorax.

c Extravascular malposition of a right subclavian catheter in the mediastinum is marked by rapid progression of mediastinal widening.

Pulmonary Artery Catheter

Pulmonary artery catheters (Swan–Ganz catheters, flow-directed catheters) are used in ICU patients to monitor cardiopulmonary function and to direct therapeutic measures. The catheter monitors the pulmonary capillary wedge pressure, which is a measure of the pressure in the left atrium. Cardiac output and other important hemodynamic variables can also be measured or calculated.

The principal indications are:

- septic shock
- severe respiratory failure (ARDS)
- heart failure
- major operations (especially cardiac surgery)

Typically, the catheter is passed through an introducer sheath into the subclavian vein or internal jugular vein and floats from there through the superior vena cava, right atrium, right ventricle, and into the main trunk of the pulmonary artery. Placement of the pulmonary artery catheter—even when characteristic pressure waveforms are obtained—should always be followed by a chest radiograph to confirm the catheter position and exclude complications.

▶ A chest radiograph should always be obtained after the insertion of a pulmonary artery catheter.

Normal Position

The normal position of the catheter tip is variable depending on its functional state (wedge position). Its position in the "resting state" ranges from the right ventricular outflow tract and main pulmonary trunk to the right or left pulmonary trunk (**Fig. 2.18a**). Ideally, the pulmonary artery catheter should be placed so that when the balloon is inflated, the catheter can easily advance into the lung for monitoring wedge pressures. While in the wedge position, the tip of the pulmonary artery catheter is located in a pulmonary artery branch and blood flow often carries the tip into a posterior area of the lung.

Malposition

The most common positioning error is a peripheral malposition in which the catheter tip is in a pulmonary artery branch located more than 2 cm from the hilum. This distal placement may result in a pulmonary infarction, or the tip may perforate a pulmonary arterial branch, causing hemorrhage. If placed too far proximally in the right ventricle, the catheter may cause arrhythmia, endothelial damage, or perforation.

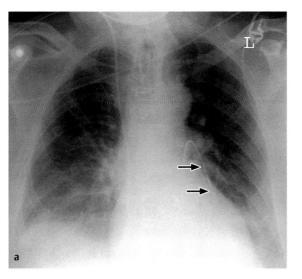

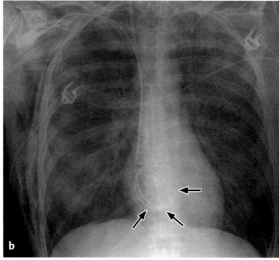

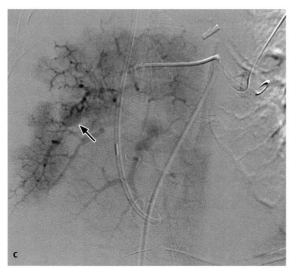

Fig. 2.18 a–c **Pulmonary artery catheter.**
a The Swan–Ganz catheter is correctly positioned with its tip in the inferior branch of the left pulmonary artery.
b Malposition of the pulmonary artery catheter, which was introduced via the right jugular vein. Looping has occurred within the right atrium. The chest radiograph also shows a right-sided pneumothorax with chest tube in place, soft-tissue emphysema, and intrapulmonary vascular congestion.
c The Swan–Ganz catheter is positioned too far distally, giving rise to an intrapulmonary aneurysm in a segmental arterial branch.

Complications

The most frequent complication visible on radiographs is *pulmonary infarction*, which may occur when the catheter has been placed too distally or the balloon has been inflated for too long. The infarcted area usually appears as a focal opacity in the lung region peripheral to the catheter. It is rare to find a classic homogeneous, wedge-shaped area of subpleural consolidation (the "Hampton hump").

Looping or coiling of the catheter within the atrium or ventricle may provoke *atrial and ventricular arrhythmias* (**Fig. 2.18b**).

A rare complication is rupture of the pulmonary artery leading to pulmonary hemorrhage. Other rare complications are pseudoaneurysms involving the pulmonary artery or a segmental branch (**Fig. 2.18c**), intracardiac knotting of the catheter, and localized thrombosis.

Intra-aortic Balloon Pump

The intra-aortic balloon pump (IABP) is a device that provides mechanical circulatory assistance. It consists of a catheter tipped with an inflatable balloon 26–28 cm long. Controlled by the patient's ECG signals, the balloon is inflated during diastole with ca. 40 mL of gas (usually helium) and is deflated during systole. A chest radiograph taken during diastole shows the IABP as an elongated gas-filled structure in the descending aorta. The balloon itself is not visible during systole because it is deflated, but its position is still indicated by a small radiopaque marker at the tip.

The IABP improves oxygen delivery to the myocardium and brain during diastole (balloon inflation) and reduces the cardiac afterload during systole (balloon deflation).

The following are indications for an IABP:
- low-output syndrome
- cardiogenic shock

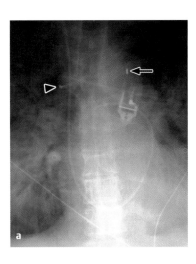 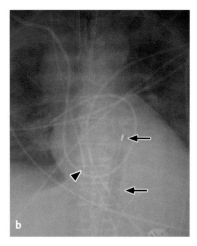

Fig. 2.19 a, b **Intra-aortic balloon pump.**
a The balloon is deflated during systole, but a metal marker at the catheter tip is projected over the aortic arch distal to the origin of the left subclavian artery, confirming correct placement. A malpositioned CVC is visible in the azygos vein (arrowhead).
b Gas makes the inflated balloon visible during diastole. The metal-tagged tip is malpositioned, being projected too far peripherally in the descending aorta. The CVC is malpositioned on the right side with its tip low in the right atrium (arrowhead).

- weaning difficulties from a heart–lung machine
- perioperative support in patients at high cardiac risk
- bridging to heart transplantation

Normal Position

Correct placement of the IABP is easily confirmed on plain radiographs. The catheter can be introduced percutaneously via the femoral artery or surgically through an arteriotomy. Transfemoral insertion, in which the catheter is advanced in retrograde fashion into the thoracic aorta, is usually performed under fluoroscopic guidance. Ideally, the tip of the catheter, bearing a radiopaque marker, is positioned just distal to the origin of the left subclavian artery in the aortic arch (junction of middle and lower thirds) in the AP chest radiograph (**Fig. 2.19a**).

In rare cases an IABP is placed intraoperatively from a proximal approach, passing through the aortic arch and into the descending aorta. In this case the small metal bead marks the distal rather than proximal end of the device. An IABP advanced into the aorta from a proximal site will also require operative removal.

The tip of the IABP catheter should be located in the aortic arch (junction of middle and lower thirds) in the AP chest radiograph.

Malposition

If positioned too far *proximally*, the IABP may occlude the left subclavian artery or the arteries supplying the brain, with consequent risk of cerebral embolism. If placed too far *distally*, the device will cause a functional deficit with risk of visceral artery obstruction (**Fig. 2.19b**).

Impella Device

The Impella device is a catheter-based cardiac-assist device with a small pump mounted at its tip. The catheter can be introduced percutaneously via the femoral artery or may be inserted directly into the aorta. The pump can be positioned in the left ventricle (or rarely in the right ventricle) to provide a temporary increase in cardiac output. The pump rotates at about 40 000 rpm and can generate a stroke volume up to 2.5 L/min, providing effective hemodynamic support. Unlike the IABP, the effectiveness of the Impella does not depend on preexisting cardiac performance. The indications for the Impella are similar to those for the IABP.

The Impella device has also been used in conjunction with the IABP or with ECMO (extracorporeal membrane oxygenation, see below).

Normal Position

As the diagram in **Fig. 2.20 a** shows, part of the Impella is distal to the aortic valve plane while the rotor-bearing part is proximal to the valve plane, that is, within the ventricle. Accordingly, the two metallic markers at the ends of the device should be located proximally and distally of the aortic value on the chest radiograph.

Malposition

Positioning the Impella too far proximally or distally (**Fig. 2.20 b**) will reduce its functional performance, and the device may injure or even perforate the ventricular wall.

Chest Tubes

Thoracostomy tubes (chest tubes) are used to evacuate air or fluid from the pleural cavity. Fluid collections tend to gravitate to posterior sites in the supine patient while air collections rise to anterior sites. Accordingly, the tube may occupy various positions depending on the indication. Chest radiographs should be obtained routinely after thoracostomy tube insertion to evaluate tube position, exclude complications (e.g., pneumothorax when draining a pleural effusion), and evaluate response.

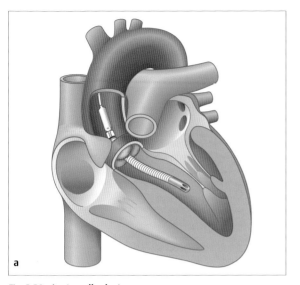

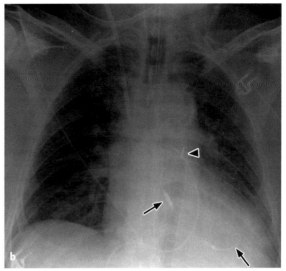

Fig. 2.20 a b **Impella device.**
Diagram of the normally positioned device (**a**) and clinical example of malposition (**b**), in which the device has been positioned too far peripherally. The proximal metal part (rotary pump) (left arrow) should be within the aorta, just distal to the aortic valve, while the distal intake tube is within the left ven- tricle (right arrow) . The radiograph also documents peripheral malposition of the IABP (arrowhead) while showing normal positioning of the endotracheal tube, Swan–Ganz catheter, Quinton catheter, and nasogastric tube.

Normal Position

The radiographic criteria for evaluating the position of a chest tube depend on the indication:

- The tip of a tube for *evacuating a pneumothorax* should be placed close to the pulmonary apex at the level of the anterior axillary line and should be direct- ed anterosuperiorly.
- The tip of a tube for *draining pleural fluid* should be placed posteroinferiorly between the sixth and eighth intercostal spaces at the level of the midaxillary line. Particular care is taken that the sideholes (appearing as breaks in the radiopaque line) are intrathoracic.
- *Loculated air or fluid collections* require atypical tube positions. The tubes are inserted separately under ultrasound guidance or, increasingly, under CT guid- ance.

Malposition

Up to 25% of thoracostomy tubes placed under emer- gency conditions are found to be malpositioned. The tube is assumed to be malpositioned if the radiograph after insertion does not show immediate release of signs of tension or gradual decrease of pneumothorax or pleural fluid, respectively. Chest tubes may be located in the in- terlobar fissures, in the lung parenchyma, or in the ex- trapleural thoracic soft tissues.

— Practical Recommendation

In cases where the chest tube is not providing adequate drainage, the posteroanterior (PA) radiograph should be supplemented by a lateral or oblique view or by CT scans (**Fig. 2.21**) for the precise localization of the chest tube. Thoracic CT is recommended in all patients with equivocal chest films.

The radio- graphic criteria for evaluating chest tube position depend on the indication.

CT scans can confirm an *intrafissural (interlobar)* position by locating the tube to the interlobar fissures.

If the tube is not closely aligned with the interlobar fissures, an *intraparenchymal* malposition should be as- sumed. In most but not all cases, this type of malposition is also associated with hematoma formation around the tube (**Fig. 2.22**). This collection, usually distributed around the tip of the tube, may also be visible on the initial chest radiograph. If a hematoma has not formed around the tip of an intraparenchymal tube, or if exten- sive consolidation is present (e. g., due to a pulmonary contusion), even CT may be unable to distinguish be- tween an interlobar and intraparenchymal malposition (note the course of the fissures).

Complications

Possible complications include bleeding due to laceration of an intercostal artery, the liver, or the spleen. Inserting the tube into the lung tissue will cause a parenchymal laceration with hematoma formation. Malpositioned chest tubes may even injure large central vessels (aorta,

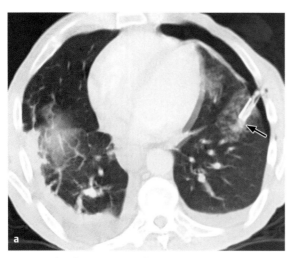

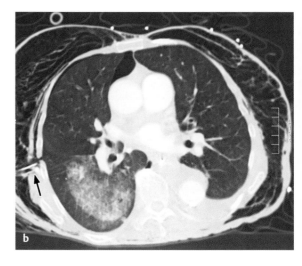

Fig. 2.21 a, b **Thoracostomy tube.**
a   Intrapulmonary malposition with surrounding hematoma.

b   Peripheral placement in the chest wall with extensive soft-tissue emphysema (chest wall fistula) and pulmonary contusion.

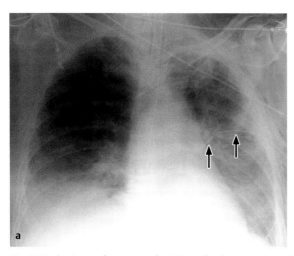

Fig. 2.22 a, b **Intrapulmonary malposition of a thoracostomy tube with parenchymal laceration.**
The malposition and the extent of the injury are poorly visualized on the chest radiograph but are well defined by CT. Note the kinked condition of the chest tube, which prevents normal drainage (with kind permission of H. Shin, Medizinische Hochschule Hannover).

vena cava, pulmonary vessels). In rare cases intraparenchymal placement may be followed by a bronchopulmonary fistula. An abscess or empyema may develop as a late complication of a malpositioned chest tube.

Feeding Tubes

Gastric, duodenal, or jejunal tubes may be used for enteral nutrition or drainage. Malposition is not uncommon and often produces no clinical signs. Thus, a chest radiograph should be obtained routinely after the insertion of a new feeding tube.

A malpositioned feeding tube often produces no clinical signs, so a chest radiograph should always be obtained after tube insertion.

Normal Position

Feeding tubes have a radiopaque stripe which aids their localization on chest films. It should be emphasized that feeding tubes are poorly visualized if the film is underexposed or the tube is not very radiopaque. Localization can be aided in these cases by opacifying the tube with radiographic contrast medium. Most feeding and drainage tubes have sideholes distributed along the distal 10 cm of the tube. The tip, then, should be located at least 10 cm distal to the gastroesophageal junction. Duodenal and jejunal tubes are generally introduced under endoscopic or fluoroscopic guidance.

Malposition

Malpositioned feeding tubes are not at all uncommon in ICU patients. The tip of a gastric tube may double back into the pharynx or esophagus, leading to the *aspiration* of nutrient solution (**Fig. 2.23a**). The feeding tube may inadvertently enter the tracheobronchial tree leading to

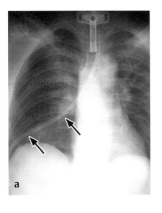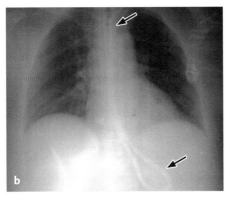

Fig. 2.23 a, b **Nasogastric tube.**
a Malpositioned in the lower lobe of the right lung.
b Tube doubled back on itself (risk of aspiration).

pneumonia or to bronchial perforation with subsequent *pneumothorax* (**Fig. 2.23b**).

Complications

Esophageal perforation is a rare complication of feeding tube insertion. It may lead to mediastinal widening and pneumomediastinum.

Cardiac Pacemakers and Defibrillators

Cardiac pacemakers. Temporary pacemaker leads in ICU patients are usually inserted by the transvenous route via the subclavian or internal jugular vein. Generally, the wire lead is placed under fluoroscopic control at the apex of the right ventricle, where the lead is anchored in the trabeculae. Cardiac surgery is usually followed by temporary epicardial pacing with leads that are placed intra-operatively and are removed after the immediate post-operative period. The leads are usually anchored in the epicardium over the right atrium and right ventricle (or bipolar leads may be placed on the right atrium). They terminate over the pericardium, typically in the right parasternal area of the chest wall, where they can be connected to a pacemaker as required.

Defibrillators. Various systems are available for defibrillation by implantable cardioverter defibrillators (ICDs). The following types are distinguished based on the nature of the components:
- epicardial patch electrodes (usually two patches)
- transvenous defibrillator lead plus a subcutaneous patch in the chest wall
- transvenous defibrillator lead without a patch electrode

The transvenous defibrillator lead usually has two wire-wrapped expansions, one of which is placed at the junction of the superior vena cava with the right atrium or in the brachiocephalic vein. The other is placed on the floor of the right ventricle. The tip of the defibrillator lead is screwed into the apical portion of the right ventricle.

Combinations. An ICD may be combined with a pacemaker. Depending on the type of arrhythmia, the tips of the pacing wires may be located in the right atrium, right ventricle, coronary sinus, and in the left ventricle with biventricular pacing.

Normal Position

Anteroposterior (AP) and lateral radiographs are both necessary for accurate localization (**Fig. 2.24**). In the AP view, the tip of the transvenous pacemaker lead is projected onto the floor of the right ventricle, just medial to the left cardiac border. In the lateral view, the pacemaker

▶ AP and lateral radiographs are both necessary for the accurate localization of cardiac pacemakers and ICDs.

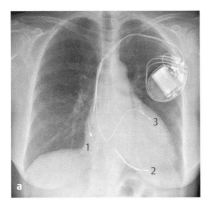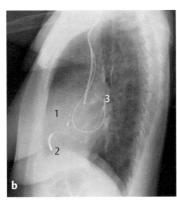

Fig. 2.24 a, b **Implantable cardioverter defibrillator.**
The tips of the wires are located in the right atrium (1), right ventricle (2), and coronary sinus (3).
a AP view.
b Lateral view.

lead should run anteriorly. Only the lateral view can show posterior deflection of the wire due to placement in the coronary sinus.

The tips of the leads for *epicardial pacing* are generally projected over the right atrium and right ventricle. The exact location depends on the surgeon and patient and is highly variable. Evaluating the position of epicardial leads always requires comparison with immediate postoperative chest radiographs.

Because the position of transvenous *defibrillator leads* is highly variable depending on the system, the radiologist should know the type of system used and its normal radiographic appearance.

Malposition

Malposition in the superior or inferior vena cava, right atrium, pulmonary trunk, or pulmonary arteries can usually be detected on the basis of abnormal impulse conduction.

Complications

Myocardial perforation may be difficult to detect unless the tip of the pacemaker lead is definitely projected outside the myocardium or epicardial fat stripe. Myocardial perforation does not cause detectable changes in most cases. Rare cases may present with hemopericardium and pericardial tamponade, or with a pneumothorax (**Fig. 2.25**).

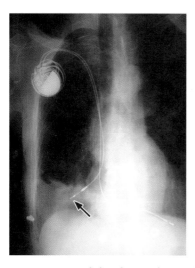

Fig. 2.25 **Myocardial perforation by a cardiac pacemaker.** The right atrium has been perforated by an atrial pacing lead with migration into the pleural space, pericardial and pleural effusion, and a basal pneumothorax.

Drains after Cardiac Surgery

Drainage tubes after cardiac surgery may be found in various types, numbers, and locations depending on the particular surgeon and patient. The drains may be located in the anterior or posterior mediastinum, pericardium, or pleural cavity.

Pericardiocentesis and Pericardial Drainage

Fluid collections in the pericardium may be acutely life-threatening in patients who develop signs of pericardial tamponade. The treatment of choice is immediate (ultrasound-guided) drainage by pericardiocentesis. The needle position should be evaluated to exclude incorrect needle placement and injury to the great vessels or cardiac chambers. After the needle has been introduced, the fluid aspirated, and the needle position confirmed, a pigtail catheter is usually inserted into the pericardial sac.

Normal Position

Correct placement of the catheter should be verified by a chest radiograph after contrast administration, or by ultrasonography.

Complications

The main risk of pericardiocentesis is injury to adjacent organs or vessels (liver, stomach, lung, pleura, internal mammary artery, coronary artery, ventricle). Rare complications are pneumothorax, cardiac arrhythmias, and infection.

Extracorporeal Membrane Oxygenation

Extracorporeal membrane oxygenation (ECMO) has assumed growing importance in recent years, especially in adults with acute respiratory failure (see also ARDS, p. 37). Two types of ECMO are used: venovenous and venoarterial.

In *venovenous* ECMO, a catheter is advanced into the right atrium via the internal jugular vein. Blood aspirated from the right atrium is oxygenated and then returned to the right atrium through a double-lumen catheter or via a large peripheral vein (usually the femoral vein).

In *venoarterial* ECMO, blood is aspirated via a catheter passed into the right atrium via the internal jugular vein. It is then oxygenated and returned to the ascending aorta through a catheter in the carotid artery.

Pulmonary Hemodynamics and Edema in ICU Patients

S. Metz-Schimmerl and C. Schaefer-Prokop

Evaluation of Hemodynamics

Radiography

The use of a standardized radiographic technique can improve evaluations of the heart and vessels and facilitates comparison with previous images. Patient position, projection, film–focus distance, depth of inspiration, and ventilation parameters in patients on mechanical ventilation will critically influence the morphology and evaluation of cardiovascular status on radiographs.

Criteria

The following criteria are useful in the radiographic evaluation of hemodynamics:

- cardiac size
- the vascular pedicle (width of the upper mediastinum)
- diameter and outlines of the intrapulmonary vessels
- parenchymal density
- thickness of the chest wall

These parameters provide qualitative information on an increase or decrease in vascular pressure and the volume of extravascular fluid in the lung parenchyma or the "third space" (pleural cavity and chest wall). This permits an indirect assessment of left-heart function and fluid balance.

Cardiac size. Even in the supine position, cardiac size can be evaluated by determining the ratio of the transverse diameters of the chest and heart. When the different magnification factor (AP versus PA) and supine patient position are taken into account, the threshold value is adjusted upward and is > 0.53 (versus < 0.5).

Vascular pedicle. The vascular pedicle in the upper mediastinal shadow can be used to estimate the intravascular volume. Consisting of the superior vena cava, azygos vein and descending aorta, it is measured as the distance between the point where the right main bronchus crosses the superior vena cava and a vertical line drawn through the origin of the left subclavian artery from the aorta (**Fig. 2.26**).

An *increase* in the width of the vascular pedicle (generally toward the right side) correlates with an increase in intravascular volume. An increase of ca. 0.5 cm corresponds to an approximate 1-L increase in the intravascular fluid volume, while a 1-cm increase corresponds to approximately 2 L. It should be noted, however, that rotating the patient to the right or changing from a sitting to supine position will also cause apparent widening of the vascular pedicle. A width of 7 cm is accepted as the upper limit of normal, although it is more meaningful to evaluate the progression of widths than the absolute value.

A *decrease* in mediastinal width may be caused by hypovolemia, a high ventilation pressure, or rotation of the patient toward the left side.

Intrapulmonary vessels. Evaluation of the intrapulmonary vessels is often difficult due to superimposed infiltrates or atelectasis, and is a highly subjective assessment. Often it is more meaningful to evaluate the progression of findings.

In bedside chest radiography, the supine position itself is sufficient to cause an equalization of vessel calibers in the upper and lower lung zones. By contrast, "vascular inversion," or an upper zone redistribution of blood flow, is a sensitive criterion that is independent of patient position. Even in supine patients it is a useful indicator of pulmonary venous hypertension. A diffuse caliber increase is suggestive of hypervolemia.

Chest wall thickness. Chest wall thickness is an important consideration because fluid is mobilized much faster from the soft tissues than from the vascular compartment. As a result, changes in chest wall thickness are a

Widening of the vascular pedicle by 1 cm corresponds to an approximate 2-L increase in the intravascular volume. Caution: patient rotation to the right or moving from sitting to supine can mimic mediastinal widening.

A standard radiographic technique and comparison with previous images will improve the evaluation of cardiovascular status.

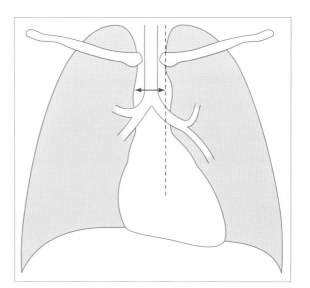

Fig. 2.26 **Upper mediastinum.**
Measuring the width of the upper mediastinum (vascular pedicle) on the chest radiograph.

more direct indicator of hydrostatic pressure changes than pulmonary vascular calibers: a 1-cm increase corresponds to an approximate 1-L increase of fluid volume in the extravascular compartment.

Edema

Pulmonary edema refers to an extravascular accumulation of intrapulmonary fluid. Initially the fluid is confined to the interstitium and may remain there (predominantly) or may spread to the alveolar spaces.

Types. Pulmonary edema is subdivided into two main pathophysiologic categories:
- *Hydrostatic edema*, which is caused by increased capillary pressure. This type leads to an excessive filtration of low-protein fluid through the capillary wall into the interstitial or alveolar spaces.
- *Permeability edema*, which is caused by increased permeability of the capillary wall. This increases the filtration of high-protein fluid into the interstitial space and alveolar wall.

This two-part classification is simplistic, as it disregards the fact that increased capillary pressure damages the capillary wall ("stress failure") and also culminates in the leakage of protein-rich fluid.

> Pulmonary edema is classified pathophysiologically as one of two types: hydrostatic edema and permeability edema.

Radiography

As with radiographs in the upright position, a distinction is made between *interstitial edema* and *alveolar edema* in bedside radiography. In communicating with clinicians, it has proven useful to classify pulmonary edema qualitatively as "mild," "moderate," or "severe," its progression as increasing or decreasing, and identify grades of edema (**Tables 2.3**, **2.4**).

Interstitial Edema

Radiographic signs of interstitial edema are as follows (**Fig. 2.27** and **Table 2.3**):
- blurring of vessel margins
- subpleural thickening
- thickened interlobar septa
- peribronchial cuffing
- septal lines

A (predominantly) interstitial fluid accumulation is characteristic of grade 2 pulmonary edema.

— Practical Recommendation —

Vessel margins *always* appear less sharp on bedside chest radiographs than on standard radiographs due to the larger focal spot and shorter film–focus distance. Acute interstitial edema can be distinguished from older preexisting interstitial changes in the lung parenchyma (e. g., due to pulmonary fibrosis) by comparison with previous radiographs taken before the acute event.

Table 2.3 Interstitial edema: pulmonary venous pressure > 25 mmHg (modified from Milne and Pistolesi 1993)

	Borderline	Mild	Moderate	Severe
Extracellular fluid volume in mL/L lung (TLC)	50–60	60–70	70–80	80–90
Central vessel margins		Indistinct	Indistinct and dilated	Very indistinct and markedly dilated
Cuffing	–		+	++
Lung density	–	Slightly increased	Moderately increased	Markedly increased
Delineation of small vessels	–	Questionable	Questionable	Poor delineation

TLC = total lung capacity.

Table 2.4 Alveolar edema: pulmonary venous pressure > 40 mmHg (modified from Milne and Pistolesi 1993)

	Borderline	Mild	Moderate	Severe	Fulminating
Extracellular fluid volume in mL/L lung (TLC)	90–100	100–120	120–140	140–180	> 180
Central vessel margins	Indistinct	Indistinct	Slightly obscured	Obscured but still definable	No longer definable
Cuffing	+	+	Slightly obscured	Obscured but still definable	No longer definable
Lung density	Gray	Grayish white	Regional opacity	Diffuse opacity	Complete opacity
Delineation of small vessels	Poor	Increasingly obscured	Obscured at the base	Diffusely obscured	Complete opacity

TLC = total lung capacity.

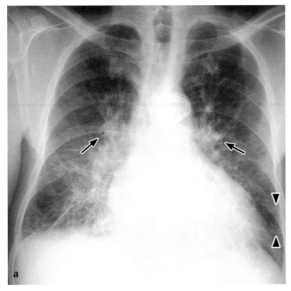
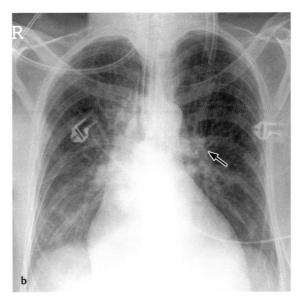

Fig. 2.27 a, b **Appearances of predominantly interstitial edema.**
Bronchial wall thickening (bronchial cuffing) (arrows), Kerley lines (arrowhead), and blurring of vascular margins due to interstitial fluid accumulation.

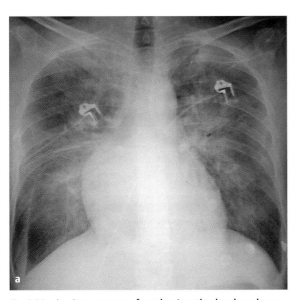
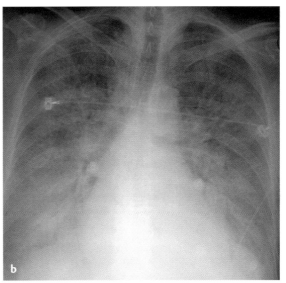

Fig. 2.28 a, b **Appearances of predominantly alveolar edema.**
Butterfly pattern of perihilar consolidation. The vessels are no longer defined. Note the absence of air bronchograms (differentiation from pneumonia) and the sparing of the subpleural space.

Alveolar Edema

Radiographic signs of alveolar edema are as follows (**Fig. 2.28** and **Table 2.4**):

- Increased density, which is often uniform and diffuse in the acute phase.
- With progression, density is mainly increased in dependent (posterobasal) lung zones.

Alveolar edema may be focal or diffuse, symmetrical or very asymmetrical, and may even show a nonuniform patchy distribution (**Fig. 2.29**). A symmetrical, predomi-

nantly perihilar distribution is known as butterfly edema (**Fig. 2.28a** and **Fig. 2.29a**). It should be noted that underlying parenchymal changes (scars, emphysema, bullae) and heart disease (e.g., mitral regurgitation) affect the distribution of edema. Given the significant interindividual variations, the presentation in a given individual is remarkably constant, and it may be helpful to compare the radiographs with images taken at earlier stages of decompensation.

A (predominantly) alveolar fluid accumulation is characteristic of grade 3 pulmonary edema.

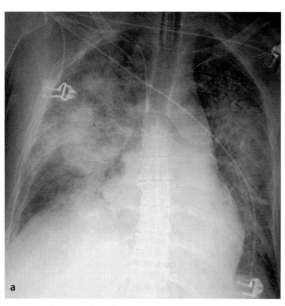 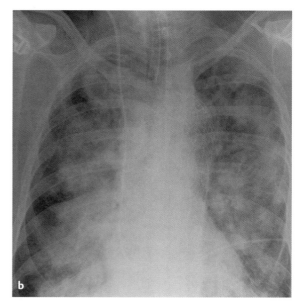

Fig. 2.29 a, b **Alveolar edema.**
Alveolar edema may be very asymmetrical (**a**) or may show an inhomogeneous patchy distribution (**b**).

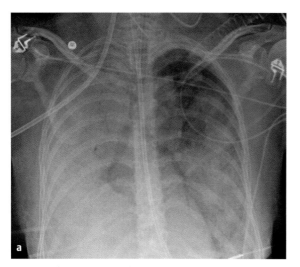 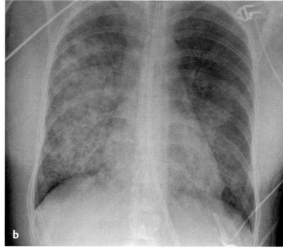

Fig. 2.30 a, b **Regression of alveolar edema.**
Alveolar hydrostatic edema (**a**) and ARDS may have identical appearances. But hydrostatic edema responds to treatment within hours, and shows marked improvement within 24 hours (**b**) compared with a time scale of several days or weeks in ARDS.

The following signs are helpful in differentiating alveolar edema from pneumonia:

- typical position dependence of the edema
- rapid onset
- prompt regression in response to therapy
- usual absence of an air bronchogram (the bronchi are often filled with fluid)

It is noteworthy that radiographic findings lag behind hemodynamic findings by up to 24 hours. Thus, edematous changes may still be radiographically visible even though the capillary venous pressure has fallen or returned to normal. A hallmark of pulmonary edema is its tendency to regress within 12–24 hours in response to therapy (**Fig. 2.30**); this contrasts with the greater persistence of infiltrates due to infection and the more gradual resolution of permeability edema (see ARDS, p. 37).

The changes of interstitial edema (grade 2) and alveolar edema (grade 3) are on a continuum, and it is common for radiographic signs of both forms to coexist. Accordingly, the findings described in the tables should be construed as "dominant" findings with various gradations rather than absolute differentiating criteria. As a rule, alveolar edema is more mobile and position-dependent than interstitial edema.

Interstitial (grade 2) edema and alveolar (grade 3) edema are on a continuum and often coexist.

Table 2.5 Criteria for distinguishing different types of edema (modified from Milne and Pistolesi 1993)

	Acute heart failure	Chronic recurrent heart failure	ARDS	Hypervolemia, renal failure
Bronchial cuffing	+++	+++	+	+++
Air bronchogram	Rare	Rare	+++	+/–
Septal lines	+	+	–	+
Widening of upper mediastinum	–	+	–	++
Dilated azygos vein	–	+	–	++
Pleural effusion	–	++	Rare; always small	++
Cardiac size	Normal	+	Normal	Normal (caution: pericardial effusion)

Differentiation of Hydrostatic (Cardiogenic) Edema from Permeability Edema (ARDS)

Besides the clinical presentation, the following radiographic signs are helpful in identifying the cause of pulmonary edema (**Table 2.5**).

- *Bronchial cuffing* is a classic sign of hydrostatic edema. It is also found in approximately one-third of patients with permeability edema, indicating a coexistence of both types in these cases.
- *Septal lines* are a rare finding and are seen in approximately one-third of patients with hydrostatic edema or hypervolemia. They almost never occur in permeability edema.
- *Air bronchograms* are very rare in hydrostatic edema, even in cases where alveolar fluid accumulation has already occurred (the bronchi are also filled with fluid). By contrast, air bronchograms are a characteristic early finding in permeability edema.
- The *width of the upper mediastinum (vascular pedicle)*, the size of the cardiac silhouette, and the diameter of the azygos vein are indicators of the circulating blood volume. This volume is normal or even reduced in permeability edema and acute heart failure, while it is increased in chronic heart failure or overhydration. A mediastinal width greater than 7 cm and cardiomegaly have proven to be the most accurate criteria for distinguishing hydrostatic edema from permeability edema (> 70% diagnostic accuracy).
- *Cardiomegaly* or a large azygos vein in a patient with permeability edema suggest that the increased hydrostatic pressure has a secondary cause (overhydration).
- *Pulmonary vascular redistribution to the upper zones* (vessel diameters larger in the upper zones than in the lower zones) is a typical sign of cardiogenic hydrostatic edema (> 50%).
- The *lung volume* is diminished in both hydrostatic and permeability edema, but it may be increased due to fluid overload in renal failure.

Edema Due to Other Causes

Table 2.6 and **Figs. 2.31, 2.32, 2.33, 2.34** list the causes and features of noncardiogenic forms of edema. The morphologic features of interstitial or alveolar edema may predominate in any given case, depending on the degree of severity. Noncardiogenic edema tends to resolve spontaneously and has a good prognosis.

Table 2.6 Criteria for distinguishing different types of edema (modified from Milne and Pistolesi 1993)

Permeability edema without diffuse alveolar damage
- Heroin overdose (often shows upper lobe predominance)
- Cytokine therapy (melanoma)
- After nutritional disorders (anorexia, refeeding syndrome)
- After bone marrow transplantation (capillary leak)

Pulmonary syndrome after hantavirus infection
- Intense immune response, diffuse capillary leak, frequent severe liver failure with an unfavorable prognosis

Neurogenic edema
- Follows severe CNS insult
- Bilateral alveolar edema, typically in the upper zones, tends to resolve spontaneously
- Does not contraindicate organ removal for transplantation

Reexpansion edema
- Follows rapid reexpansion of the lung after a pneumothorax or large effusion (lung compression for > 3 days); alveolar edema is typically unilateral, rarely bilateral due to blood-borne mediators

Postobstructive edema
- Bilateral perihilar edema that resolves within 24 hours
- Follows clearing (!) of an upper airway obstruction (e. g., laryngospasm, epiglottitis, strangulation, impacted foreign body)
- Broad vascular pedicle (increased pulmonary venous return after elevated intrapulmonary pressure falls with expiration)

Tocolytic therapy (μ-adrenergic agonists)
- Multifactorial cause (vascular volume overload and/or decreased plasma protein content, corticosteroid therapy); good prognosis

After pulmonary embolism
- Massive pulmonary embolism (> 50% obstruction) causes edema to develop in lung areas that are still perfused.

After lung transplantation
- Caused by impaired lymphatic drainage; typically begins at 24 hours, followed by spontaneous resolution over the next 10 days.

After pneumonectomy
- Caused by hyperperfusion of residual lung (see Chapter 3)

A mediastinal width > 7 cm and cardiomegaly are signs of hydrostatic edema (aid differentiation from permeability edema).

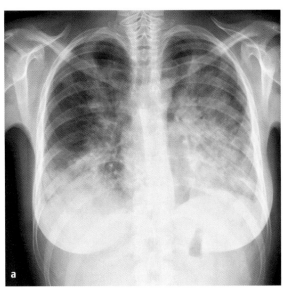

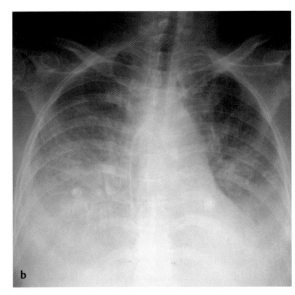

Fig. 2.31 a, b **Permeability edema without diffuse alveolar damage.**
a Refeeding syndrome in a girl with anorexia.

b Capillary leak after bone marrow transplantation.

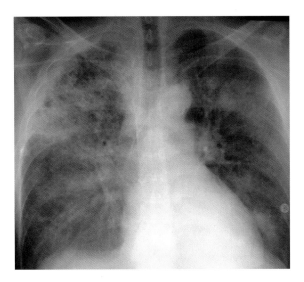

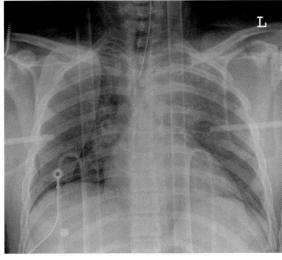

Fig. 2.32 **Neurogenic edema.**
Upper lobe predominance of edema following head trauma.

Fig. 2.33 **Postobstructive edema.**
Upper lobe predominance of edema following strangulation.

Computed Tomography

Pulmonary edema is evaluated on chest radiographs and is rarely an indication for CT.

On the other hand, edema should always be included in the differential diagnosis of thoracic CT findings in ICU patients and mainly requires differentiation from consolidation due to infection. The radiologist should therefore be familiar with the highly variable CT morphology of edema.

The CT features of intrapulmonary edema (**Fig. 2.35**) are as follows:

■ Increased parenchymal density combined with superimposed thickened (fluid-filled) interlobular and intralobular septa ("crazy paving" pattern; **Fig. 2.35a**). Like radiographs, CT scans also show thickening of the central bronchovascular interstitium (bronchial cuffing).

■ The increased density ranges from ground-glass opacity (parenchymal architecture and vessels are still visible) to dense consolidation (completely obscuring the parenchymal architecture), depending on the degree of intra-alveolar fluid accumulation. The degree of opacity correlates with the extravascular fluid volume (**Fig. 2.35b**).

▨ Edema requires differentiation from infection during the interpretation of thoracic CT in ICU patients.

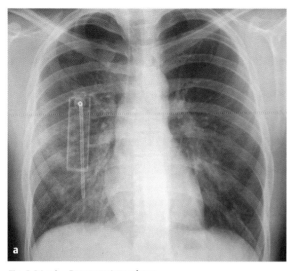
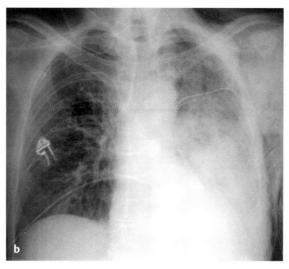

Fig. 2.34 a, b **Reexpansion edema.**
a   Reperfusion edema following a right-sided pneumothorax.
b   Reexpansion edema following a massive left-sided pneumothorax.

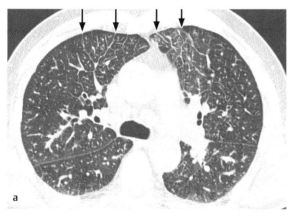
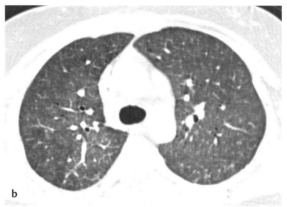

Fig. 2.35 a, b **Edema as seen by CT.**
Pulmonary edema can have a range of appearances on CT scans.
a   Interstitial edema with thickened interlobular septa (Kerley
lines).
b   Diffuse ground-glass opacity due to alveolar fluid accumulation.

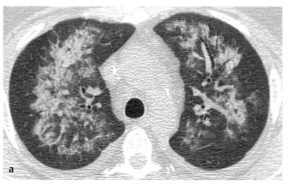
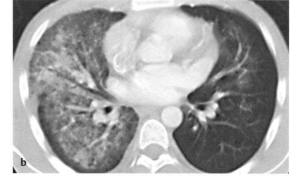

Fig. 2.36 a, b **"Infiltrative" spread of pulmonary edema.**
Edema, like consolidation, may show an "infiltrating" pattern of involvement. Note the asymmetrical distribution and sparing of the
subpleural space.

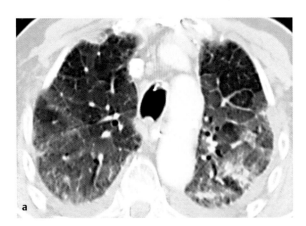

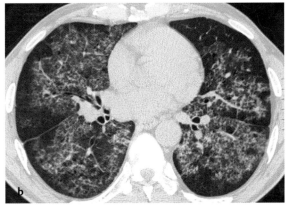

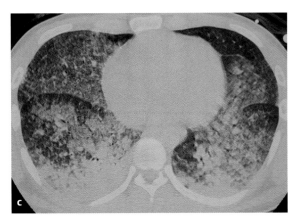

Fig. 2.37 a–c **Differential diagnosis of edema.**
Diffuse alveolar opacities are nonspecific in themselves and may result from a range of conditions.
a   ARDS.
b   Alveolar proteinosis ("crazy paving").
c   Parenchymal hemorrhage in Goodpasture syndrome (antero-posterior gradient).

- The subpleural space is typically spared or less severely involved (**Fig. 2.36a**). Sometimes the opacities show a geographic pattern in which they are sharply demarcated by interlobular septa.
- Alveolar edema is gravity-dependent. As a result, ground-glass opacity and consolidation are most pronounced in the dependent portions of the pulmonary lobes (increased lobar anterodorsal density gradient). Thickened interlobular septa, on the other hand, are most clearly defined in anterior lung regions.
- The opacities are generally bilateral but are not necessarily symmetrical. As on radiographs, the edema pattern may be very patchy and inhomogeneous, sharply delineated from areas of nonconsolidated lung (**Fig. 2.36b**).

The clinical presentation, course, and distribution of opacities can help narrow the differential diagnosis. Edema should always be considered in the differential diagnosis of ICU patients.

Differential Diagnosis

Pulmonary edema does not have specific radiographic or CT features. It presents with the relatively nonspecific morphologic findings of intra-alveolar transudate or exudate (alveolar filling). This material, consisting of fluid and cells, is cleared by lymphatic and venous drainage,

creating a superimposed pattern of reticular and septal opacities. This "crazy paving" pattern is found in various other conditions such as:
- permeability edema / diffuse alveolar damage (DAD, ARDS; **Fig. 2.37a**)
- pneumonia
- alveolar proteinosis (**Fig. 2.37b**)
- pulmonary hemorrhage (**Fig. 2.37c**)

The clinical presentation (e.g., inflammatory markers, hemoptysis), course (change within hours or days), and distribution of the opacities (gravity-dependent, subpleural sparing, diffuse or patchy) are helpful in narrowing the differential diagnosis. Especially in ICU patients, it is often important to include edema in the differential diagnosis rather than interpret all pulmonary opacities as pneumonia.

Adult Respiratory Distress Syndrome

I. Noebauer-Huhmann,
L. Kramer, and
C. Schaefer-Prokop

Definitions

Clinical parameters. Adult respiratory distress syndrome (ARDS) is a clinical diagnosis prompted by severe, acute respiratory failure in an adult patient. It is the most severe form of acute lung injury (ALI; PaO_2/FIO_2 < 300 mmHg) and was defined at a 1994 consensus conference by the following criteria:

- hypoxia with PaO_2/FIO_2 < 200 mmHg, requiring mechanical ventilation
- bilateral diffuse infiltrates on the frontal chest radiograph
- pulmonary artery wedge pressure < 18 mmHg

The mortality rate of ARDS is ca. 50% and depends on the age of the patient and the severity of the condition. Despite advanced intensive care measures, it is only recently that mortality has been reduced as a result of new ventilation strategies with optimized parameters, measures such as ECMO (extracorporeal membrane oxygenation), prone positioning, and improvements in the prevention and treatment of infection.

Radiographic findings. The definition of ARDS established by the American–European Consensus Conference (AECC) takes into account clinical parameters in addition to the radiographic finding of "diffuse bilateral infiltrates." Infiltrates are defined as ill-defined lung opacities not associated with tissue destruction or displacement, while "diffuse" means greater than 80% involvement of the radiographic lung area.

It should be emphasized, however, that the criterion of "bilateral infiltrates consistent with pulmonary edema" is *not sufficient* for the diagnosis of ARDS. Instead, the diagnosis of ARDS is based on a combination of clinical and radiographic findings. A lung opacity that remains stable or increases over a period of several days may be consistent with ARDS if the clinical respiratory parameters conform to the above definitions. Conversely, a diagnosis of ARDS is unlikely if the radiographic findings change within a matter of hours or there is no evidence of (increasing) consolidation.

Etiology

ARDS may have a variety of causes. A basic distinction is drawn between direct and indirect risk factors (**Table 2.7**). It is common for multiple risk factors to coexist in the same patient. They may immediately precede the acute respiratory failure or may antedate it by hours or days.

Pathophysiology

Pathophysiologically, ARDS represents the most severe form of *permeability edema*, in which diffuse alveolar damage (DAD) supervenes and dictates the further course of the syndrome.

Permeability edema alone is found only during the initial phase of ARDS. This condition is marked by damage to the *capillary* endothelium, allowing fluid to pass into the interstitium. The dominant and decisive mechanism, however, is diffuse damage to the *alveolar* epithelium. This causes flooding of the alveoli with proteinaceous fluid, leading to cell necrosis and inciting a hyperplastic inflammatory reaction of the alveolar epithelium with atelectasis and hyaline membrane formation. This process may culminate in end-stage fibrosis.

While the lung damage was once thought to be inhomogeneous, today it is believed that the entire lung is *uniformly* affected. Much as in a sponge, the edematous fluid increases the density and weight of the lung tissue, leading to the compression and atelectasis of dependent lung areas.

Phases of Adult Respiratory Distress Syndrome

The pathophysiology of ARDS is characterized by the following phases:

Early or exudative phase (24 hours). This phase develops within hours of the pulmonary insult and is characterized by edema of the interstitium and alveolar wall. The alveoli fill with a proteinaceous exudate containing red blood cells. This is accompanied by capillary congestion with the formation of fibrin thrombi in the capillaries, arterioles, and venules.

Intermediate phase (days 2 to 7). The alveolar edema becomes more compact and contains leukocytes and macrophages. Hyaline membranes are formed. As cellular proliferation increases, the edema is absorbed and areas of atelectasis develop.

▨ ARDS consists of an early or exudative phase, an intermediate phase, a late or proliferative phase, and an end stage.

▨ ARDS is a "clinical" diagnosis based on a combination of clinical and imaging findings.

Table 2.7 Etiology of adult respiratory distress syndrome (ARDS).

Direct insults	Indirect insults
▪ Aspiration	▪ Sepsis
▪ Severe pneumonia	▪ Extrathoracic trauma
▪ Near drowning	▪ Transfusion reaction
▪ Toxic inhalation	▪ Hypotension (shock)
▪ Lung contusion	▪ Burns
	▪ Disseminated intravascular coagulation
	▪ Pancreatitis, circulating toxins
	▪ Air or fat embolism

Late or proliferative phase (> 1 week). This phase is characterized by the proliferation of fibroblasts and myelofibroblasts in the alveolar and interstitial spaces. There is a mixed pattern of resolution and irreversible parenchymal destruction.

End stage. Patients who survive ARDS develop varying degrees of interstitial fibrosis. Only a small percentage of patients with a benign course have a good recovery with no impairment of pulmonary function.

Diagnostic Strategy

Radiography. The chest radiograph is part of the diagnostic workup and is used for follow-ups. Chest radiographs have a diagnostic accuracy of ca. 84% for detecting the presence of ARDS, but they are much less sensitive in detecting complications.

Computed tomography. CT has assumed an increasingly important role in the evaluation of ARDS patients. This is due mainly to the higher sensitivity of CT in detecting pulmonary complications such as pneumonia, abscesses, interstitial emphysema and hyperinflation, and mediastinal pathology (**Table 2.8**). At the same time, CT has contributed greatly to understanding the pathophysiology of ARDS and its response to mechanical ventilation. In the future, CT may play an even greater role in documenting the effects of various ventilation techniques.

Imaging

Radiography

ARDS is a clinical diagnosis. The nature, distribution, and extent of radiographic lung opacities are highly variable (**Fig. 2.38a, b**).

It should be noted that the clinical manifestations of ARDS may precede radiographic findings by more than 12 hours. Patients may already be markedly hypoxemic and still have a relatively normal-appearing chest film. This can be a useful differentiating feature from cardiogenic edema, in which radiographic changes tend to be synchronous with clinical manifestations.

Phases

Radiographs can demonstrate the successive phase of ARDS, although today the disease is usually modified by intensive care and rarely takes a "classic" course. The phases are described as exudative, proliferative, and fibrotic (**Table 2.9**).

Early or exudative phase (24 hours, stage I). The only initial finding in the chest radiograph may be elevation of the hemidiaphragm as a result of microatelectasis. Very little exudation occurs initially, and respiratory failure is due mainly to reduced compliance. These initial changes are soon followed by interstitial edema with thickening of vascular and bronchial walls and blurring of the pulmonary hila.

Intermediate phase (days 2 to 7, stage II). The early intermediate phase (days 2–4) is characterized by increased opacities spreading to all regions of the lung as the interstitial edema progresses to alveolar edema. The mediastinal shadow and diaphragm leaflets become less distinct and eventually are completely obscured (**Fig. 2.38a, b**). Extreme cases develop a densely opacified "white lung" with a positive air bronchogram. The patient is extremely hypoxic at this stage (**Fig. 2.38c**). The right ventricle and pulmonary arteries may be enlarged.

In the *late* intermediate phase (days 4–7) the opacities become more inhomogeneous and show a less compact distribution as focal and patchy opacities alternate with

Table 2.8 Indications for the CT examination of ARDS patients

- Detection or exclusion of complications (pneumothorax, abscess) in patients with equivocal radiographs
- Detection of clinically apparent but radiographically occult complications
- Discrepancy between radiographic and clinical findings
- Lack of treatment response not adequately explained by radiographs
- Quantification and characterization of parenchymal lung changes
- Quantification of atelectasis in dependent lung areas (selecting patients who would benefit from prone positioning, optimizing ventilation therapy)
- Help differentiate an extrapulmonary cause from primary pulmonary ARDS
- Detect and quantify barotrauma effects in patients who survive ARDS

Table 2.9 Phases of ARDS in the chest radiograph

I Early or exudative phase (24 hours)
- Hypovolemia and elevation of the hemidiaphragm
- Interstitial edema with thickened vascular and bronchial walls and increased hilar density with blurred margins

II Intermediate phase (days 2–7)
- Increasing alveolar edema with diffuse or patchy confluent opacities and air bronchograms
- Increased opacities spreading to all lung areas. Heart and diaphragm are no longer visualized; "white lung" in extreme cases
- Focal and patchy opacities; increased linear and reticular markings may be seen

III Late or proliferative phase (> 1 week)
- Inhomogeneous pattern with coarse reticular and patchy opacities and bullous hyperinflation

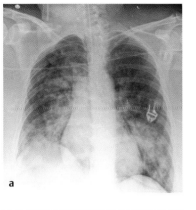
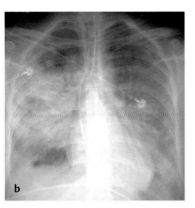
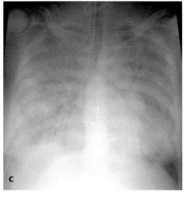
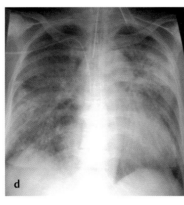

Fig. 2.38 a–d **Radiographic progression of ARDS in two patients.**

a, b Day 2: the extent and distribution of intrapulmonary opacities are highly variable. Both patients were diagnosed with ARDS based on their respiratory function.

c Day 4 (patient in **b**): dense opacification (white lung). Cardiac size and mediastinal width are normal.

d Day 6: increased opacities with a more patchy, inhomogeneous distribution. (Note the increasing cardiac size.)

increased linear and reticular markings (**Fig. 2.38d**). Regional lucencies due to mechanical ventilation and foci of pneumonia produce a heterogeneous pattern.

Pleural effusions are not a feature of ARDS per se. They may signify complications such as pneumonia or pulmonary embolism, they may be caused by clinically necessary infusion therapy, or they may result from fluid retention in a setting of acute renal failure.

Late or proliferative phase (> 1 week, stage III). Radiographs show a variable pattern consisting of coarse reticular, linear, and patchy opacities along with areas of bullous hyperinflation.

Scoring and Standards

Lung Injury Score. The Lung Injury Score (LIS)—also used in traumatology—is based on the number of quadrants showing alveolar consolidation on the chest radiograph. "Consolidation" is defined as increased lung density with little or no signs of volume loss and with the (potential) presence of an air bronchogram. The location of the central pulmonary arteries defines the boundary between the upper and lower quadrants.

Interpretation standards. The interpretation of radiographs varies considerably in the diagnosis of ARDS. This is particularly true in settings that involve different readers. For example, only moderate agreement was found between two ICU physicians and one radiologist in the reading of 728 radiographs in 99 ICU patients (kappa = 0.68–0.80). However, consensus training (definition of standard interpretive criteria, discussion of controversial readings, discussion of borderline cases) was followed by significant improvement in inter-reader agreement (kappa = 0.88–0.94). This supports the use of standards for chest radiograph interpretation in ARDS patients.

Scoring systems. Two scoring systems for ARDS have been described in the literature (after Pistolesi, **Table 2.10**; and after Haplerin, **Table 2.11**). Both systems have shown a high correlation with the distribution of CT attenuation values, but neither has become established for the rou-

Pleural effusions are not a primary feature of ARDS but result from disease- or treatment-related complications.

A standard protocol should be followed for chest radiograph interpretation in ARDS.

Table 2.10 Scoring system of Pistolesi et al. Each lung is evaluated individually to yield a total score between 0 and 52

Criterion	Score
Right heart enlargement	2.4
Hilar enlargement	1.2
Air bronchogram	2.4
Pulmonary opacity	
▪ Central opacity	1.2
▪ Peripheral opacity	2.4
▪ Diffuse opacity	3.6
▪ Central consolidation	2.4
▪ Peripheral consolidation	5.1
▪ Diffuse consolidation	7.1
▪ White lung	20

Table 2.11 Scoring system of Halperin et al. Each lung is evaluated individually and divided into three regions (upper, lower, and perihilar). The total score is between 0 and 390

Criterion	Score
Normal	0
Pulmonary congestion	
■ Mild	10
■ Moderate	20
■ Severe	30
Interstitial edema without septal lines	40
Interstitial edema with septal lines	45
Mixed interstitial and alveolar edema	
■ With regional sparing	50
■ Affecting the whole lung	55
Alveolar edema	
■ With regional sparing	60
■ Affecting the whole lung	65

Typical ARDS (caused by extrapulmonary injury in ca. 80% of cases) shows a characteristic AP density gradient.

tine evaluation of ARDS. One system is based on the scoring of lung opacity, the other on the distribution pattern of lung edema.

Computed Tomography

CT is far superior to radiography in the visualization of parenchymal densities. In particular, the inhomogeneity of the changes is displayed more clearly in sectional images than in projection radiographs.

Phases

As with radiographs, pulmonary opacities in patients diagnosed with ARDS take on a variety of appearances on CT.

Early or exudative phase. The dominant findings are ground-glass opacities and thickened interstitial septa.

Intermediate phase. The intermediate phase is characterized by increasing opacification, which may present various patterns:

- Typical ARDS (caused by extrapulmonary injury in ca. 80% of cases) shows a characteristic AP density gradient with areas of consolidation (= atelectasis) in the posterior lung, ground-glass opacities in the mid-lung, and well-ventilated areas in the anterior lung (**Fig. 2.39b**. Another possible pattern is diffuse homogeneous opacification throughout the lung parenchyma with no apparent density gradient (**Fig. 2.39a**).
- "Atypical" ARDS (most common after direct lung injury) is characterized by very nonuniform, patchy areas of consolidation that also involve the anterior lung and areas of apparent normal lucency and aeration. This form is considerably more difficult to ventilate (**Fig. 2.39c**).

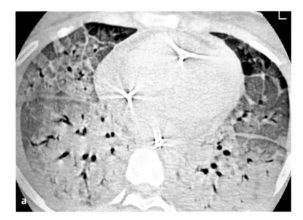

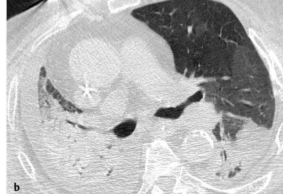

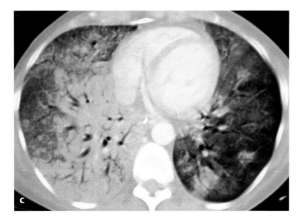

Fig. 2.39 a–c **Typical and atypical ARDS.**
The CT appearance of ARDS is variable and ranges from symmetrical bilateral consolidation (**a**) to symmetrical opacities with an anteroposterior gradient ("typical" ARDS, more common with an extrapulmonary cause) (**b**) or asymmetrical, patchy, inhomogeneous opacities ("atypical" ARDS, more common with a pulmonary cause) (**c**).
A CT slice in typical ARDS (**b**) shows an AP gradient across three lung compartments: aerated anterior lung, ground-glass opacities in the mid-lung, and dense consolidation (atelectasis) in the posterior lung. (The lung behaves like a "wet sponge.")

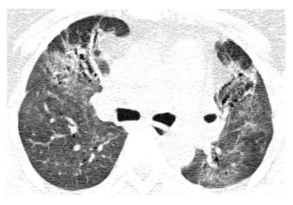 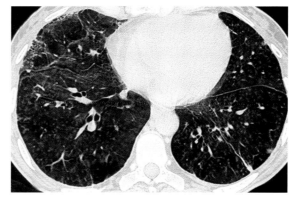

Fig. 2.40 a, b **Late phase of ARDS.**
Patients who survive ARDS develop fibrotic parenchymal changes in anterior lung regions, which are subjected to the greatest shear forces during ventilation.

Areas of moderate "ground-glass" opacity merit special attention because they are potentially recruitable in response to positive end-respiratory pressure (PEEP) ventilation. The variable location and extent of ground-glass opacities and consolidated areas explains why some patients respond well to PEEP while others (nonresponders) show little improvement of respiratory function. Patients with a patchy, inhomogeneous alternation of aerated and atelectatic lung areas (atypical ARDS) are particularly difficult to ventilate.

Late phase. Patients in the late phase (and patients who survive ARDS) show increasing signs of parenchymal destruction with coarse reticular markings, dilated bronchi, and hyperinflated lung areas. Fibrotic changes are found predominantly in anterior (nondependent) lung areas (**Fig. 2.40**). This is attributable to the protective effect of consolidated areas in the posterior lung, which serve to prevent lung damage from ventilation-induced shear forces and hyperinflation.

CT Densitometry in Acute Respiratory Distress Syndrome Patients

CT has provided new insights into the pathophysiology of ARDS and has greatly improved our understanding of how ARDS responds to mechanical ventilation. Despite the detection of regional density variations, it is widely accepted today that all portions of the lung—including areas that appear relatively normal at CT—are damaged and that the edematous changes caused by endothelial injury are distributed throughout the lung parenchyma. The accumulation of extravascular water significantly increases (triples) the weight of the lung parenchyma, leading to compression atelectasis in gravity-dependent regions of the lung. Air content is reduced to 20–30% while the total lung volume (air and tissue) is essentially unchanged.

Recruitment by PEEP. An increased respiratory pressure can at least partially reopen the collapsed alveoli, making them available for ventilation. Ventilating the patient with a positive end-expiratory pressure (PEEP) ensures that the alveoli remain open, even at end-expiration, and reduces the harmful effects of shear forces at the interfaces between aerated and atelectatic lung areas. Recruitment takes place against an anteroposterior and craniocaudal gradient, meaning that high volumes and pressures are needed to reach the posterior and inferior lung regions. This carries an associated risk of relative hyperinflation of anterior and superior lung areas (see Barotrauma, p. 46). Strong correlations exist between the size of the atelectatic areas on CT, the degree of intrapulmonary shunting, and the degree of oxygen tension reduction.

CT monitoring of response. CT attenuation measurements (CT densitometry) can be used to visualize and quantify the response to ventilation therapy (**Fig. 2.41**). This method is based on a somewhat simplified model quantifying lung compartments with regard to their air content and their associated CT attenuation value. Three ranges of values are distinguished:

- well-aerated lung areas with CT attenuation values between −900 and −500 HU
- moderately aerated areas with attenuation values between −500 and −100 HU
- atelectatic areas with attenuation values from −100 to +100 HU

The intermediate range from −500 to −100 HU corresponds to potentially recruitable areas, while the consolidated areas (−100 to +100 HU) are not recruited, even with high ventilatory pressures. CT can document the increasing alveolar recruitment with rising PEEP (recognized by an increase in the well-aerated lung compartment) (**Fig. 2.41**). Studies have established a significant

Moderate "ground-glass" opacities may by recruitable in response to PEEP.

CT densitometry can be used to document and quantify response to ventilation therapy.

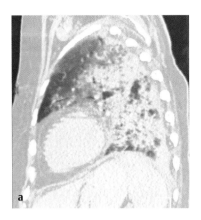 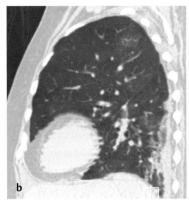

Fig. 2.41 a, b **Visualization of the effects of high PEEP ventilation.**
Coronal reconstructions of low-dose thoracic CT scans.
a   Without PEEP.
b   With PEEP. The posterior atelectatic areas are recruited. The effects can be appreciated within a few minutes.

correlation between PaO$_2$, alveolar recruitment, and the density compartments of the lung that are quantifiable by CT. While these compartments were formerly quantified in selected CT slices, today we have sophisticated software that can quantitate the density distribution throughout the lung volume.

Hyperinflated lung areas. Different values have been published for the limits at which a lung area should be considered "hyperinflated." Thus, attenuation values between −1000 HU and −900 HU have been classified as hyperinflated in healthy subjects, while other studies state attenuation values between −950 and −910 HU as the cutoff between normal ventilation and hyperinflation. It should be noted that lung attenuation values are already increased owing to the greater proportion of extravascular fluid, and that this effect may mask preexisting hyperinflation. The measured ventilatory pressures and pressure–volume curves in themselves cannot predict whether a given patient will sustain barotrauma because these parameters are additionally influenced by chest wall pressures.

PEEP ventilation can open microatelectatic areas, resulting in improvement of compliance, functional residual capacity, and gas exchange.

Technique of densitometry. Regarding the optimum technique for the measurement of CT attenuation values, it is still unclear at present whether it is sufficient to perform discrete density measurements at selected levels, whether continuous volumetry of the lung would be preferred, or whether dynamic measurements in one plane during one respiratory cycle would yield the best results.

Effect of Therapeutic Measures on Radiographic Findings

Ventilation with Positive End-Expiratory Pressure

Patients with ARDS are invariably placed on mechanical ventilation, usually with a PEEP. **Table 2.12** reviews various forms of mechanical ventilation.

— **Practical Recommendation** —————————————

Ventilation parameters critically influence the radiographic appearance of ARDS. This must be considered in image interpretation, and any changes in ventilator settings must be taken into account (**Fig. 2.42**). At some institutions the ventilator settings are indicated on the chest radiographs.

Pathophysiologically, the compliance of the lung depends on the volume of aerated (nonconsolidated) lung. Since consolidation may involve up to 80% of the lung volume, the normally compliant residual lung is also referred to as the "baby lung." Unlike compliance, the degree of hypoxia is independent of the consolidated lung volume and is caused by intrapulmonary shunting.

Effects. The goal of PEEP ventilation is to recruit the less severely damaged alveoli that are only temporarily atelectatic. The effect of PEEP, besides opening microatelectatic areas, is to redistribute the edema from the alveolar space to the interstitium, reducing the thickness of the alveolar fluid film. This in turn will improve compliance, functional residual capacity, and gas exchange.

The following points should be noted in ARDS patients on PEEP ventilation:

- PEEP causes an initial increase in lung volume, depression of the diaphragm, and an apparent increase in lung lucency.

Table 2.12   Various types of mechanical ventilation

Type of ventilation	Characteristics
PEEP (positive end-expiratory pressure)	Increases functional residual capacity (FRC) by opening areas of micro- and macroatelectasis
CPAP (continuous positive airway pressure)	Used in patients who can breathe spontaneously
IPPB (intermittent positive pressure breathing)	Used in patients who cannot breathe spontaneously

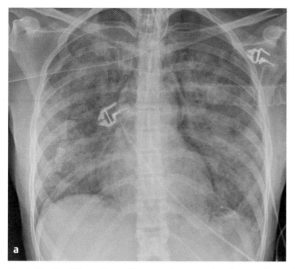 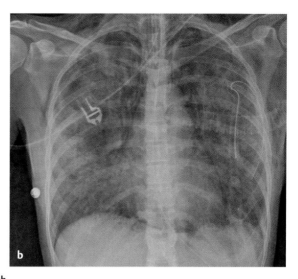

Fig. 2.42 a, b **Effect of ventilator settings on the chest radiograph.**
A 35-year-old woman with ARDS after COP (cryptogenic organ-
izing pneumonia) and barotrauma; the same patient as in
Fig. 2.46).

a PEEP 8.
b PEEP 12. Radiograph 1 day later shows apparent rapid
   "clearing" of lung opacities at the higher PEEP level.

- Hyperinflation of the bronchial system may produce
  an air bronchogram extending into the peripheral
  lung.
- The increased intra-alveolar pressure may convert alveolar edema to *interstitial edema with no actual
  change* in the intrapulmonary fluid content (apparent
  improvement).

Extracorporeal Membrane Oxygenation

Extracorporeal membrane oxygenation (ECMO) is used in
cases where optimum mechanical ventilation can no longer provide adequate oxygenation. It also serves to minimize ventilation injury and promote healing of the lungs.

Types. Venovenous ECMO (femoral vein) is used patients
with an isolated disturbance of gas exchange, while venoarterial ECMO (femoral artery and vein) can be used in
patients who are also in heart failure. Blood is withdrawn
from the inferior vena cava via bilateral inguinal catheters (connected externally by a Y-piece) and is reinfused
into the superior vena cava through a jugular vein catheter. Oxygen is introduced through the exchange membrane while carbon dioxide is removed (some degree of
hypercapnia is often allowed).

Other strategies are aimed chiefly at CO_2 removal to
reduce the volumes and rates of respiration (*ECCO₂R*).
Oxygen delivery in these cases takes place mainly
through the lung.

Effects. Overall results to date have not been encouraging.
Despite more than 20 years' experience with ECMO in
ARDS patients, a definite benefit has been demonstrated
only in newborns. The benefits that might be achieved in
adult patients are overshadowed by complications such
as bleeding and a greater need for transfusions.

ECMO can provide adequate oxygenation at a low ventilation pressure. As a result, the radiographic density of
the lung parenchyma is increased at the start of treatment due to an increase in atelectasis and alveolar edema. This initial increase in lung density does not signify
actual deterioration. On the other hand, the progression
of opacities from the peripheral to central lung or complications of barotrauma are considered to be poor prognostic signs. A new pleural effusion may be a hemothorax
resulting from anticoagulation. Care should be taken that
the ECMO cannulas are correctly positioned.

Positional Changes

The supine patient may be turned prone in an effort to
counteract the increased pressure load on posterior lung
areas from the weight of the nondependent lung
("soaked sponge" effect). This measure has been found
to improve oxygenation in ca. 65% of patients.

Effects. Turning the patient prone alters the distribution
of lung density within 10 minutes with no further significant change occurring after 45 minutes. Although the
reduction of posterobasal lung density is accompanied by
the appearance of new anterior opacities, the greater
vascularity of the posterior lung appears to play a decisive role. One study found that it took 12 hours for oxygenation (PaO_2/FIO_2) to improve, and even longer for a
reduction of extravascular lung fluid and shunt fraction.

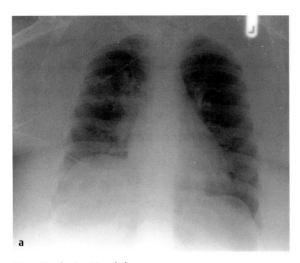
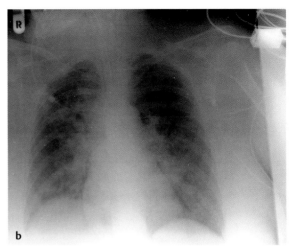

Fig. 2.43 a, b **Positional change.**
Patient with a clinical diagnosis of ARDS in the prone position (**a**) and in the supine position several days later (**b**). Note the different positions of the scapulae and clavicles and the change in cardiac shape.

Early prone positioning was found to produce a more rapid improvement of oxygenation in just 60–90 minutes. Studies have consistently shown that turning the patient back to the supine position reverses the positive effect (to a large degree), and that returning to the prone position restores the benefit. Prone positioning may even reduce the risk of infection in the posterior lung.

The prone position should be indicated on chest radiographs to avoid errors of interpretation, as this position will cause the heart, mediastinal shadow, and pleural effusions to appear larger on x-ray films (**Fig. 2.43**).

> When the patient is turned prone, the heart, mediastinal shadow, and pleural effusions appear larger on the chest radiograph.

Liquid-Assisted Gas Exchange

Partial or complete "flooding" of the lung with organic liquid (*fluorocarbon liquid-assisted gas exchange*) is still in the testing stage. This liquid can bind 17 times more oxygen than saline solution. It has a low surface tension and is rapidly distributed over the airway epithelium.

Effects. It is hoped that the heavy fluid will gravitate into the more severely affected posterior lung areas and that the weight of the fluid will redistribute ("squeeze") the blood from these regions into regions with better ventilation. Initial results with partial fluid ventilation appear promising.

The radiographic appearance resembles that of a white lung *without* an air bronchogram (see **Fig. 2.38c**).

Inhalation Therapy

Surfactant. The damage to type II pneumocytes in ARDS leads to a depletion of surfactant and an influx of fluid into the alveoli. This effect is compounded as the intra-alveolar fluid inactivates endogenous surfactant. An al-

tered lipid composition also makes the surfactant less effective.

Aerosolized surfactant may be administered by inhalation in an effort to lower the surface tension, thereby reducing atelectasis and improving ventilation. Studies to date have not shown a significant benefit with this therapy, presumably due to an uneven distribution of the surfactant, a less-than-optimum surfactant composition, and the diminished response of inflammatory fibrotic lung tissue to the medication. To date, respiratory improvement with surfactant has been documented only in newborns and preterm infants (especially after meconium aspiration).

NO ventilation, prostacyclin, prostaglandin. Vasodilating agents can be selectively administered by inhalation (NO ventilation, prostacyclin [PGI_2] or prostaglandin [PGE_1]) into aerated lung regions with the goal of improving perfusion and the ventilation–perfusion ratio. The various agents differ in their systemic side effects and their efficacy in improving oxygenation and lowering the pulmonary arterial pressure.

Differential Diagnosis in ICU Patients

Hydrostatic cardiogenic edema. The following criteria are helpful in differentiating cardiogenic hydrostatic edema from noncardiogenic permeability edema (**Table 2.13**):

- A predominantly peripheral distribution of lung opacities is typical of ARDS but is found in less than 50% of cases.
- Classic ARDS is not characterized by interstitial densities such as septal lines, peribronchial cuffing, or thickened fissures and there is no pleural effusion.

Table 2.13 Differentiation of cardiogenic hydrostatic edema from noncardiogenic permeability edema

	Cardiogenic hydrostatic edema	Noncardiogenic permeability edema
Kerley lines	Common	Uncommon
Pleural effusions	Common	Uncommon
Cardiomegaly	Common	Uncommon
Opacities	Diffuse, central	Patchy, peripheral
Air bronchogram	Uncommon	Common
Unsharp hilar vessels	Common	Uncommon
Peribronchial opacities	Common	Uncommon

Cardiac size is normal, and the vascular pedicle is not widened.
- The ARDS patient is almost always intubated for severe hypoxia. Generally this is unnecessary with hydrostatic edema.
- Hydrostatic edema changes quickly with an improvement in hemodynamic status.
- Note: Mixed forms are common, and often the findings cannot be referred to one type of edema.

Preexisting changes. In the absence of serial examinations, it can be very difficult to distinguish between pre-existing changes in the lung parenchyma (e.g., fibrosis) and ARDS-associated or barotrauma-induced changes.

Drug-induced or immunologic lung disease. These conditions should also be considered in the differential diagnosis of acute respiratory failure with increased radiographic density. The radiographic (and CT) appearance of diffuse alveolar damage (DAD) is characterized by increased lung density with superimposed reticular opacities (crazy paving, **Fig. 2.44a**). Especially in long-term ICU patients, it is common to find immune-related changes in the lung parenchyma, probably triggered by multiple causative agents, with features of DAD or organizing pneumonia and without a demonstrable cause.

Diffuse pulmonary hemorrhage. Diffuse intrapulmonary hemorrhage (e.g., in the setting of Goodpasture syndrome, vasculitis, SLE pneumonitis) can mimic the radiographic appearance of ARDS. Hemoptysis and a less severe hypoxemia, which may not require mechanical ventilation, suggest the correct diagnosis.

Pneumonia. Pneumonia should always be excluded (**Fig. 2.44 b**). Note that ARDS may also be very asymmetrical and confined to one lobe, at least initially (e.g., on

ARDS may be very asymmetrical or initially confined to one lobe, making it difficult to distinguish from pneumonia.

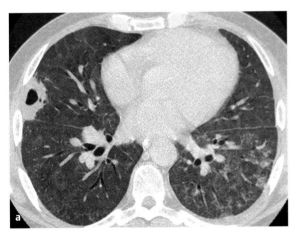

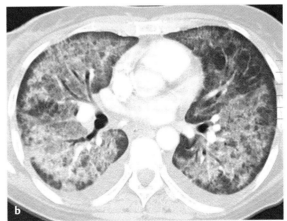

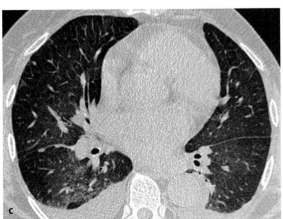

Fig. 2.44 a–c **Differential diagnosis.**
Conditions that can mimic ARDS on CT scans (note the absence of an AP gradient!).
a Patient with drug-induced diffuse alveolitis (histologic diagnosis of diffuse alveolar damage, DAD) and a cavitating subpleural infarction after pulmonary embolism. It is common to find diffusely increased lung density in long-term ICU patients, probably as a response to multiple causative factors.
b *Pneumocystis jirovecii* infection in an HIV-positive patient.
c Patient with bilateral hydrostatic edema. Note the sparing of the subpleural space (see also **Fig. 2.36**) and the anterior Kerley B lines.

the affected side after a direct pulmonary insult or on the contralateral side after lobectomy).

Hydrostatic edema. Every case of hydrostatic edema, whether cardiogenic or caused by hypervolemia, may present radiographically as ARDS. Important differentiating features are thickened interlobular septa, symmetry, and sparing of the subpleural space (**Fig. 2.44c**).

Complications

Barotrauma and Volutrauma (Ventilator-Induced Lung Injury)

Based on reports in the literature, the incidence of ventilator-induced lung injury in ARDS is higher than 50% and correlates directly with the type of ventilation, ventilation volume and inspiratory pressure, airway pressure level, patient age, and the presence of underlying lung disease. The damage is attributed to shear forces at the interfaces between atelectatic and aerated lung areas and to the repetitive opening and closing of small bronchioles and alveoli at a low end-expiratory pressure (the latter is believed to prevent optimum PEEP ventilation).

Extra-alveolar air. A high end-inspiratory volume and high PEEP can lead to alveolar overdistension in aerated lung regions with increased permeability and increased leakage of fluid, proteins, and blood into the interstitium. The rupture of marginal alveoli permits air to enter the extra-alveolar interstitial space and to spread along the interlobular septa and bronchovascular perivascular interstitium toward the hilum and mediastinum and also into the subpleural space and subcutaneous tissue (Macklin effect). Extra-alveolar air may present as (**Fig. 2.45**):

- pulmonary interstitial emphysema (PIE)
- subcutaneous emphysema and subpleural cysts

Extra-alveolar air may appear radiographically as PIE, subcutaneous emphysema, subpleural cysts, pneumothorax, pneumomediastinum, and in some cases pneumoperitoneum and pneumoretroperitoneum.

- pneumothorax
- pneumomediastinum
- pneumoperitoneum and pneumoretroperitoneum by continued air dissection

Radiographs have low sensitivity for the detection of PIE. In most cases the complications of barotrauma are not radiographically visible until mediastinal emphysema or subcutaneous emphysema has developed (**Fig. 2.46**). This underscores the importance of recognizing early signs of impending barotrauma in thoracic CT (**Fig. 2.47**).

Pulmonary interstitial emphysema. PIE appears radiographically as streaky lucencies radiating from the hila toward the periphery of the lung. Unlike bronchi, these lucent streaks do not branch and do not show peripheral tapering. A tangential section of a vessel and surrounding air-filled perivascular interstitium displays characteristic ringlike structures or double outlines called perivascular halos (**Fig. 2.47c, d**). The further progression of PIE is marked by cystic air collections, some only millimeters in size and located mainly in the subpleural lung. These peripheral bullae predispose to the development of pneumothorax. Subpleural emphysema appears as a lucent band extending over the diaphragmatic leaflets or along the chest wall (**Fig. 2.47a**).

PIE in adults is virtually invisible on chest radiographs. Superimposed, air-filled secondary lobular septa create a fairly disordered pattern that is best appreciated in the peripheral lung as a "negative" of the Kerley B lines.

Additional signs. The following additional radiographic signs suggest an increased risk of barotrauma:

- The longitudinal lung diameter is greater than 25 cm (compare with prior radiographs!)

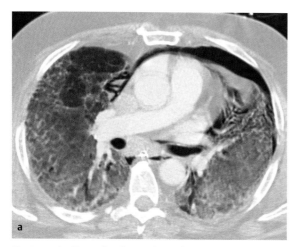
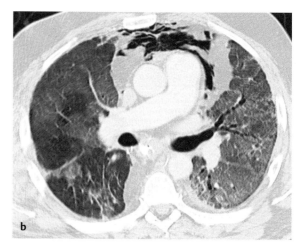

Fig. 2.45 a, b   **Extra-alveolar air due to barotrauma in an ARDS patient.**
Differentiating signs: a pneumothorax appears as a "featureless space" (**a**), and mediastinal emphysema contains septa (**b**).

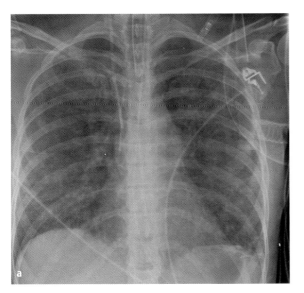 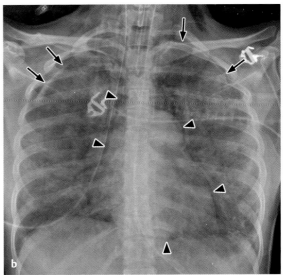

Fig. 2.46 a, b **ARDS and barotrauma.**
A 35-year-old woman with ARDS after COP; same patient as in
Fig. 2.42.
a No evidence of barotrauma (PEEP 12).

b Radiograph 3 days later show bilateral pneumothorax
(arrows) with mediastinal emphysema (arrowheads) and
subcutaneous emphysema (PEEP 8).

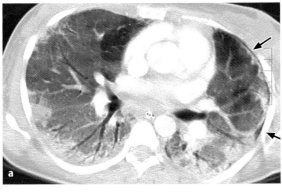 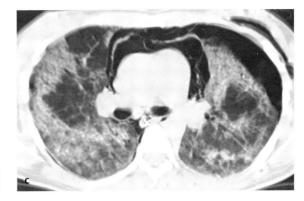

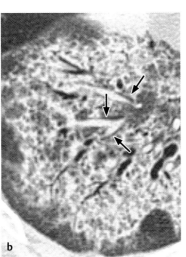 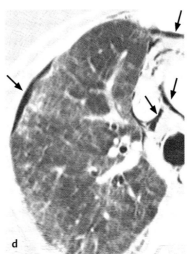

Fig. 2.47 a–d **Signs of impending barotrauma.**
a, b Peripheral hyperinflated areas, subpleural emphysematous
bullae, and interstitial emphysema.

c, d Both patients 2 days later: obvious barotrauma with
pneumothorax and mediastinal emphysema.

It is important to detect even a small pneumothorax in ventilated ARDS patients, as it may progress rapidly to a tension pneumothorax.

- The anterior part of the sixth rib is projected over lung tissue (not over the upper abdomen, as is normally the case—check the projection).

Pneumothorax and Pneumatoceles

Approximately one-third of ARDS patients develop a pneumothorax or bullae (pneumatoceles). Approximately 10% develop a pneumomediastinum.

Pneumatoceles. Pneumatoceles are cysts or bullae, usually up to 5 mm in size, that often have a subpleural or perihilar location. They may also form "interstitial air tracks" with a peribronchovascular distribution. Presumably they are not only a result of ventilator-induced barotrauma and air-trapping but are also caused by pulmonary ischemia and are considered a poor prognostic sign. They are difficult to distinguish from emphysematous changes and microabscesses on chest films, and they may even form a nidus for superinfection and microabscess formation.

Central pneumatoceles may persist or regress during ARDS. Subpleural pneumatoceles predispose to the development of a (tension) pneumothorax. Larger emphysematous bullae may be mistaken for a loculated pneumothorax, especially since they have similar functional effects.

Pneumothorax. The detection of a pneumothorax on a supine radiograph is less straightforward than on an upright radiograph (see also Pneumothorax, p. 74). The familiar pattern of a visceral pleural line with no lung markings beyond it is frequently absent. Recurrent pneumothoraces are not uncommon (up to 30%), even with a thoracostomy tube in place, and are more commonly observed when the pleural drain runs along the interlobar fissure.

The *anteromedial pleural recess* is the most common site of occurrence of pneumothorax in the supine patient, followed by the basal *subpulmonic recess*. The only radiographic sign of an anteromedial pneumothorax may be a circumscribed lucent area in the cardiophrenic angle. This may result in sharp outlining of the cardiac or mediastinal borders or deepening of the costodiaphragmatic recess ("deep sulcus" sign).

The less common *posterolateral pneumothorax* occurs predominantly on the left side and may lead to sharp delineation from the medial visceral lower lobe pleura and sharp outlining of the paraspinal line, descending aorta, or posterior costophrenic angle.

One-third of pneumothoraces are missed on the supine chest radiograph. It is important to detect even a small pneumothorax, however, because it may progress rapidly to a tension pneumothorax in the mechanically ventilated patient.

Tension pneumothorax. Tension pneumothorax in ARDS patients displays several distinctive features. The following signs of tension pneumothorax may be absent as a result of bilateral reduced lung compliance and pleural adhesions:

- pulmonary volume loss
- ipsilateral depression of the diaphragm
- contralateral mediastinal shift

The following signs are suggestive of tension pneumothorax in ARDS patients:

- flattening of the diaphragm compared with previous examinations
- flattening of the cardiac border (due to a combination of increased intrathoracic pressure and impaired venous return)
- contralateral displacement of the anterior junction line
- displacement of the azygoesophageal recess

Pneumonia in Adult Respiratory Distress Syndrome

Pneumonia is a frequent complication of ARDS (>70%) and is more life-threatening than the respiratory failure itself. While respiratory failure alone is responsible for less than 25% of deaths, the mortality rate rises to more than 70% in ARDS patients who develop pneumonia.

Nosocomial lung infection is difficult to diagnose clinically and radiologically in ARDS patients. Fever, cough, purulent sputum, and leukocytosis are not useful diagnostic criteria in mechanically ventilated ICU patients.

Radiographic criteria. While the diagnosis of pneumonia is often based on radiographic criteria, these criteria are ultimately nonspecific or greatly limited because ARDS-related opacities may be superimposed on the pneumonic infiltrates or may mask their presence. Although a new opacity appearing during the course of uncomplicated ARDS is a theoretical indicator of superimposed pneumonia, the diagnostic accuracy of chest radiographs is very low in practice. One study found that portable chest radiographs were only 52% accurate in diagnosing pneumonia in ventilated patients—comparable to the flip of a coin. Referral to previous chest radiographs and knowledge of clinical data were not helpful in improving accuracy.

Computed tomography criteria. CT can correctly diagnose pneumonia in only 60% of affected ARDS patients (true positive) and can exclude it in 70% (true negative). The following criteria are helpful:

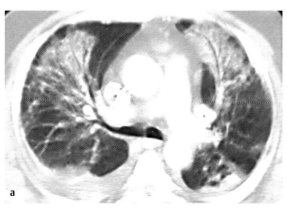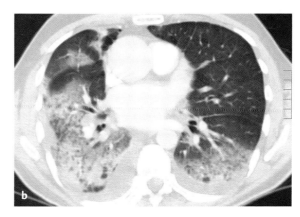

Fig. 2.48 a, b **Pneumonia in ARDS.**
Anterior (!) opacities with air bronchograms not attributable to compression or edema should always raise suspicion of pneumonia. Consolidation due to infection (**a**) and ARDS-related consolidation (**b**) are indistinguishable on CT scans.

- Consolidated areas in nondependent lung regions are detectable in more than 90% of ARDS patients with pneumonia, but are also found in up to 60% of patients without pneumonia (**Fig. 2.48**).
- When scans are performed after injection of contrast medium, atelectasis shows intense homogeneous contrast enhancement while pneumonia shows a relatively lower and inhomogeneous enhancement.
- Nosocomial diseases are often accompanied by micro-abscesses. These lesions should not be misinterpreted as pneumatoceles.

Sepsis Syndrome, Multiorgan Failure

Sepsis may be a cause or a result of ARDS. Liver failure is a particularly common cause of multiorgan failure. It may be that an intact liver protects the lung by eliminating mediators of lung injury via the reticuloendothelial system.

Fibrosis

Dilated bronchi. Bronchial dilatation in ARDS patients appears to suggest progression to irreversible fibrotic parenchymal destruction, just as bronchiectasis in areas of ground-glass opacity indicates fibrosing alveolitis. On the other hand, bronchial dilatation in the setting of infectious pneumonia is a reversible condition.

Barotrauma. Studies on the late sequelae of ARDS have shown that barotrauma and high-dose oxygen during mechanical ventilation promote the development of fibrotic lung changes. The fibrotic involvement of anterior lung areas was significantly more common in patients who were not turned prone but were ventilated only in the supine position. The posterior lung areas of supine patients are atelectatic during the acute phase, which appears to protect the lung.

It is difficult to diagnose pneumonia on chest radiographs and CT scans in ARDS patients.

Pneumonia

C. Schaefer-Prokop and E. Eisenhuber-Stadler

Classification

Most pulmonary infections in ICU patients are hospital-acquired (nosocomial). They differ from community-acquired (outpatient) pneumonias in the spectrum of causative organisms and in their course.

By definition, *nosocomial infections* develop at least 72 hours after the patient has been hospitalized. Nosocomial infections of the upper and lower respiratory tract are among the most important contributors to morbidity and mortality in ICU patients.

Multiple factors contribute to the high incidence of nosocomial pneumonia, which is ca. 10% in medical or surgical ICU patients and up to 60% in ARDS patients (**Table 2.14**). The mortality of nosocomial pneumonia is high (35%), regardless of the causative organism, and is even higher in patients with respiratory failure (55%).

Table 2.14 Factors responsible for the high incidence of pneumonia in ICU patients

- Underlying disease: diabetes, cancer, chronic airway diseases, hematologic diseases, immunosuppression
- Antibiotic therapy
- Steroid therapy
- Alteration of pharyngeal flora
- Presence of tubes and lines
- Rise of gastric pH with bacterial colonization
- Aspiration of gastric contents

By definition, *nosocomial infections* develop at least 72 hours after the patient has been hospitalized.

Table 2.15 Modified criteria of the American Thoracic Society for "severe" community-acquired pneumonia with a high complication rate (after Neuhaus et al. 2001)

Minor criteria (present on admission)
- Respiratory rate $\geq$ 30/min
- Respiratory failure (PaO$_2$/FIO$_2$ < 250) on admission
- Radiographic infiltrates in at least two lobes
- Systolic blood pressure < 90 mmHg

Major criteria (present on admission or later in the hospital stay)
- Need for mechanical ventilation
- Septic shock
- Acute renal failure or renal insufficiency (creatinine > 2 mg/dL)

Table 2.16 Risk factors associated with infection by certain types of bacteria

Risk factors	Bacteria
COPD, chronic lung disease	*Haemophilus*
Chronic lung disease, diabetes, alcohol abuse	*Legionella*, pneumococci, gram-negative bacteria
Venous catheterization (nosocomial infection)	*Staphylococcus aureus, Staphylococcus epidermis*
Immune suppression: myeloma, CLL, lymphoma, GvHD, HIV, organ transplantation (especially the heart)	*Haemophilus*
Leukemia or lymphoma	*Nocardia*
Granulocytopenia, chronic granulomatous diseases	*Staphylococcus aureus*
Post-influenza	*Staphylococcus aureus* (bacterial superinfection)

CLL, chronic lymphoblastoid leukemia; COPD, chronic obstructive pulmonary disease, GvHD, graft-versus-host disease.

Table 2.17 Risk factors for pathologic oropharyngeal colonization and nosocomial pneumonia (modified from Caven et al. 1992)

Endogenous risk factors
- Malnutrition
- Chronic illness
- Immunodeficiency
- Alcohol, nicotine abuse
- Impaired consciousness
- Aspiration
- Previous infection or antibiotic therapy
- Previous surgery (neck, lung, abdomen)

Exogenous risk factors
- Cross-contamination
- Hospitalization
- Medication (sedatives, immunosuppressants, antacids)
- Intubation (tracheostomy tube, endotracheal tube, nasogastric tube)

Nosocomial pneumonia in ICU patients requires differentiation from *community-acquired pneumonia* which requires immediate ICU admission and mechanical ventilation because of its severity and extent or occurrence in a lung with underlying disease such as pre-existing fibrosis or severe chronic obstructive pulmonary disease (COPD).

Table 2.15 reviews the criteria for *"severe"* pneumonia with a high complication rate requiring early hospitalization and intensive care to reduce complications such as ARDS, pneumosepsis, and abscess formation. Some patients are more susceptible to certain infectious organisms because of their comorbidity (**Table 2.16**) and are predisposed to a particularly severe clinical course.

Opportunistic organisms are infectious for all patients but are a particular threat to immunocompromised patients.

Pathogenesis

Nosocomial pneumonia in ICU patients, unlike community-acquired pneumonia, is commonly caused by infection with *gram-negative* organisms or anaerobes (*Pseudomonas, Enterobacter, Klebsiella, Escherichia coli*). Gram-positive organisms (*Staphylococcus aureus* and *Streptococcus pneumoniae*) are causative in less than 20% of cases (**Table 2.17**).

Half of patients with nosocomial pneumonia are found to be infected by more than one organism (*polymicrobial pneumonia*). Antibiotic-resistant organisms pose a serious, growing problem in ICU patients with nosocomial infections.

Gram-negative and polymicrobial infections are characterized by a high rate of complications such as abscess formation, empyema, and bronchopulmonary fistulae

Classification of Pathogens

The clinical diagnosis of pneumonia is often difficult in ICU patients because the classic signs of lung infection such as fever, leukocytosis, sputum production, positive sputum culture, and radiographic infiltrates may be absent. Moreover, fever and leukocytosis often have an extrapulmonary or noninfectious cause. Errors are very common in the clinical and radiologic diagnosis of pneumonia in ICU patients.

Direct identification of causative organisms. The growing list of causative organisms that have become resistant to a range of therapeutic agents has led to the more conscientious use of antibiotics and a greater reliance on hospital hygiene. Given the poor diagnostic accuracy of clinical and imaging findings and the growing number of multiresistant strains, various strategies have been developed for direct identification of the causative organisms (**Table 2.18**). Designed to aid in selecting a specific antibiotic therapy for the offending organism, these methods are based on quantitative cultures:

- *Aspirated tracheal secretions.* The diagnostic threshold is relatively high, at 10^5–10^6 CFU/mL (colony-forming units), to increase specificity.

Gram-negative and polymicrobial infections have a higher complication rate than gram-positive infections.

Table 2.18 Methods for the identification of infecting organisms

Method	Characteristics
Sputum Gram stain	Material must be sampled from the lower respiratory tract. Useful for *Streptococcus pneumoniae* but does not identify atypical organisms.
Blood culture	Low sensitivity, but still included in ATS Guidelines for hospitalized patients.
Sputum culture	Takes too long, depends on sampled material; included in ATS Guidelines.
Serologic tests	Moderate sensitivity but high specificity; take too long (require 4-fold titer increase). Exception: high IgM levels with *Mycoplasma pneumoniae*
Polymerase chain reaction (PCR)	High sensitivity and specificity, available for multiple pathogens such as mycobacteria, *Pneumocystis jirovecii*, viruses, *Aspergillus*, *Legionella* species, etc.
Thoracocentesis Aspiration bronchoscopy Transthoracic needle aspiration Lung biopsy	Invasive procedures

ATS = American Thoracic Society.

- Material sampled by *protected brush bronchoscopy* (PBB). The threshold for distinguishing between colonization and pneumonia is 10^3 CFU/mL.
- Material sampled by *conventional or protected bronchoalveolar lavage* (BAL). The threshold is $> 10^4$ CFU/mL.
- Another method is *cytologic evaluation* of the material under a microscope.

Serologic tests are available as an alternative to invasive methods (polymerase chain reaction, monoclonal antibodies).

Imaging

Radiography and Computed Tomography

Chest radiography is the imaging study of first choice in patients with suspected pneumonia. Portable chest radiographs are particularly useful for the post-therapeutic follow-up of ICU patients.

Parenchymal opacity. Opacity of the lung parenchyma is the radiographic hallmark of pneumonia. The spectrum of findings ranges from subtle focal opacities to extensive consolidation throughout the lung. An air bronchogram is *not* seen in all cases of pneumonia and is present only when air-filled bronchi are surrounded by uniformly opacified lung parenchyma. For example, lobar pneumonia (e.g., pneumococci) typically forms an air bronchogram (**Fig. 2.49a**) whereas lobular bronchopneumonia causes patchy confluent opacities without an air bronchogram (e.g., *Staphylococcus aureus*) (**Fig. 2.49b**). Interstitial pneumonia (e.g., *Pneumocystis jirovecii*, viral pneumonia) is characterized by bilateral interstitial or nodular opacities (**Fig. 2.49c**).

The presence of an air bronchogram positively identifies an opacity as an intrapulmonary infiltrate (as op-

posed to, say, a pleural effusion). Other important differentiating signs are increased lung volume (unlike atelectasis) and radiographic change occurring over a period of days (unlike edema, which changes within hours).

Signs of specific organisms. Table 2.19 reviews the imaging findings that are commonly associated with certain infectious organisms. Note, however, that the imaging findings are *not* specific and are meant only as a guide for narrowing the spectrum of causative organisms.

The following points have proven useful in practice:
- Pneumococci are the "classic" causative agent of lobar pneumonia. They produce a positive angiogram sign on CT scans (high intravascular contrast with low parenchymal enhancement, **Fig. 2.50a**).
- *Klebsiella* infections tend to increase the affected lung volume (caution: abscess formation) (**Fig. 2.50b**).
- Staphylococci are the classic organisms of bronchopneumonia and septic pneumonia. They may produce cavitating and cystic lesions (**Figs. 2.51, 2.53a, b**).
- Pseudomonas infections present as bronchopneumonia and are usually widespread. Caution: abscesses (**Fig. 2.53c, d**).
- A "tree-in-bud" pattern of peribronchiolar infiltrates may be found in the setting of *any* bacterial or atypical infection (**Fig. 2.52**).
- Fungal infections are usually bilateral and appear as focal opacities arranged in a bronchovascular distribution. Invasive aspergillosis produces a halo sign, especially around larger infiltrates. *Aspergillus* and *Candida* infections are indistinguishable from each other (aspergillosis is more common) (**Fig. 2.56**)
- Atypical infections (*Mycoplasma*) and viral infections may start with tree-in-bud and ground-glass opacities but may then develop extensive consolidated areas (often mixed infections with bacterial superinfection) (**Figs. 2.54, 2.55**).

The presence of an air bronchogram definitely identifies an opacity as *pulmonary* and distinguishes it from a pleural cause. This sign is not always present, however.

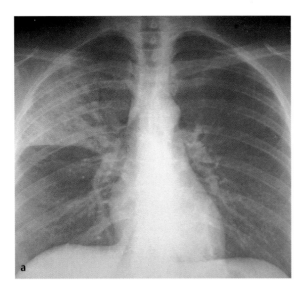

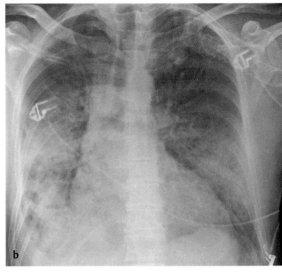

Fig. 2.49 a–c **Various opacification patterns found in pneumonia.**
a Homogeneous opacification with an air bronchogram (lobar pneumonia).
b Patchy confluent bronchopneumonia without an air bronchogram (lobular pneumonia).
c Reticulonodular opacities in bilateral "interstitial" pneumonia.

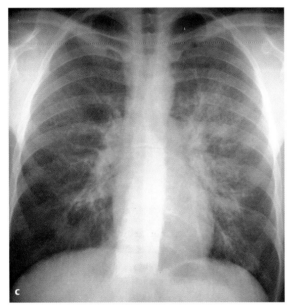

■ Pneumocystis infections are highly variable in their appearance (ground-glass, microcystic, reticular), depending on the duration of the infection. Subpleural sparing is common (**Fig. 2.57**).

■ Preexisting changes in the lung parenchyma (emphysema, COPD) will alter the imaging appearance (**Fig. 2.58**).

■ Note that the lungs of sick patients often presents with a combination of overhydration, pneumonia, pleural effusion, and possible immune reactions evoked by multiple insults to the lung (drugs, mechanical ventilation, sepsis, etc.) (**Fig. 2.59**).

Note also that typical pulmonary opacities may be absent depending on the patient's immune status and degree of hydration (**Table 2.20**). A negative chest radiograph does *not* exclude pneumonia, therefore. The chest radiograph fails to show pneumonic infiltrate in up to 40% of cases, especially in immunosuppressed patients..

Indications for computed tomography. Table 2.21 summarizes the indications for CT scanning in patients with confirmed or suspected pneumonia.

Differential Diagnosis

The most common "mimics" of pneumonia are:
■ atelectasis
■ aspiration
■ focal pulmonary edema
■ intrapulmonary hemorrhage
■ cryptogenic organizing pneumonia (COP)

A negative chest radiograph does not exclude pneumonia, especially in immunosuppressed patients.

Table 2.19 Summary of imaging findings commonly associated with certain infectious organisms. Caution: whereas imaging findings can help narrow the spectrum of causative organisms, they are not specific!

Causative organism	Patient group	Imaging findings
Streptococcus pneumoniae	Causes up to 45% of CAPs with a fatal outcome	▪ Lobar pneumonia with an air bronchogram; may also cause patterns like those seen in bronchopneumonia ▪ Rare effusion ▪ Cavitation suspicious for superinfection ▪ On CT: positive angiogram sign (**Fig. 2.50a**)
Klebsiella pneumoniae	Nosocomial infection > CAP	▪ Air bronchogram ▪ Volume increase (**Fig. 2.50b**) ▪ Cavitation and abscess more common than with pneumococci ▪ Effusion in ~70%
Legionella pneumophila	Approximately 25% of CAP and 40% of nosocomial infections	▪ Initially subsegmental and peripheral, spreads quickly to entire lobe and adjacent lobes, often bilateral ▪ Abscess and cavitation in immunosuppressed patients ▪ Rare lymphadenopathy
Staphylococcus aureus	In endocarditis, sepsis, catheter-related infection, post-viral infection	▪ Bronchopneumonia ▪ Volume loss, no air bronchogram with tree-in-bud ▪ Frequent abscessation with cavitation and pneumatocele formation (**Figs. 2.51, 2.53**)
Streptococcus pyogenes		▪ Like *S. aureus*, but rarely causes pneumatoceles ▪ Large pleural effusion
Haemophilus influenzae	Mainly nosocomial	▪ 60% like bronchopneumonia, 40% like lobar pneumonia ▪ Effusion in > 50% ▪ Rare empyema; cavitation in < 10%
Pseudomonas aeruginosa	In ARDS, AIDS	▪ Bronchopneumonia involving all lobes (especially lower lobes) ▪ Rare multinodular or reticular pattern ▪ Pulmonary vasculitis with infarctions ▪ Necrosis and cavitation are common, even initially (**Fig. 2.53c, d**)
Escherichia coli	Mainly nosocomial	▪ Bronchopneumonia, especially in lower lobes ▪ Effusion is common, empyema rare
Mycoplasma pneumoniae	Frequent extrapulmonary symptoms	▪ Highly variable (**Fig. 2.54**) ▪ Reticular pattern ▪ Patchy bronchopulmonary infiltrates, or ▪ Larger consolidated areas
Pneumocystis jirovecii	Immunosuppression including AIDS	▪ Ground-glass opacities, diffuse or in a mosaic pattern (**Fig. 2.57**) ▪ Subacute stage: reticular, septal and fine nodular opacities, bronchial wall thickening, parenchymal retraction, (reversible) cysts
Influenza virus	Potentially fatal hemorrhagic pneumonitis	▪ Interstitial reticular pattern or consolidated areas, depending on bacterial superinfection (effusion, cavitation) (**Fig. 2.55c, d**)
CMV	Post-transplantation	▪ Ground-glass opacities or consolidated areas in a mosaic pattern, diffuse or confined to one lobe (**Fig. 2.55a, b**) ▪ May also form nodules with halos ▪ Tree-in-bud pattern (rare)
Varicella	Follows 2–5 days after skin changes	▪ Confluent perihilar nodules 5–10 mm in size (tracheobronchitis) ▪ Rare effusion ▪ Frequent lymphadenopathy
Mycobacteria	Immunosuppression	▪ Primary: lymphadenopathy with consolidation in > 90%, most common in segments 1, 2 (early infiltrate) ▪ Postprimary: tree-in-bud (endobronchial), rosette sign, thick-walled cavitation, consolidated areas
Nontuberculous mycobacteria (MOTT)	Preexisting lung diseases, also in AIDS and immunocompromised patients	▪ Like tuberculosis, but with smaller, thin-walled cavitation and less upper lobe predominance
Candida	Opportunistic (oral flora)	▪ Candidiasis: miliary pattern, peribronchovascular focal opacities (**Fig. 2.56e**)
Aspergillus	Opportunistic (oral flora)	▪ Vascular: CT shows halo sign (DD: CMV, herpes, Wegener granulomatosis, Kaposi sarcoma) (**Fig. 2.56a–d**) ▪ Endobronchial: atelectasis, bronchial wall thickening and peribronchiolar infiltrates
Cryptococcus		▪ Nodules 0.5–4 cm in size, sometimes with halos as in angioinvasive aspergillosis; may mimic neoplasms ▪ Lymphadenopathy is rare but massive when present ▪ Miliary pattern and pleural effusion with disseminated infection
Nocardia species	Opportunistic in transplantation and lymphoma patients, rare in AIDS	▪ Frequent cavitation and empyema formation

CAP, community-acquired pneumonia; CMV, cytomegalovirus; DD, differential diagnosis; MOTT, mycobacterium other than tuberculosis

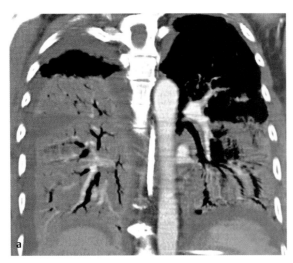

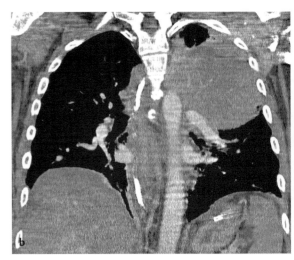

Fig. 2.50 a, b **Bilateral lobar pneumonia.**

a Pneumococcal pneumonia with a positive air bronchogram and positive angiogram sign.

b *Klebsiella* pneumonia. The volume increase had caused bulging of the interlobar fissure.

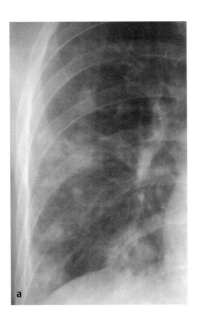

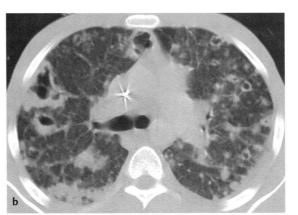

Fig. 2.51 a, b **Septic pneumonia (*Staphylococcus aureus*) with multiple focal opacities, some showing cavitation.**

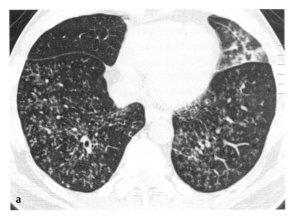

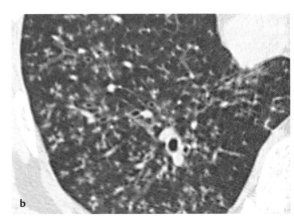

Fig. 2.52 a, b **Tree-in-bud sign.**
Thick-walled bronchioles, filled with secretions, produce a "tree-in-bud" pattern of branches and nodular opacities, appreciated most clearly in the peripheral lung. This is a nonspecific sign found in acute bacterial infections, atypical infections, and endobronchial tuberculosis.

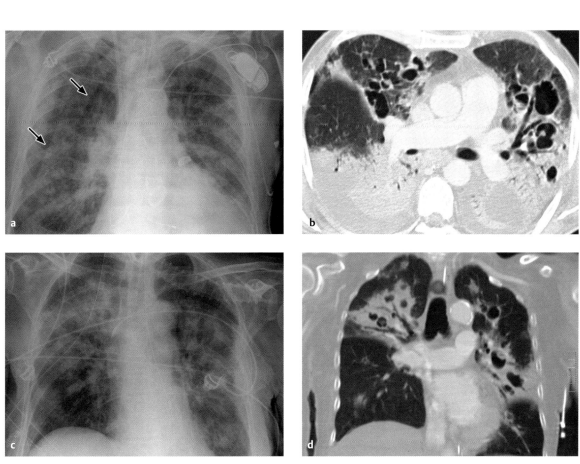

Fig. 2.53 a–d Cavitating bacterial infection.

a, b   Staphylococcal bronchopneumonia with peribronchial focal opacities (skin folds visible on the right side). CT shows cystic cavitation (late sign).

c, d   Extensive, patchy peribronchial infiltrates in *Pseudomonas* pneumonia. Cavitations are visible on CT.

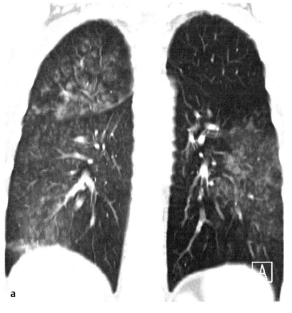
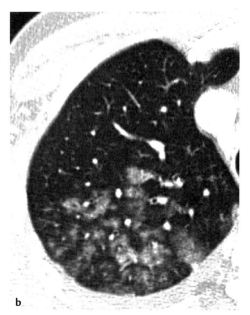

Fig. 2.54 a, b Atypical infections.
Patchy peribronchial infiltrates in *Mycoplasma* pneumonia.

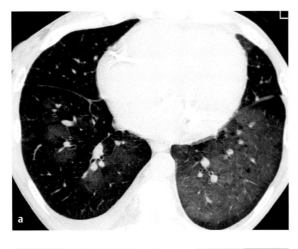

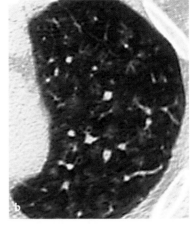

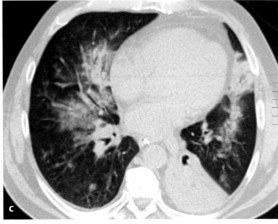

Fig. 2.55 a–d **Atypical infections.**

a, b Viral infections (in this case CMV) produce acinar or diffuse ground-glass opacities.

c, d Viral infections (in this case influenza virus) may also cause consolidation.

 When pneumonia is suspected, a diagnosis can often be established only by invasive procedures, serial examinations, and correlation with clinical findings.

In many cases an accurate diagnosis can be made only by performing additional imaging studies, serial examinations, invasive diagnostic procedures, and by correlation with clinical findings (**Table 2.22**).

Aspiration and Aspiration Pneumonia

 Intubation or tracheotomy bypasses normal defenses to aspiration. Patients with a tracheostomy tube have twice the aspiration risk as patients with an endotracheal tube.

Pneumonia in ICU patients is often secondary to aspiration (**Table 2.23**). Infectious material may be aspirated from the paranasal sinuses, pharynx, or tracheobronchial tree.

The posterior, gravity-dependent lung regions are most commonly affected. Sites of predilection in bedridden patients are the apical and posterior segments of the lower lobes and the posterior segments of the upper lobes (**Fig. 2.60**). Chronic or recurrent aspiration in an up-

right position (e.g., due to swallowing difficulties) most commonly affects the basal segments of the lower lobes.

Causes. Approximately 90% of post-aspiration pneumonias and pulmonary abscesses are caused by gram-negative bacteria (*Klebsiella, Pseudomonas, Proteus, Escherichia coli*; **Fig. 2.50b** and **Fig. 2.53**).

Mendelson syndrome is a special form of aspiration in which a large amount of pure gastric juice enters the lung, inciting a chemical pneumonitis with acute damage to the lung parenchyma.

It should be noted that patients with an endotracheal tube or tracheostomy tube are not protected from aspiration: Tracheal intubation interferes with glottic closure, while a nasogastric tube interferes with gastroesophageal closure. Patients with a tracheostomy tube have twice the aspiration risk of patients with an endotracheal tube.

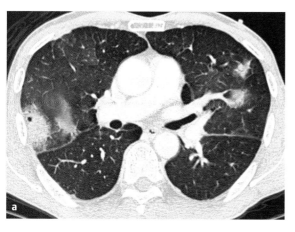

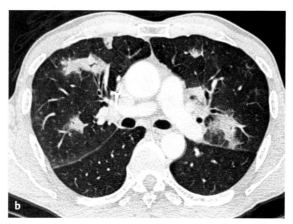

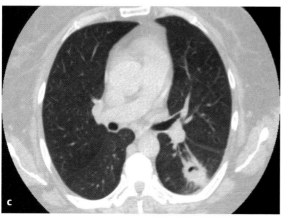

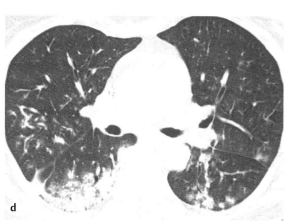

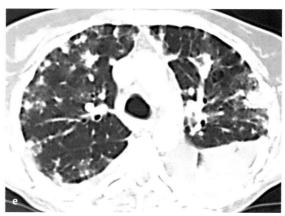

Fig. 2.56 a–e **Fungal infections.**

a, b Angioinvasive *Aspergillus* infection with bilateral patchy consolidation. The consolidated areas are surrounded by ground-glass halos (hemorrhage).

c An air crescent is pathognomonic for an angioinvasive *Aspergillus* infection, with evidence of an initial immune response.

d Peribronchial infiltrates in an endobronchial *Aspergillus* infection.

e Bilateral patchy consolidation in a *Candida* infection. Some of the consolidated areas are rimmed by halos.

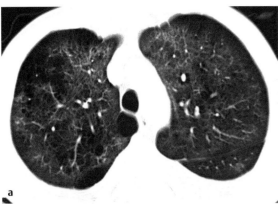

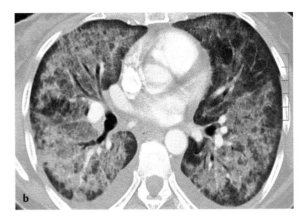

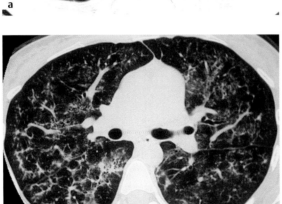

Fig. 2.57 a–c **Pneumocystis jirovecii infection.**
a Ground-glass opacities, accompanied here by underlying emphysematous changes.
b Diffuse ground-glass opacities with superimposed reticular opacities (note the sparing of the subpleural space, similar to the pattern found in edema).
c *Pneumocystis* infection: late stage following prolonged treatment, which is characterized by more septal interstitial opacities.

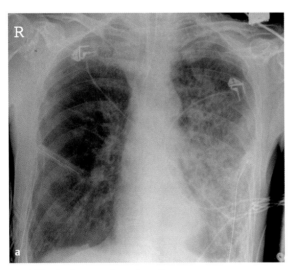

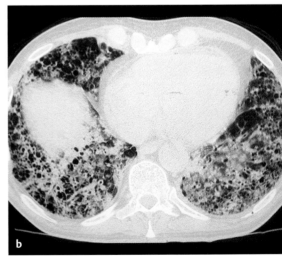

Fig. 2.58 a, b **Pneumonia and emphysema.**
Pneumonia in lungs with (pronounced) preexisting emphysematous changes produces a more reticular, weblike pattern of opacities rather than larger areas of consolidation.

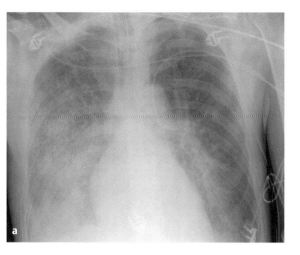

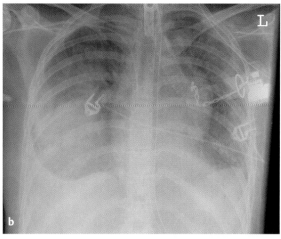

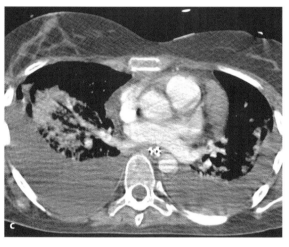

Fig. 2.59 a–c **Consolidation caused by multiple superimposed pathologies.**
This is a common finding on chest radiographs in ICU patients.
a   Right-sided pneumonia and congestion.
b, c   Right-sided pneumonia and bilateral pleural effusions.

Table 2.20 Reasons for a negative radiograph despite clinical manifestations of pneumonia

- Age > 65 years
- Neutropenia
- Dehydration (!), especially in elderly patients
- COPD and bullous lung changes
- Pulmonary fibrosis, heart failure (mask pneumonia)

Table 2.21 Indications for CT in patients with confirmed or suspected pneumonia

- Discrepancy between radiographic and clinical findings
- Investigation of unusual or indeterminate radiographic findings
- Suspected complications (abscess, cavitation, liquefaction)
- Suspected infection in an immunosuppressed patient with a normal chest radiograph
- Differentiation of effusion, empyema, atelectasis, and infiltration
- Characterization of infiltrates and to narrow the spectrum of causative organisms
- Localization of infiltrates prior to bronchoscopy or lavage
- Defining the extent of infiltration
- Evaluating treatment response
- Exclusion of underlying or associated lung diseases (tumor, bronchiectasis, anomalies of the central tracheobronchial system)

Pathogenesis

Significant pathogenetic factors are the amount of material aspirated, the pH of the material, its osmolality, and its content of solid constituents. Material with a pH less than 2.5 can lead to severe bronchospasm and inflammatory lung changes within a few minutes after aspiration. As the pH rises, the pulmonary changes become less extensive and less severe.

Imaging

Radiography

Mendelson syndrome (aspiration of gastric juice only) is characterized radiographically by extensive multifocal patchy opacities that show a perihilar and basal distribution. The opacities do not show a predilection for dependent lung areas and are unrelated to patient position at the time of the aspiration. The infiltrates gradually clear over a period of 7–10 days unless other complications arise.

Table 2.22 Differential diagnosis of pneumonia in ICU patients

Diagnoses	Characteristics
Pulmonary edema	▪ Changes within a few hours in response to therapy
Atelectasis	▪ Signs of volume reduction; CT shows homogeneous enhancement ▪ Changes within a few hours after (bronchoscopic) removal of causal obstruction (usually an endobronchial mucus plug) ▪ Atelectasis has sharper margins than pneumonia, even when it involves only segments or subsegments
Pulmonary embolism and infarction	▪ Pleural-based (wedge-shaped) consolidation, may subsequently cavitate ▪ Direct visualization of thrombus by CT
Drug reaction	▪ May present as COP, NSIP, or hemorrhagic area
Intrapulmonary hemorrhage	▪ Detection of blood by bronchoscopy
Alveolitis (allergic/idiopathic)	▪ Patchy or diffuse ground-glass opacities ▪ Signs of parenchymal retraction due to incipient fibrosis
ARDS	▪ Clinical diagnosis: oxygen tension $PaO_2/FIO_2 < 200\,mmHg$

COP, cryptogenic organizing pneumonia; NSIP, nonspecific interstitial pneumonia.

Table 2.23 Predisposing factors for aspiration

- Decreased level of consciousness (general anesthesia, alcohol, drugs)
- Absent or diminished cough reflex
- Swallowing difficulties (neuromuscular diseases, diseases of the esophagus, postoperative)
- Nasogastric tube
- Intubation

Chest radiographs following the aspiration of gastric juice *and* particulate food material show unilateral or bilateral patchy opacities, usually in the basilar lung, which become confluent over time. Initially they tend to increase for several days but generally show rapid improvement thereafter.

If initial improvement is followed by a further progression of findings, this usually signifies a bacterial

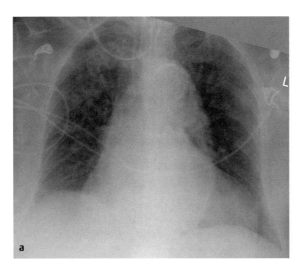

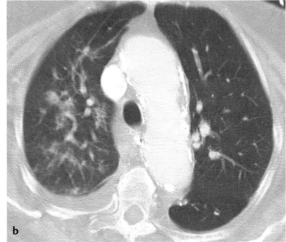

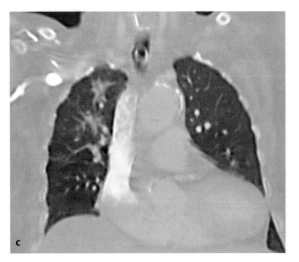

Fig. 2.60 a–c **Aspiration pneumonia in the right upper lobe with patchy peribronchial infiltrates, accompanied by cardiomegaly and a small, right-sided pleural effusion.**

Table 2.24 Radiographic findings for various aspirated materials

Aspirated material	Radiographic findings
Gastric juice	Edema
Bland fluid (small volumes)	No change
Gastric juice and particulate food material	Pneumonia

superinfection of the lung, the development of ARDS, or a pulmonary embolism.

Chronic recurrent aspiration incites an increasingly fibrotic reaction with septal fibrosis and occasional larger areas of fibrosis, secondary hyperinflated lung areas, and architectural distortion of the lung. The fibrotic changes in particular are appreciated more clearly on CT and HRCT (high resolution) scans than on chest radiographs.

Differential Diagnosis

The appearance of *Mendelson syndrome* can mimic that of cardiogenic pulmonary edema or fully developed ARDS. Resolution is much slower than in cardiogenic edema.

The aspiration of gastric juice *and* particulate food material produces changes similar to those in basal bronchopneumonia (**Table 2.24**). The history and clinical findings are helpful in narrowing the differential diagnosis.

Pneumonia during Mechanical Ventilation

Differential Diagnosis

The radiologic diagnosis of pneumonia is often quite difficult in patients on mechanical ventilation. The radiographic diagnosis of pneumonia is hampered by several other conditions that have a similar appearance on chest films:
- atelectasis
- infarction
- aspiration
- focal pulmonary edema
- intrapulmonary hemorrhage

A positive air bronchogram has the best predictive value for pneumonia-related lung changes but is not specific. An air bronchogram may also occur in association with other pulmonary opacities (e. g., atelectasis, intrapulmonary hemorrhage) or is missing in pneumonia if the bronchi are filled with secretion.

Changes in radiolucency. The goal of mechanical ventilation, especially with PEEP, is to induce the partial reinflation of atelectatic lung areas (see **Table 2.12**). The associated increase in lung volume leads to the following changes on the chest radiograph:
- an increase in lung lucency
- descent of the diaphragm
- A reduction of pulmonary opacities caused by infiltration or edema. The lung appears more radiolucent, mimicking a regression of pulmonary infiltration. These lucency changes are reversible and will disappear when the ventilation pressure is lowered.

On the other hand, when the patient is weaned from the respirator and respiratory function improves to a point where the patient can be extubated, chest radiographs taken during the initial hours of spontaneous breathing will often show paradoxical worsening with an increase in pulmonary opacities.

To avoid misinterpretation of the chest radiograph, any changes in ventilator settings should be reported to the radiologist and noted on the radiograph itself. The position of the patient (e. g., prone) also significantly influences the interpretation of lung opacities in ICU patients (see also **Fig. 2.43**).

Pathogenesis

Ventilator-associated pneumonia (VAP) develops in up to 30 % of ICU patients as a complication of mechanical ventilation. By definition, VAP occurs more than 48 hours after intubation and the start of mechanical ventilation. The risk of pneumonia is three to ten times higher in ventilated ICU patients than in nonventilated ICU patients, the risk increasing with the duration of ventilation. **Table 2.25** lists risk factors for VAP that have been identified in numerous studies.

Early- and late-onset ventilator-associated pneumonia. VAP is classified as early or late onset based on the timing of its occurrence during mechanical ventilation. Early-onset VAP occurs during the first four days of ventilation, late-onset VAP after that period.

While early-onset VAP is caused chiefly by *Haemophilus influenzae*, *Streptococcus pneumoniae*, *Staphylococcus aureus*, and *Enterobacter* species, late-onset VAP most

New progression following initial improvement usually signifies a bacterial superinfection, the development of ARDS, or pulmonary embolism.

Changes in ventilator settings or patient position should be charted to avoid misinterpretations.

Table 2.25 Various risk factors for the development of ventilator-associated pneumonia (VAP)

- Age >60 years
- Underlying disease: COPD, other lung diseases, ARDS, burns, trauma, community-acquired, organ failure
- Antibiotic therapy
- Mechanical ventilation >2 days
- Stress ulcer prophylaxis
- Change in gastric pH with bacterial colonization
- Bacterial colonization of the upper respiratory tract
- Aspiration of gastric contents
- Reintubation
- Sinusitis

Table 2.26 Main causative organisms of VAP

- *Pseudomonas aeruginosa*
- *Acinetobacter* spp.
- *Proteus* spp.
- *Escherichia coli*
- *Klebsiella* spp.
- *Haemophilus influenzae*
- *Staphylococcus aureus*
- *Streptococcus* spp.
- *Streptococcus pneumoniae*

commonly occurs after previous antibiotic therapy and is caused mainly by infection with *Pseudomonas aeruginosa*, *Acinetobacter*, MRSA (methicillin-resistant *Staphylococcus aureus*), and other multiresistant gram-negative organisms, with a correspondingly worse prognosis (**Table 2.26**).

The longer the patient is on the ventilator, the higher the incidence of infection with MRSA and gram-negative bacteria. Previous antibiotic therapy, especially with broad-spectrum antibiotics, increases the risk of infection by problem organisms (*Pseudomonas aeruginosa*, MRSA, *Enterobacter baumannii*, *Streptococcus maltophilia*).

Local (facility-specific) factors also play a crucial role, and individual institutions have responded to this problem with systematic epidemiologic evaluations.

Clinical Aspects and Imaging

The clinical diagnosis of VAP is based on:

- leukocytosis
- fever
- purulent sputum
- new infiltrate(s) on the chest radiograph (**Fig. 2.61**)

The combination of clinical signs and symptoms with an abnormal chest radiograph has high sensitivity, exceeding 75%, but a specificity of only 35%. When all four factors are required to make a diagnosis of VAP, the sensitivity drops to values below 50%.

Clinical Pulmonary Infection Score. The Clinical Pulmonary Infection Score (CPIS) devised by Pugin is based on 0–2 points for:

- fever
- leukocytosis
- oxygenation
- quantity and quality of purulent tracheal secretions
- sputum culture and gram stain
- an abnormal chest radiograph

According to the authors, a CPIS of greater than 6 has a sensitivity of 93% and a specificity of 100% for the diagnosis of VAP.

According to one study which took into account multiple *CT criteria*, the detection of opacities in nondepen-

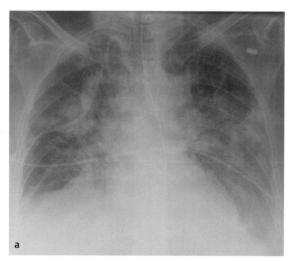
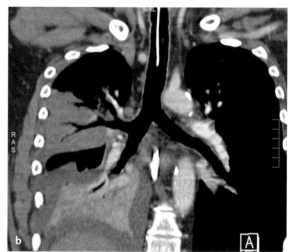

Fig. 2.61 a, b **Ventilator-associated pneumonia (VAP).**

a   New bilateral, patchy opacities that are nongravity-dependent are suspicious for pneumonia.

b   VAP in the upper lobe (slight contrast enhancement) compared with atelectasis (intense homogeneous enhancement).

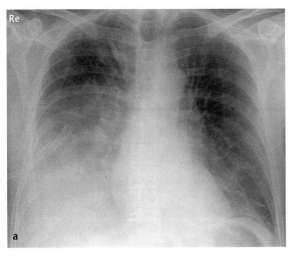

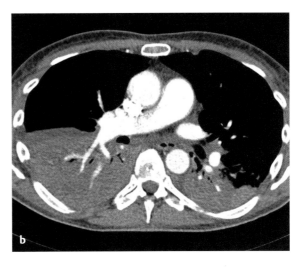

Fig. 2.62 a, b **Bilateral lower lobe pneumonia.**

a Chest radiograph shows consolidated areas in the lower lobes of both lungs with only a faint central air bronchogram. It is difficult to distinguish atelectasis and effusion from pneumonia based on radiographic findings.

b Both lower lobes show a positive angiogram sign, an air bronchogram, and relatively slight parenchymal enhancement indicative of infiltration and not (!) atelectasis (despite involvement of dependent lung).

dent lung areas creates a particularly high index of suspicion for pneumonia (7-fold increase in statistical probability) (**Fig. 2.61 b**). All other criteria (e. g., focal versus diffuse opacities, interstitial versus alveolar pattern, ground-glass opacity versus consolidation, associated findings such as effusion, lymphadenopathy, cavitation, nodules, pneumatoceles, etc.) have proven to be nonspecific. Another helpful CT criterion is slight, inhomogeneous enhancement of pneumonic consolidation after IV contrast administration, as opposed to the intense homogeneous enhancement that occurs in atelectasis (**Figs. 2.61 b**, **2.62**).

It should be noted that while an *air bronchogram* definitely signifies an intrapulmonary (not pleural or extrapulmonary) opacity, an air bronchogram is not always present in pneumonia (**Figs 2.61**, **2.62**). It is absent when the bronchi are completely filled with secretions. Findings are also changed by the presence of pleural effusion, congestion, or preexisting lung disease (see **Fig. 2.49b** and **Fig. 2.59**).

ARDS and Pneumonia

Pneumonia is twice as common in ARDS patients as in patients without ARDS. Typically, ventilator-associated pneumonia in ARDS patients develops approximately 1 week after the start of mechanical ventilation. The spectrum of causative organisms is basically the same as in ventilated patients without ARDS. Many cases are caused by problem organisms such as methicillin-resistant *Staphylococcus aureus* and multiresistant gram-negative organisms (*Enterobacter* spp., *Pseudomonas*).

Imaging

Imaging studies have very low accuracy for diagnosing pneumonia in ARDS patients. In a series of 141 autopsied patients who died in ICUs, half of the patients had histologically confirmed pneumonia but only 26% of cases had been correctly diagnosed from antemortem imaging studies (sensitivity 29%, specificity 77%).

Any new or increasing opacity on the chest radiograph of an ARDS patient should be considered suspicious for pneumonia. Adding clinical information did *not* improve the accuracy of chest radiograph interpretation. Even with CT or HRCT, imaging is of limited value for diagnosing pneumonia in ARDS.

Septic Pneumonia

Septic emboli are a common finding in drug-dependent and immunosuppressed patients. The principal sources are an intravenous catheter, an infected tricuspid valve (IV drug abuse), an infected cardiac pacemaker wire, or septic thrombophlebitis. In principle, sepsis always carries a risk for the development of pneumonic foci. The main causative organism is *Staphylococcus aureus*.

Lesions may be detectable by radiography or CT before positive blood cultures are obtained. Images may show multiple pulmonary nodules or wedge-shaped, pleural-based consolidation (e. g., infarction) showing varying degrees of liquefaction in more than 50% of cases (see **Fig. 2.51**). A concomitant pleural effusion or empyema is common. A feeding-vessel sign is suggestive but not specific.

Any new or increasing radiographic opacity in an ARDS patient is suspicious for pneumonia.

Helpful CT criteria are opacities in nondependent lung areas and slight, inhomogeneous enhancement of pneumonic consolidation after IV contrast administration.

Pneumonia in Immunodeficient or Immunosuppressed Patients

Pathogenesis

A complex interaction of mechanical, humoral, and cellular host defenses is normally sufficient to prevent a pulmonary infection. Functional disturbances of these defense mechanisms are associated with heightened vulnerability to certain infectious organisms (**Table 2.27**).

Neutropenia predisposes to infection with pyogenic or extracellular bacteria and fungi (e.g., streptococci, staphylococci, *Pseudomonas*, *Klebsiella*, *Escherichia coli* and *Aspergillus*, *Mucor*, *Candida*). Impaired humoral immunity predisposes to infection with gram-negative or encapsulated bacteria (e.g., streptococci, *Haemophilus*, staphylococci), and impaired T cell immunity increases host vulnerability to opportunistic organisms like cytomegalovirus (CMV) and *Pneumocystis* and *Nocardia* species.

HRCT is the modality of choice for the early diagnosis of pulmonary infection in immunosuppressed patients. Images may show typical findings that are suspicious

within the clinical context as well as nonspecific patterns that are difficult to interpret, even when the clinical parameters are known (**Tables 2.19** and **2.28**).

Specific Immune Dysfunctions

Organ transplantation. Patients with impaired cellular immunity due to organ transplantation are highly susceptible to infection with (gram-negative) bacteria (e.g., *Pseudomonas* and *Legionella*) during the first four postoperative weeks (phase I, days 1–28). After that period (phase II, days 19–180) they are more susceptible to viral infections (e.g., CMV) and *Pneumocystis*. The majority of infections are reactivated viral infections in patients who were already seropositive before the transplantation and develop a disseminated infection with respiratory manifestations. Fungal infections are relatively rare but are potentially very dangerous.

Bone marrow transplantation and severe neutropenia. Pulmonary complications that develop in patients with severe neutropenia following bone marrow transplantation tend to follow a timeline (**Fig. 2.63**). Approximately

> HRCT is the method of choice for early confirmation of pneumonia in immunosuppressed patients.

Table 2.27   Immune dysfunctions that predispose to infection by certain organisms

Type of immune disorder	Etiology	Infectious organisms*

Neutropenia (granulocytopenia and/or granulocyte dysfunction)	• Leukemia
	• CT, radiotherapy, steroids
	• Bone marrow transplantation
	• Sarcoidosis
	• Diabetes
	• Alcohol abuse
	• Hepatic cirrhosis
	• Lupus erythematosus
		Bacteria:
		• Staphylococci*
		• Gram-negative bacteria
		  – *Escherichia coli*
		  – *Klebsiella* spp.
		  – *Pseudomonas*
		  – *Enterobacter* spp.
		Fungi:
		• *Aspergillus*
		• *Candida*
		• *Mucor*

Cellular immune dysfunction (T cell immunity)	• Lymphoma • Steroids, immunosuppression, organ transplantation • Congenital (e.g., thymic aplasia or agammaglobulinemia) • HIV, AIDS	Bacteria: • Mycobacteria* • *Nocardia* spp.* • *Salmonella* • *Legionella* spp.* Viruses: • Varicella • Herpes • CMV* Fungi: • Cryptococci • Histoplasma • Coccidioidomycosis Protozoa: • Cryptosporidia • *Pneumocystis jirovecii* • Toxoplasmosis
Humoral immune dysfunction (B cell immunity)	• Lymphoma, CLL, multiple myeloma • Steroids, immunosuppression • GvHD • Splenectomy • Nephrotic syndrome	Encapsulated bacteria • Streptococci* • *Haemophilus* • Staphylococci* Viruses: • CMV • RSV Protozoa: • *Pneumocystis jirovecii*

* The most common organisms are marked with an asterisk. CLL, chronic lymphocytic leukemia; CMV, cytomegalovirus; GvHD, graft-versus-host disease; RSV, respiratory syncytial virus.

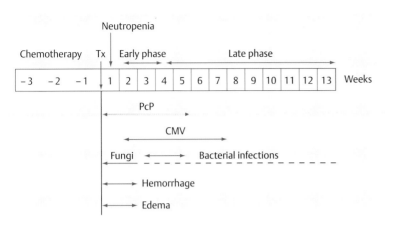

Fig. 2.63 **Timeline of pulmonary complications after bone marrow transplantation (BMT).**
PcP, Pneumocystis pneumonia; CMV, cytomegalovirus.

Table 2.28 Common radiologic findings in opportunistic infections caused by specific groups of organisms

Organisms	Timing, incidence	Radiologic findings
Bacterial pneumonia	During neutropenia (20–50%)	Consolidated areas or ground-glass opacities in an acinar or lobular distribution
Pneumocystis jirovecii	Incidence declining due to prophylaxis (< 10%)	Mosaic pattern of ground-glass opacity, interstitial pattern with thickened septa and reticular opacities
Fungi	In neutropenia	Peribronchovascular focal opacities <ul><li>*Aspergillus*: CT halo sign, crescent sign</li><li>Candidiasis and mucormycosis: multiple nodules</li></ul>
Cytomegalovirus	> 40 days after BMT (> 70%)	Patchy or diffuse ground-glass opacities or consolidated areas
Tuberculosis	Any time	Nonsegmental opacities or nodules, diffuse ground-glass opacities

Table 2.29 Differential diagnosis of pulmonary opacities following bone marrow transplantation (BMT)

Cause	Timing, incidence	Radiologic characteristics
Drug-induced lung changes	During chemotherapy or after radiotherapy	<ul><li>Diffuse ground-glass opacities or consolidation</li><li>Same pattern as in BOOP</li><li>Fibrotic reticular and linear opacities with foci of bronchiectasis</li></ul>
Leukemic infiltrates	Rarely, immediately after BMT	<ul><li>Thickening of bronchovascular interstitium, peribronchovascular patchy consolidation or ground-glass opacities, nodular opacities</li></ul>
Intrapulmonary hemorrhage	In > 20%, most frequent cause of noninfectious lung consolidation	<ul><li>Consolidated areas or ground-glass opacities</li><li>"Crazy paving": ground-glass opacities with superimposed reticular pattern</li></ul>
Edema	Any time	<ul><li>Perihilar consolidation or ground-glass opacity sparing the subpleural parenchyma, thickened septa and thickened bronchovascular interstitium, pleural effusion</li></ul>
Idiopathic pneumonia syndrome	Histologic: diffuse alveolar damage (DAD), > 10% during early phase	<ul><li>Diffuse ground-glass opacities, predominantly in dependent lung areas</li></ul>
Bronchiolitis obliterans and organizing pneumonia (OP reaction*)	> 10% during late phase, GvHD	<ul><li>Air trapping (expiratory images), mosaic pattern</li><li>Subsequent bronchiectasis, tree-in-bud pattern</li><li>In OP: sharply defined focal opacities with air-filled ectatic bronchi</li></ul>

* OP reaction was formerly called a BOOP-like reaction.

75% of deaths are due to respiratory infections, especially with gram-negative bacteria (> 50%) or fungi (invasive *Aspergillus*).

It is significant that radiographs in neutropenic patients often show ground-glass opacity instead of consolidation. Besides infectious pneumonia, the *differential diagnosis* of these findings should include infiltrates in the setting of an underlying neoplastic disease (usually leukemia), drug-induced changes, pulmonary edema (common in overhydration), intrapulmonary hemorrhage, and idiopathic pneumonia syndrome (**Table 2.29**).

Neutropenic patients receive broad antimicrobial coverage (including *Pseudomonas* species) appropriate for the duration and intensity of their neutropenia. Antifungal therapy should be added in patients with persistent fever (72–96 hours after the start of treatment). Hematology and oncology departments employ the following guidelines for adding antifungal therapy:

Radiographs of neutropenic patients with pneumonia often show ground-glass opacity rather than consolidation.

- lack of response to antimicrobial therapy
- new or persistent pulmonary infiltrates during antimicrobial therapy
- pulmonary infiltrates with a presumed or confirmed fungal etiology

Viral and opportunistic infections in AIDS patients tend to regress with antiviral therapy (HAART) while bacterial and mycobacterial infections tend to increase.

Human immunodeficiency virus and AIDS. Opportunistic lung infections represent 65% of all AIDS-associated diseases. More than 70% of AIDS patients have at least one respiratory infection during the course of their disease.

Since the advent of highly active antiretroviral therapy (HAART) several years ago, there has been a shift in the spectrum of infecting organisms in AIDS patients. Viral and opportunistic infections are less frequent while bacterial and mycobacterial infections are more prevalent. *Pneumocystis jirovecii* pneumonia (see **Fig. 2.57**) has the second highest incidence after bacterial infections (staphylococci, streptococci, and *Haemophilus*) and has the highest mortality rate (**Tables 2.30**, **2.31**).

Bacteria are the most common infecting organisms in patients who are still immunocompetent (CD 4 count > 200). Protozoa (especially *Pneumocystis jirovecii*) are most important in patients with impaired immune function (CD 4 count between 100 and 200), while fungi (*Aspergillus*) and atypical mycobacteria are the dominant organisms in patients with severe immune deficiency (CD 4 count < 50). Tuberculosis may develop at any time, the spectrum of causative organisms again correlating with the patient's immune status (CD 4 count > 200: typical mycobacteria, CD 4 count < 200: atypical mycobacteria, CD 4 count < 50: *Mycobacterium avium* complex).

Table 2.30 Spectrum of causative organisms and immune status in HIV patients

Organism	Incidence	CD 4 cell count (cells/mm³)
Bacteria	Very common	At any status
Mycobacteria	Common	At any status
MAC	Common	< 100
Fungi		
• *Cryptococcus*	Common	< 100
• *Aspergillus*	Rare	< 50
Pneumocystis jirovecii	Very common	< 200
Protozoons, MAC, fungi (*Aspergillus*)	Rare	< 100
CMV	Rare	< 100 (end stage)

MAC, *Mycobacterium avium* complex.

Table 2.31 Imaging patterns of pulmonary diseases in HIV patients (modified from Maki 2000)

Chest radiograph	Causative organism	Typical CT findings
Normal	PCP	Ground-glass opacities
	Mycobacteria	Miliary pattern or small nodules
	Disseminated fungal pneumonia	Miliary pattern or small nodules
Lymphadenopathy (LN)	Lymphoma	Nonspecific
	Mycobacteria	Rim enhancement, hypodense LN
	Kaposi sarcoma	Hypervascular LN
	Fungal infection	Nonspecific
Pleural effusion	Heart failure	Nonspecific
	Empyema	Thickened pleura
	Fungi, *Nocardia*, mycobacteria	Possible loculated effusion
	Lymphoma	Nonspecific
	Kaposi sarcoma	Nonspecific
Alveolar or interstitial opacities	PCP	Ground-glass opacities, cysts, septa
	CMV	Ground-glass opacities
	Tuberculosis	LN, effusion
	Kaposi sarcoma	Peribronchovascular opacities
	Bacterial pneumonia	Nonspecific consolidation
	LIP	Diffuse ground-glass opacities with cysts
Nodules	Lymphoma	Solitary or multiple, peribronchovascular
	Fungal infection	Miliary or peribronchovascular with halo
	Kaposi sarcoma	Peribronchovascular opacities, +LN, effusion
	Mycobacteria	Miliary or endobronchial
	Septic emboli	Foci of liquefaction
Focal infiltrates	Bacterial pneumonia	Nonspecific
	Mycobacteria	+LN
	Fungal pneumonia	+LN
	PCP	Rare
	Lymphoma	Nonspecific, LN, effusion

CMV: cytomegalovirus, LIP: lymphoid interstitial pneumonia, PCP: *Pneumocystis pneumonia*, LN: lymph nodes.

Complications of Pneumonia

Complications of pneumonia may involve the lung parenchyma or the pleural space and consist of:

- pulmonary abscess formation
- pneumatocele
- pleural empyema
- bronchopulmonary fistula

ARDS may develop from pneumonia in some patients.

Pulmonary Abscess, Cavitation

A pulmonary abscess is a circumscribed area of intrapulmonary necrosis caused by infection. It appears radiographically as a focal lucent zone located within a pneumonic infiltrate. CT scans can demonstrate this zone with much greater sensitivity than chest radiographs.

One should be careful not to misinterpret relative hypodensities within a consolidated area as abscesses (wide CT window). Following contrast administration, the nonenhancing necrotic area will become more clearly demarcated relative to the enhancing parenchyma that is still perfused (**Fig. 2.64a**).

Necrotizing pneumonia (due to infection with gram-negative bacteria, anaerobic bacteria, *Staphylococcus aureus*, or streptococci) is characterized by the formation of multiple, sometimes small, foci of liquefaction or *microabscesses*. If the abscess communicates with the bronchial tree, the necrotic area will fill with air and cause *cavitation* (**Fig. 2.64b**). Large areas of ischemic necrosis develop in patients with vasculitis or vascular thrombosis (e. g., *Klebsiella pneumoniae*).

Differential diagnosis. Liquefaction in a pulmonary abscess requires differentiation from:

- a dilated air-filled bronchus

- preexisting emphysema (see **Fig. 2.58**)
- a pneumatocele, which has a markedly thinner and smoother wall

Treatment. Pulmonary abscesses, especially those with broad pleural contact, are accessible to percutaneous drainage (7–14F catheter) with published success rates of 73–100 % within 10–15 days. Complete evacuation and collapse may take 4–5 weeks, depending on peripheral granulations. Decompression should proceed slowly to avoid vascular ruptures. Surgery is indicated for cases with bleeding or extensive necrosis.

Pneumatocele

A pneumatocele is a localized air collection, generally transient, which may be solitary or multiple and usually has a subpleural location. It is caused by rupture of the alveolar walls, especially as a result of *Staphylococcus aureus* infection (see **Fig. 2.52**), and occurs predominantly in children.

Empyema

Parapneumonic pleural effusions are not uncommon and are observed in ca. 40 % of patients with bacterial infections. Pleural empyema with pus in the pleural space occurs in less than 5 % of cases, however.

Besides clinical signs and symptoms, the diagnosis of empyema is based on a *laboratory analysis* of the effusion:

- leukocytosis > 500 cells/mm^3
- protein content > 2.5 g/dL
- specific gravity > 1018

Typical causative organisms are anaerobes, streptococci, and gram-negative bacteria. Published mortality rates for empyema vary widely from 1 % to 20 %. The mortality rate

> Relative hypodensities within an area of pneumonic consolidation should not be mistaken for abscesses.

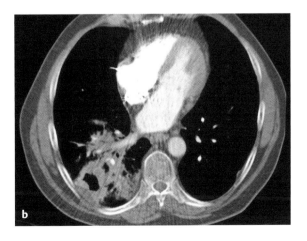

Fig. 2.64 a, b **Pneumonia with abscess formation.**
Postcontrast CT shows inhomogeneous enhancement (**a**) and air inclusions (**b**) too large to be localized to the airways.

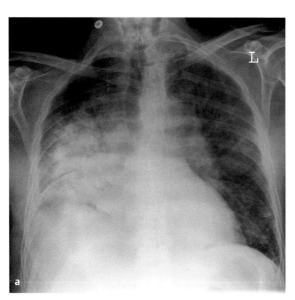
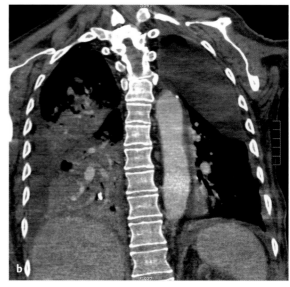

Fig. 2.65 a, b **Empyema.**
An infected pleural effusion (exudate or empyema) is assumed to be present in extensive bacterial pneumonia, even when classic CT signs such as pleural thickening or air inclusions are absent.

Table 2.32 CT criteria for differentiating between empyema and abscess

Empyema	Abscess
▪ Crescent shape	▪ Rounded shape
▪ Obtuse angle with the chest wall	▪ Acute angle with the chest wall
▪ Thickened pleural layers	▪ Irregular margins
▪ No air in the wall	▪ Air in the wall
▪ Bronchopleural fistula	▪ Communicates with bronchi
▪ Compression of adjacent lung	▪ Distortion of adjacent lung
▪ Changes shape with position changes	▪ Does not change shape with position changes

Central air inclusions (depending on causative organism) and peripheral rim enhancement are found in empyema and abscesses.

Ultrasonography is better than CT for detecting septation and loculation of an effusion or empyema. CT is better for defining the size and location of the effusion.

is substantially higher (40–70%) in patients over 65 years of age with comorbid conditions.

Imaging findings. The following are typical CT signs of pleural empyema (**Fig. 2.65**):
▪ wall-thickened (2–5 mm) pleura that is hyperdense on plain scans and enhances markedly after contrast administration
▪ effusion with a biconvex lenticular shape
▪ CT attenuation > 20 HU

It should be noted, however, that all of the above CT criteria may be absent, even when an infected exudate, rather than a sterile transudate, is present. The diagnosis ultimately relies on percutaneous aspiration and analysis of the sampled material. The differentiation of empyema from abscess is also difficult on chest radiographs and is

not always possible even on CT scans (**Table 2.32** and **Fig. 2.66**).

Ultrasonography is a simple bedside examination that can detect septation and increased echogenicity of the effusion with high confidence. Both of these findings suggest the presence of an infected exudate or empyema. While CT can more clearly define the size and location of the parapneumonic effusion/empyema, ultrasound is better for detecting septa and encapsulation in a "complicated" effusion (**Fig. 2.67**).

Treatment. If thoracostomy is indicated (**Tables 2.33, 2.34**), the drainage tube should be introduced under CT or sonographic guidance. While large-gauge tubes (28–36F) were once preferred, recent publications have described favorable results with smaller, less traumatizing catheters (16F) or double-lumen suction drains. The early placement of multiple drains is recommended for effusions loculated by septa and for multiple fluid collections.

Drainage alone is often inadequate for effusions with increasing fibrinous septation in the fibropurulent stage. The addition of local *chemical fibrinolysis* (**Table 2.35**) may be very successful in some patients, despite highly divergent success rates reported in the literature.

The drains should be removed when the drainage volume falls below 50 mL/day with minimal residual effusion.

Bronchopleural Fistula

A bronchopleural fistula is formed by air entering the pleural space not from the outside (as in a pneumotho-

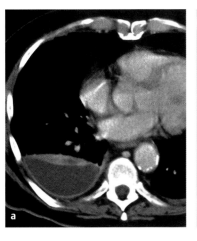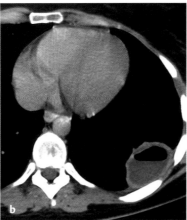

Fig. 2.66 a, b **Pleural empyema versus intrapulmonary abscess.**
Note the overall shape of the collection, which is lenticular in empyema (**a**) and round in intrapulmonary abscess (**b**). The angle formed with the chest wall is obtuse (**a**) or acute (**b**).

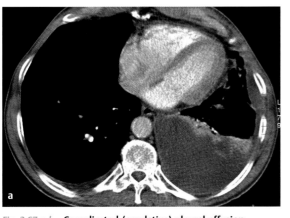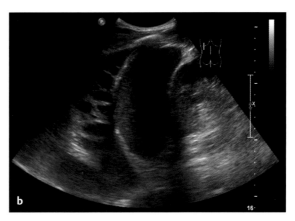

Fig. 2.67 a, b **Complicated (exudative) pleural effusion.**
Compared with CT (**a**) the multiple septa are defined more clearly by ultrasound scan (**b**).

Table 2.33 Developmental stages and treatment of pulmonary empyema (after Light 1985)

Stage	Characteristics	Treatment
Exudative	Normal pH and glucose level, low LDH Free-flowing effusion	No drainage
Fibropurulent	Low pH and glucose level, high LDH Increasing loculation or septation, viscous cellular fluid	Drainage (7–30F catheter)
Organization	Fibroblast invasion, increasing fibrosis prevents collapse of pleural space and reexpansion of lung Complication: pleuritis necessitatis with perforation toward the chest wall or bronchopleural fistula with perforation toward the lung	Surgical decortication

LDH, lactate dehydrogenase.

Table 2.34 Risk categories and drainage recommendations based on the ACCP Consensus Conference (after Colice et al. 2000)

Risk category	Pleural space	Bacteriology*	pH	Drainage
1	Minimal effusion	Unknown	Unknown	No
2	Moderate, free-flowing effusion (<½ hemithorax)	Negative	>7.2	No**
3	Large (>½ hemithorax) or loculated effusion or thickened pleura on CT	Positive	<7.2	Yes
4		Pus		Yes

* Culture and Gram stain.
** With a symptomatic effusion or if clinical condition deteriorates, repeat thoracentesis and reclassify.

Table 2.35 Local fibrinolysis for pleural empyema: technique and contraindications

Technique	Contraindications
▪ 250 000 IU streptokinase or 100 000 IU urokinase ▪ Dissolve in 100 mL NaCl, instill via the drain every 12 or 24 h ▪ After instillation, clamp the drain for 2–3 h and reposition the patient at frequent intervals ▪ Continuous suction thereafter	▪ Hypersensitivity to fibrinolytic agents ▪ Hemorrhagic diathesis ▪ Prior cerebral hemorrhage ▪ Intracranial tumor ▪ Previous surgery or trauma ▪ Bronchopleural fistula

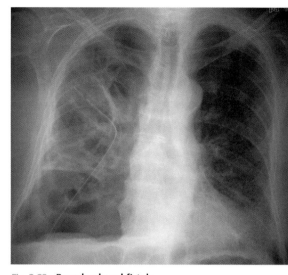

Fig. 2.68 **Bronchopleural fistula.**
New or persistent air inclusions (not iatrogenic) in a pleural effusion or empyema should raise suspicion of a bronchopleural fistula.

rax) but from the inside due to a communication between the pleural space and airways (**Fig. 2.68**). Suspicion of this fistula is raised by the new occurrence of multiple bubblelike air collections that are located at various levels in the pleural space and are *not* gravity-dependent.

Besides postsurgical (see p. 97) and iatrogenic causes, a bronchopleural fistula may form as a result of necrotizing pneumonia or pleural empyema. Rarely can the fistula be directly visualized, and more often it is suggested by an intrapleural air collection with no other demonstrable cause.

▶ An intrapulmonary air collection *without* a demonstrable cause is suspicious for a bronchopleural fistula.

Acute Respiratory Distress Syndrome

Today, efforts are being made to define factors prospectively that would predict a particularly severe course of pneumonia with risk for developing respiratory failure (ARDS) or septic shock so that these patients can be referred early for intensive care.

Besides age and comorbid conditions, increasing attention is also being given to genetic factors (see **Table 2.14**).

E. Eisenhuber-Stadler

Atelectasis

Atelectasis refers to the partial or complete collapse of a pulmonary lobe or segment. It is characterized functionally by a decrease in the area available for gas exchange and a shunting of blood flow leading to hypoxia, whose severity depends on the extent of the atelectasis.

Pathogenesis

Two main types of atelectasis are distinguished based on their *pathogenic mechanism:*
▪ poststenotic obstructive or resorptive atelectasis
▪ compression atelectasis

▶ Atelectasis is a very common pulmonary change in ICU patients. The posterobasal region of the left lung is most commonly affected.

Ventilation defects due to atelectasis are among the most common pulmonary changes in ICU patients. They are observed in up to 30% of patients after upper abdominal surgery, 5% after lower abdominal surgery, and more than 90% after thoracic surgery (**Table 2.36**). Due to gravity and decreased respiratory excursions, the posterobasal lung regions are sites of predilection for atelectasis, with most cases occurring on the left side. Frequent (usually partial) atelectasis of the left lower lobe results from a combination of cardiac compression and gravitational forces. Additionally, (blind) suctioning of the intubated patient generally reaches only the right lower lobe bronchus owing to anatomical constraints.

Plate atelectasis or *discoid atelectasis* is a partial collapse that occurs predominantly in hypoventilated middle or lower lung zones at the subsegmental level (**Fig. 2.69**).

Table 2.36 Causes of atelectasis in ICU patients

▪ Hypoventilation due to central respiratory depression, sedation, general anesthesia, or pain
▪ Previous abdominal or thoracic surgery
▪ Trauma
▪ Increased bronchial secretions (e. g., due to inflammation) with mucus plugging
▪ Malpositioned endotracheal tube
▪ Intubation with decreased bronchial clearance
▪ Aspiration
▪ Compression atelectasis due to pneumothorax, pleural effusion, or hemothorax

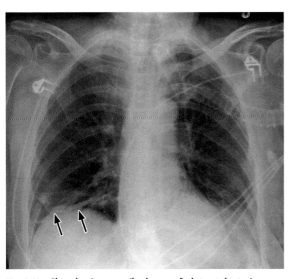

Fig. 2.69 **Sharply circumscribed area of plate atelectasis.**

Segmental, lobar, and *complete atelectasis* are often caused by obstruction of the corresponding bronchus. The cause may be a malpositioned endotracheal tube or partial or complete obstruction due to a mucus plug, blood clot, or aspirated foreign material (**Fig. 2.70**).

Large pleural effusions may cause the *compression atelectasis* of entire pulmonary lobes (most commonly the lower lobes).

Imaging

Radiography

Atelectasis is manifested on portable chest radiographs less by a decrease in lung lucency (often masked by other opacities) than by the *displacement of pulmonary fissures* or other indirect signs (**Table 2.37**; **Figs. 2.70, 2.71**).

The radiographic correlates of plate atelectasis are triangular or bandlike *parenchymal lung opacities* with relatively sharp margins (**Fig. 2.69**). These areas undergo rapid and frequent changes in their location and orientation, sometimes changing from day to day.

Atelectasis of the left lower lobe (**Fig. 2.72**) is common in supine patients and is recognized by increased opacity of the retrocardiac lung and loss of the diaphragm silhouette. The presence of an *air bronchogram* is suggestive of compression atelectasis and is not characteristic of resorptive atelectasis. In resorptive atelectasis (especially due to a longstanding obstruction), the bronchi are filled

Table 2.37 Direct and indirect signs of atelectasis

Direct signs of atelectasis	Indirect signs of atelectasis
Triangular or wedge-shaped lung opacities directed toward the pulmonary hilum, with or without an air bronchogram	Elevation of the hemidiaphragm on the affected side, more pronounced with lower lobe atelectasis than with upper lobe atelectasis
Displacement of interlobar fissures toward the atelectasis: • Minor fissure (when viewed tangentially) appears as a horizontal line between the ipsilateral hilum and 6th rib • Major fissures run obliquely and are not visible in an AP supine radiograph	Mediastinal shift toward the affected hemithorax: • Upper mediastinum (trachea) is shifted by upper lobe atelectasis • Basal mediastinum (heart) is shifted by lower lobe atelectasis
Vascular displacement: • With lower lobe atelectasis, the lower lobe artery may disappear in the mediastinal shadow (right > left). The diaphragm silhouette is (at least partially) absent • With upper lobe atelectasis, the lower lobe artery is displaced cephalad	Compensatory hyperinflation of unaffected lung areas

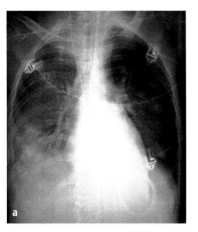
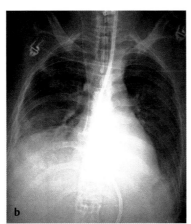
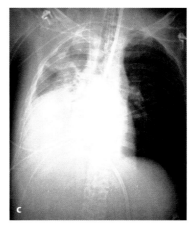

Fig. 2.70 a–c **Progression of findings in lower lobe atelectasis of the right lung.**
Note the progressive increase in opacity and decrease in volume.

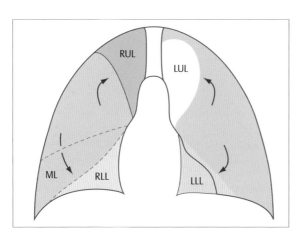

Fig. 2.71 **Diagrammatic representation of direct and indirect signs of atelectasis on the chest radiograph.**
RUL: right upper lobe
RLL: right lower lobe
ML: middle lobe
LUL: left upper lobe
LLL: left lower lobe

with secretions (mucoid impaction) and therefore do not produce an air bronchogram (**Fig. 2.73**).

Interpretation is aided by displacement of the interlobar fissures (diminished volume), the silhouette sign (loss of the diaphragmatic and cardiac contour), and the displacement of vascular structures (best appreciated in a side-to-side comparison).

An air bronchogram is *not* useful for differentiating atelectasis from pneumonia, as it may occur in compression atelectasis as well as pneumonia (**Fig. 2.74**).

Computed Tomography

CT may show a homogeneous density conforming to the location and configuration of the atelectasis, depending on the size of the affected area. Concave displacement of the interlobar fissures with signs of diminished volume is helpful in distinguishing atelectasis from pneumonic infiltrates.

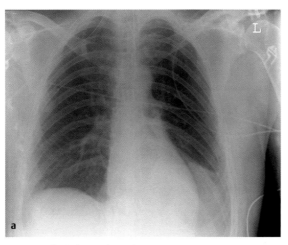
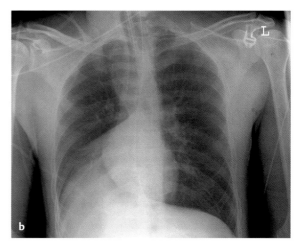

Fig. 2.72 a, b **Lobar atelectasis.**
Left lower lobe atelectasis (a) and right lower lobe atelectasis with mild middle lobe atelectasis (b). Note the distortion of the interlobar fissures and compensatory hyperinflation of the ventilated upper lobes.

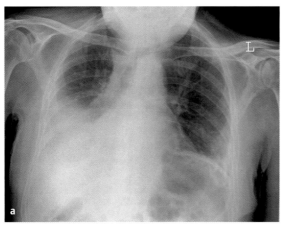
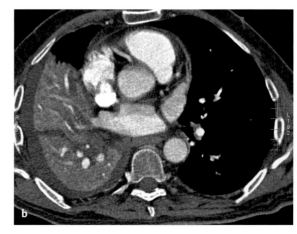

Fig. 2.73 a, b **Postobstructive atelectasis.**
Middle and lower lobe atelectasis of the right lung is associated with moderate volume loss but pronounced mucoid impaction of the bronchi (no air bronchogram).

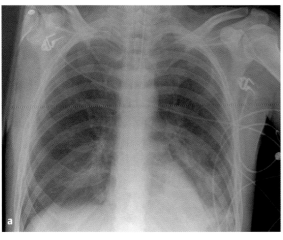 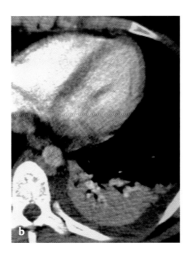

Fig. 2.74 a, b **Compression atelectasis.**
Typical posterobasal location of compression atelectasis with a positive air bronchogram. Note the intense, homogeneous enhancement of the atelectasis on CT.

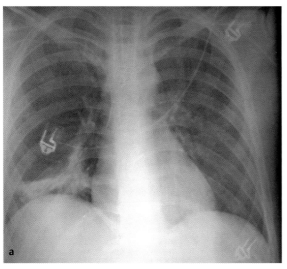 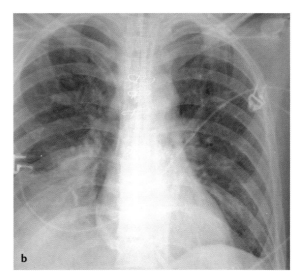

Fig. 2.75 a, b **Pneumonia versus atelectasis.**
The sharply circumscribed atelectasis (**a**) progresses to form a larger, poorly circumscribed infiltrate (**b**).

The presence or absence of an air bronchogram is helpful in recognizing the cause of the atelectasis:

- An air bronchogram is generally absent in *poststenotic obstructive atelectasis* (e.g., caused by an endobronchial mucus plug, tumor, or foreign body). The impacted bronchi appear as hypodense (but not air-filled) ringlike or tubular structures (**Fig. 2.73b**).
- A positive air bronchogram is usually preserved in *compression atelectasis* (e.g., caused by a large pleural effusion or pneumothorax) (**Fig. 2.74b**).

The presence or absence of an air bronchogram within the atelectatic consolidation is of key importance in therapeutic decision-making: in the absence of an air bronchogram, the patient is more likely to benefit from bronchoscopy (obstructive atelectasis); whereas patients with a positive air bronchogram often do not show respiratory improvement after bronchoscopy.

Differential Diagnosis

Pleural effusion versus atelectasis. It is often difficult to distinguish between pleural effusion and atelectasis on supine radiographs because a large pleural effusion may obscure or offset the classic signs of atelectasis. The differentiation of atelectasis and effusion is the domain of ultrasonography, which can detect a pleural effusion, determine its extent, and locate the optimum site for percutaneous pleural drainage.

Pneumonia versus atelectasis. It may not be possible to distinguish between lobar atelectasis and lobar pneumonia or between (segmental) atelectasis and circumscribed

Patients with obstructive atelectasis (no air bronchogram) will often benefit from bronchoscopy, whereas patients with compression atelectasis (positive air bronchogram) will not.

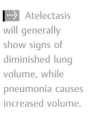 Atelectasis will generally show signs of diminished lung volume, while pneumonia causes increased volume.

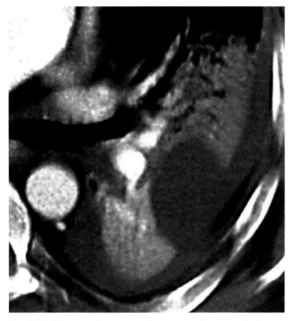

Fig. 2.76 **Pneumonia versus atelectasis—enhancement characteristics.**
Atelectasis shows intense homogeneous enhancement (posterior) contrasting with the slight, inhomogeneous enhancement of the infiltrate (anterior).

pneumonic consolidation on chest radiographs when there are no signs of diminished volume (atelectasis) or increased volume (pneumonia). Both conditions—atelectasis and infectious infiltration—may be responsible for lobar consolidation.

The following points are helpful:

- If an opacity interpreted as atelectasis becomes larger and more ill defined over time, it is more likely to be a pneumonic infiltrate. Any atelectasis that does not resolve within a matter of days is also suspicious for infectious infiltration (**Fig. 2.75**).
- CT can differentiate atelectasis and pneumonic consolidation by their different enhancement characteristics after contrast administration: Atelectatic lung shows intense homogeneous enhancement while pneumonic lung tissue shows much weaker, inhomogeneous enhancement (**Fig. 2.76**).
- A positive air bronchogram may be found in both atelectasis and pneumonia, so it is *not* a useful differentiating sign. The absence of an air bronchogram in atelectasis signifies a central bronchial obstruction due to mucoid impaction (see **Fig. 2.73b**).

E. Eisenhuber-Stadler and S. Metz-Schimmerl

Pneumothorax

Pneumothorax is a relatively common and important finding in the ICU, especially in ventilated patients. Pneumothorax may have an iatrogenic cause in ICU patients and may result from surgery, barotrauma, or catheter-related complications (**Table 2.38**). Rare causes of pneumothorax are blunt or penetrating thoracic trauma and mediastinal emphysema with the secondary development of a pneumothorax.

A pneumothorax may develop hours or even days after successful (or unsuccessful) pleural drainage. It may also result from suboptimal placement of a thoracostomy tube.

A pneumothorax may still develop hours or days after a tube thoracostomy.

Treatment. An acute pneumothorax (without septations) can be drained through an 8–10F catheter which is usually placed in the second intercostal space in the midclavicular line (anterior) or in the sixth to eighth intercostal space in the midaxillary line. With a loculated pneumothorax, the drains should be placed under CT or ultrasound guidance.

Diagnostic Strategy

The method of first choice is the *portable chest radiograph*. If the frontal view does not yield a clear diagnosis, other options are to obtain a lateral chest radiograph (difficult to position), a lateral decubitus view, or a tangential view.

The most rewarding imaging modality in patients with clinical suspicion of an occult pneumothorax is *computed tomography.*

Increasingly, *ultrasonography* is being used as a bedside study for the diagnosis of pneumothorax.

Table 2.38 Causes of pneumothorax in ICU patients

Iatrogenic (common):
- Barotrauma
- Central venous catheter
- Thoracentesis, thoracostomy
- Cardiac massage

Blunt or penetrating thoracic trauma (rare):
- Mediastinal emphysema with secondary pneumothorax
- Tracheobronchial injuries
- Tracheotomy
- Barotrauma
- Tracheal or esophageal perforation

Imaging

Radiography and Computed Tomography

Localization. In the supine patient, the classic signs of pneumothorax are seen only with a relatively large intrapleural air collection and a compliant lung (**Fig. 2.77**). Air in the supine patient tends to be distributed in the anterior and basal portions of the pleural space (**Table 2.39**). Sites of predilection in supine patients are anteromedial and subpulmonic (**Fig. 2.78**). Anterior air collections on the AP chest radiograph may easily escape direct detection. Watch for these signs:

- a sharp diaphragm silhouette
- a rounded or oval-shaped area of increased lucency ("black oval")
- an avascular area

Volume estimation. The extent of a pneumothorax is difficult to estimate on portable chest radiographs. Suction

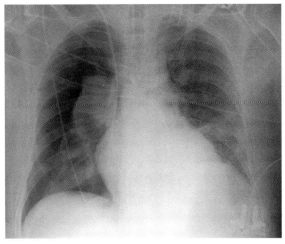

In a supine patient with pneumothorax, the air tends to be distributed in the anterior and basal portions of the pleural space.

Fig. 2.77 **Pneumothorax.**
The classic radiographic signs of pneumothorax are seen only with a large air collection and a compliant lung.

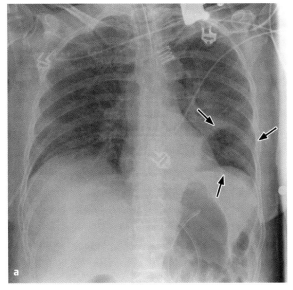

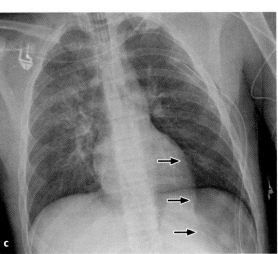

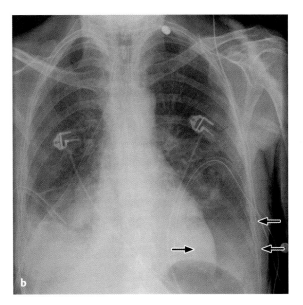

Fig. 2.78 a–c **Anterior or anterobasal pneumothorax.**
An anterior or anterobasal pneumothorax is often manifested only indirectly by a rounded hyperlucent area with well-defined margins (**a**), an avascular area (**b**), or sharp outlining of the cardiac borders or diaphragm (**c**).

Table 2.39 Location and radiographic signs of pneumothorax in the supine patient

Location	Indirect signs of pneumothorax

Anteromedial pneumothorax	**Suprahilar**
	▪ Sharp outlining of:
	  – superior vena cava
	  – azygos vein
	  – left subclavian artery
	  – superior pulmonary vein
	▪ Contralateral displacement of anterior pleural reflection
	
	Infrahilar
	▪ Sharp outlining of:
	  – cardiac border
	  – inferior vena cava
	  – cardiophrenic angle
	  – medial part of diaphragm below cardiac silhouette
	  – pericardial fat pad

Subpulmonic pneumothorax (chest radiograph must include the upper abdomen)	▪ Hyperlucent upper quadrant ▪ Deep costophrenic sulcus (deep sulcus sign) ▪ Sharp outlining of the diaphragm ▪ Appearance of a second diaphragm shadow ("double diaphragm sign") ▪ Delineation of inferior vena cava
"Classic" apicolateral pneumothorax	▪ Lack of contact between the minor fissure and chest wall

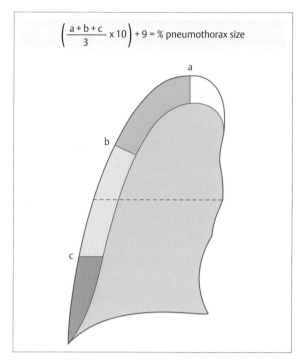

$$\left(\frac{a+b+c}{3} \times 10\right) + 9 = \%\text{ pneumothorax size}$$

Fig. 2.79 **Estimation of pneumothorax size using the formula of Choi et al. (1998).**

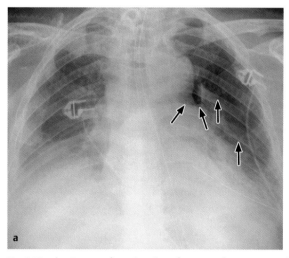
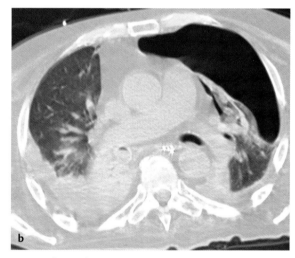

Fig. 2.80 a, b **Gross underestimation of pneumothorax size in the supine radiograph.** Chest radiograph (**a**) and CT scan (**b**) of the same patient taken 2 hours apart.

drainage is indicated if more than 35% of the lung volume is affected. The indication for drainage depends on clinical manifestations, a visual volume assessment on the chest radiograph, and on tension signs.

Choi et al. (1998) described a formula for estimating the volume of a pneumothorax. The average interpleural distances are measured at apical, lateral, and laterobasal locations and are used in the following formula:

([a + b + c]/3 × 10) + 9 = percentage pneumothorax size (**Fig. 2.79**)

One limitation of this formula is that the pneumothorax must extend along the lateral chest wall and must be

defined there. We know from experience, however, that the anterior pneumothorax in supine patients may reach a considerable size without displaying clear outlines, resulting in a gross underestimation of pneumothorax size on the chest film (**Fig. 2.80**). If radiographic findings are equivocal, CT should be used for the detection, localization, and quantification of pneumothorax, even in preparation for chest tube placement.

Barotrauma. The detection or exclusion of pneumothorax may be difficult or impossible when subcutaneous empyema (e.g., due to barotrauma) is superimposed on the

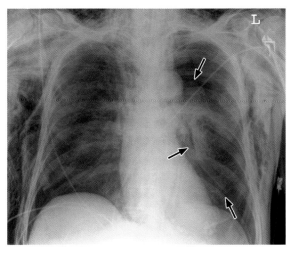

Fig. 2.81 **Pneumothorax with superimposed soft-tissue emphysema.**
A pneumothorax is particularly difficult to detect when accompanied by soft-tissue emphysema.

radiograph (**Fig. 2.81**), and CT may be appropriate in these cases. Premonitory signs of barotrauma are interstitial emphysema after the rupture of interstitial septa, which may be followed by air dissection to the mediastinum (mediastinal emphysema) and into the soft tissues (soft-tissue emphysema; see p. 46).

The risk of pneumothorax in barotrauma is significantly increased when the hemidiaphragm is lower than the sixth anterior rib segment or when the craniocaudal extent of the lung is greater than 25 cm.

Ultrasonography

In the absence of pneumothorax, the ultrasound scan shows *lung sliding* along the echogenic pleural interface during inspiration and expiration. It also shows *comet tail artifacts*, which are high-level reverberations extending from the pleural line to the lower edge of the screen (**Fig. 2.82**). With pneumothorax, both criteria are absent because of air in the pleural space. The absence of lung sliding during respiration is considered to have a negative predictive value of 90–100% and a false-positive rate of 10%.

Ultrasonography can be a useful diagnostic aid in bed-confined patients with equivocal radiographic findings.

Differential Diagnosis

Skin folds. Mistaking skin folds for pneumothorax on chest radiographs is most likely to occur in elderly and cachectic patients. Skin folds typically extend beyond the chest wall, are often multiple or bilateral, disappear suddenly, and are traversed by vascular structures (**Fig. 2.83**). Other signs of skin folds are indistinct margins, an associated soft-tissue shadow, and nonparallel alignment relative to the chest wall. Skin folds are easy to recognize as a rule, and only rarely do they require repeating the chest radiograph under controlled conditions or proceeding with CT.

Other air collections. The following intra- and extrathoracic air collections may not be misinterpreted as pneumothorax: lung cysts, emphysematous bullae, pneumatoceles, air collections in the mediastinum, pericardium or thoracic soft tissues, intrathoracic hernias (**Fig. 2.84**).

There is significant risk of pneumothorax due to barotrauma when the craniocaudal extent of the lung exceeds 25 cm and the diaphragm leaflets are lower than the sixth anterior rib segment.

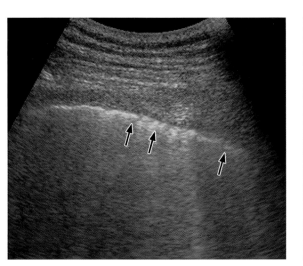

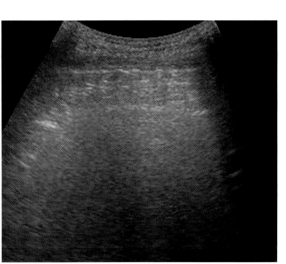

Fig. 2.82 a, b **Ultrasonographic appearance of pneumothorax.**
A characteristic feature of pneumothorax by ultrasound scan is the lack of the comet tail caused by absence of the pleural line

(a) compared with normal findings (b) (with kind permission of F. Gleeson, Oxford, UK).

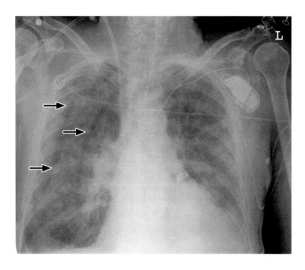

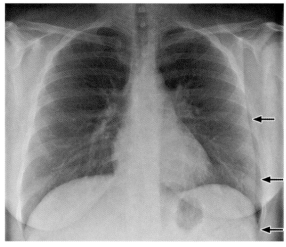

Fig. 2.83 a–c **Skin folds on the chest radiograph.**
Skin folds are a frequent mimic of pneumothorax. Usually they can be traced beyond the chest wall or mediastinum.

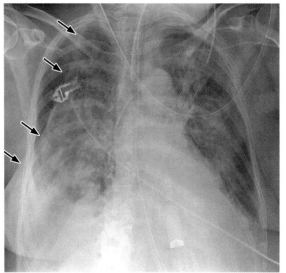

— Practical Recommendation ——————————

Unlike mediastinal emphysema or pericardial air, which outlines the cardiac border past the midline on the AP chest radiograph (**Fig. 2.85**), the pleural air of a pneumothorax keeps to the ipsilateral side and does not cross the midline.

Tension Pneumothorax

Any pneumothorax may become a tension pneumothorax in mechanically ventilated patients, even with a small air collection that appears loculated by pleural adhesions. A tension pneumothorax may even develop while a thoracostomy tube is in place.

A tension pneumothorax may develop even while a chest tube is in place.

Imaging

The radiographic signs of tension pneumothorax may be quite subtle in patients with diffuse bilateral lung changes (e. g., ARDS).

The cardinal signs of tension pneumothorax are a shift of mediastinal structures (tracheal shift!) toward the opposite side (**Fig. 2.86c**), herniation of the collapsed or retracted lung toward the mediastinum, and inversion of the diaphragm. The most reliable, and often the only, radiographic sign of tension pneumothorax is flattening and depression of the hemidiaphragm on the affected side (**Fig. 2.86b**). At higher pressures the hemidiaphragm becomes inferiorly convex and is associated with blunting and deepening of the costophrenic sulcus (**Fig. 2.86a**). A tension pneumothorax on the left side causes flattening of the cardiac border.

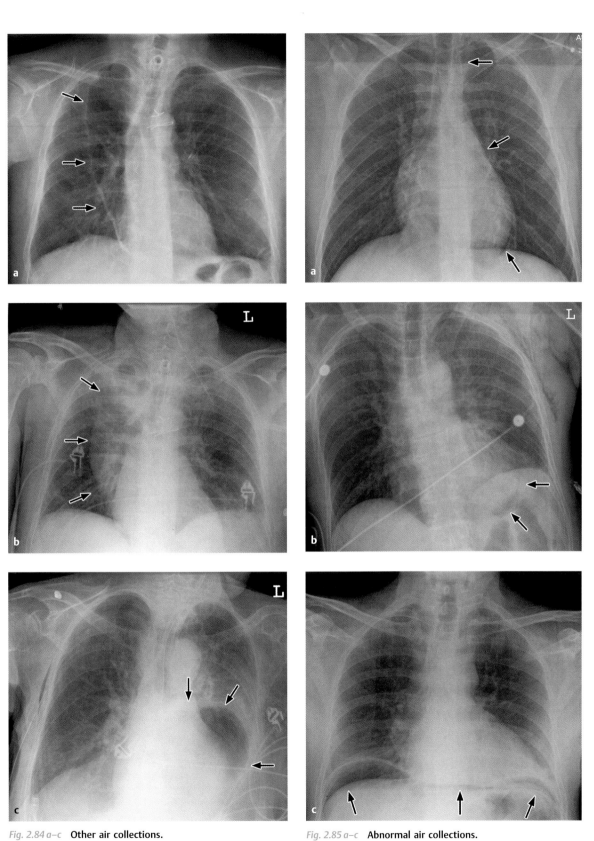

Fig. 2.84 a–c **Other air collections.**
Air collections like those following a gastric transposition (**a, b**) or occurring in a hernia (**c**) should not be mistaken for a pneumothorax.

Fig. 2.85 a–c **Abnormal air collections.**
Air collections that are abnormal but not located in the pleural cavity.
a Mediastinal emphysema (streaky and intramediastinal).
b Pericardial air (follows the heart contour).
c Subdiaphragmatic air (continuous diaphragm sign).

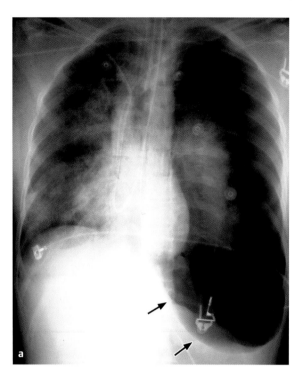

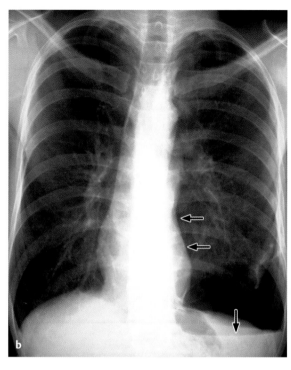

Fig. 2.86 a–c **Tension pneumothorax.**
a Deep sulcus sign.
b Flattening and displacement of the cardiac border and diaphragm.
c Contralateral mediastinal shift.

Differential Diagnosis

The low diaphragm position that results from obstructive lung disease (emphysema, COPD) or an asthenic body habitus should not be mistaken for a deep sulcus, especially on the left side. Doubts are resolved by comparison with older or preoperative images.

C. Schaefer-Prokop

Pleural Effusion

More than 60% of ICU patients have a pleural effusion. Small effusions are difficult to diagnose and accurately quantify on *supine radiographs*. The portable chest radiograph has a reported accuracy of only ca. 65% in the diagnosis of pleural effusion.

Ultrasound scans are superior to chest radiographs for the quantification and characterization of effusions (loculated versus nonloculated) at the bedside. The effusion is aspirated under ultrasound guidance at the level of the fifth or sixth intercostal space in the midaxillary line.

Pathogenesis

While heart failure, pneumonia, hepatic cirrhosis, hypoalbuminemia, and malignant diseases are the main causes of pleural effusion in medical patients, the leading causes in postsurgical patients are hemothorax and chy-lothorax. In a febrile patient with a unilateral (often loculated) pleural effusion an empyema has to be excluded, especially in the absence of other recognized causes for a pleural effusion.

Imaging

Radiography

Free pleural fluid tends to flow cephalad in the supine patient, causing uniform decreased lucency over the affected lung relative to the opposite side, poor or absent delineation of the hemidiaphragm, and opacity in the lateral costophrenic angle (**Fig. 2.87**).

The supine radiograph is relatively insensitive for the detection of effusions. The effusion volume must be greater than 200 mL to cause visible opacity on the chest radiograph (**Fig. 2.88**). The effusion may occupy up to one-third of the chest before it is detectable on the supine radiograph. Effusions are frequently missed on supine radiographs, especially in obese patients. A comparison with CT studies has shown that up to one-third of pleural effusions go undetected on portable chest radiographs.

Free-flowing effusions may collect in the major and minor *lobar fissures* (**Fig. 2.89**):

- Effusions flowing into the *major* fissure form a curvilinear opacity that becomes less dense laterally and superiorly.
- Effusions flowing into the *minor* fissure may form wedge-shaped opacities in the right midzone with their base directed toward the chest wall, or they may form acute biconvex (lemon-shaped) opacities (**Fig. 2.90**). The latter should not be mistaken for intrapulmonary masses.

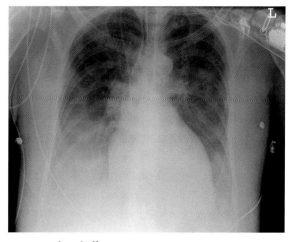

Fig. 2.87 **Pleural effusion.**
Nondelineation of the diaphragm, obliteration of the pleural sinus, and increasing basilar opacity (without an air bronchogram!) are the classic signs of pleural effusion on the supine chest radiograph.

Loculated effusions that are confined by adhesions, infiltrates, or atelectasis may assume a globular shape, depending on their volume, and may form a convex bulge impressing on the lung (**Fig. 2.91**). Loculated effusions in the major and minor fissures can mimic a "pseudotumor" or pneumonia (no air bronchogram!).

With a pure *subpulmonic* effusion, the opacity of the effusion mimics elevation of the hemidiaphragm.

Ultrasonography

Ultrasonography is very helpful for localizing the collection to the lung or pleura, quantifying the pleural effusion, and characterizing its internal structure (septa, echogenicity). In particular, ultrasound scanning is easily performed as a bedside examination in ICU patients (**Fig. 2.92**).

> A pleural effusion must have a volume greater than 200 mL to cause visible opacity in the portable chest radiograph.

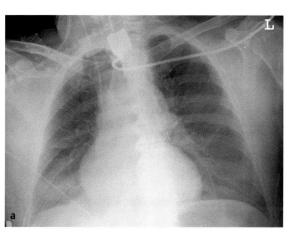
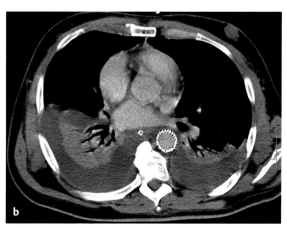

Fig. 2.88 a, b **Effusion volume.**
The supine radiograph may grossly underestimate the size of a pleural effusion. Radiograph (**a**) and CT scan (**b**) of the same patient taken 2 hours apart.

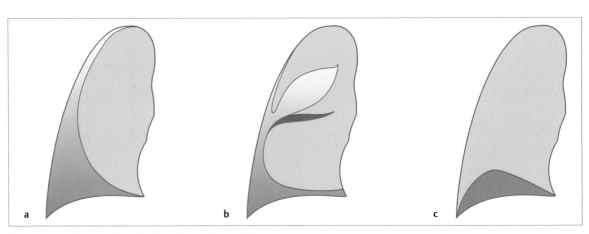

Fig. 2.89 a–c **Sites for the collection of free pleural effusions.**
a Posterior collection of a free-flowing effusion.
b Collection of effusion in the major and minor fissures.
c Subpulmonic effusion.

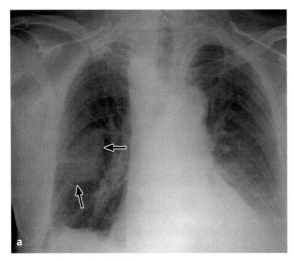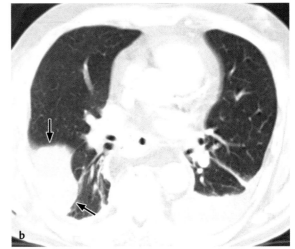

Fig. 2.90 a, b **Loculated effusion.**
An effusion loculated in the interlobar fissure may assume the shape of a pulmonary nodule (pseudotumor) or a biconvex "lemon" opacity.

Differential Diagnosis

The homogeneous opacity of the "grid effect" should not be confused with the decreased lucency caused by a pleural effusion. A grid effect is recognized by noting concomitant opacification of the soft tissues (see **Fig. 2.6**).

Effusion versus atelectasis. The complete opacification of a hemithorax requires differentiation between effusion (= mass effect) and atelectasis (= volume reduction). An effusion is indicated by a shift of the mediastinum (tra-

cheal border) toward the opposite side and by widening of the basal intercostal spaces (**Fig. 2.93**).

Effusion versus pneumonia. An air bronchogram is helpful in differentiating an effusion from pneumonia, as the presence of an air bronchogram proves that the opacity is intrapulmonary (**Fig. 2.94**).

Computed tomography. CT can more easily differentiate among hemothorax, parapneumonic effusion or empyema and transudate based on attenuation values and pleural thickness (**Fig. 2.95**; see also Chapter 3).

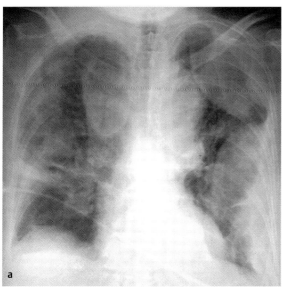

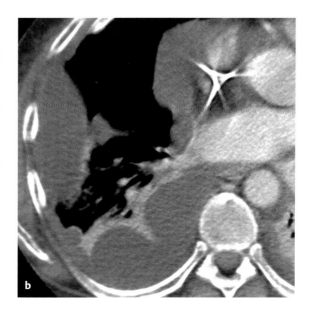

Fig. 2.91 a, b **Complicated effusion.**
With a "complicated" pleural effusion, the fluid may collect in multiple loculated pockets that exert a mass effect. The pockets do not communicate with one another and may have to be drained separately.

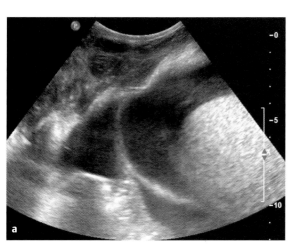

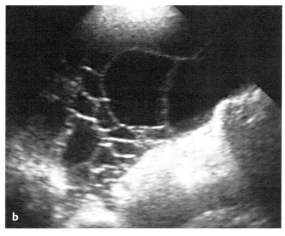

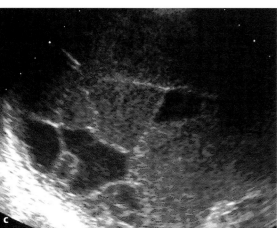

Fig. 2.92 a–c **Ultrasonography of a septated pleural effusion.**
The septa located within a complicated pleural effusion and the nature of the fluid (clear vs. corpuscular) are most accurately evaluated by ultrasound scan (with kind permission of F. Gleeson, Oxford, UK).

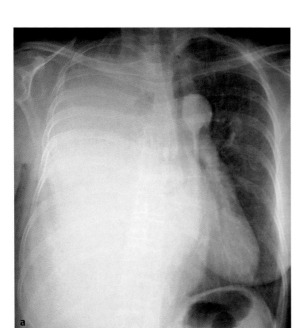

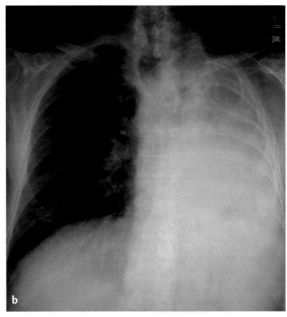

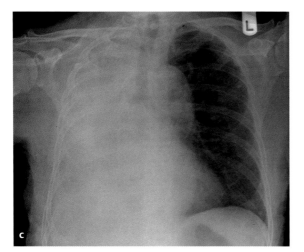

Fig. 2.93a–c **Differential diagnosis of unilateral lung opacity.**
a Contralateral mediastinal shift caused by the mass effect from an expansile pleural effusion.
b Massive ipsilateral mediastinal shift following a left pneumonectomy.
c Moderate ipsilateral mediastinal shift due to complete atelectasis of the right lung.

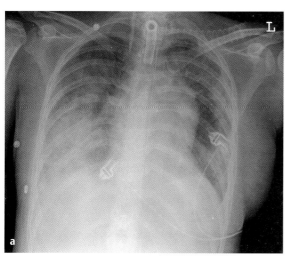

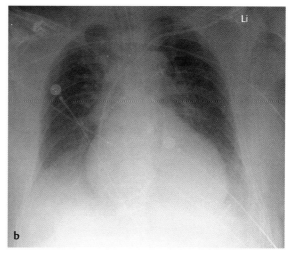

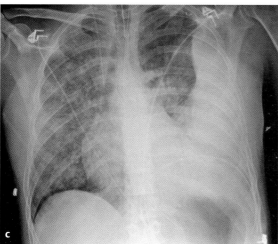

Fig. 2.94 a–c **Differential diagnosis of opacities, aided here by an air bronchogram.**

a   The presence of an air bronchogram localizes the opacity to the lung. Possible causes include pneumonia and pulmonary congestion.

b, c   Homogeneous opacity without an air bronchogram may signify a free-flowing (b) or loculated pleural effusion (c).

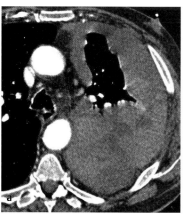
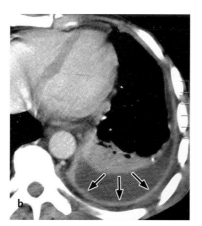
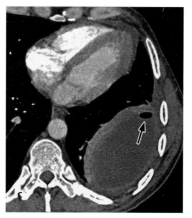

Fig. 2.95 a–c **Differential diagnosis of pleural effusions imaged by CT.**

a   Hyperdense hemorrhagic effusion.
b   Longstanding chronic effusion with pleural thickening (arrows).
c   Expansile pleural empyema with pleural thickening and an air inclusion (arrow).

Acute Pulmonary Embolism

S. Metz-Schimmerl and C. Schaefer-Prokop

Pulmonary embolism (PE) refers to the partial or complete occlusion of one or more pulmonary arteries by thromboembolic material.

Acute PE is a common and potentially life-threatening condition that has a high mortality (ca. 30%) in untreated cases. It is the third leading cause of death after cardiovascular disease and cancer. Because clinical manifestations and laboratory and ECG findings are often nonspecific and nondiagnostic, imaging studies play a particularly important role.

Risk factors. Certain situations such as prolonged immobilization (e.g., in the ICU) or surgical interventions increase the risk of acute PE. Other risk factors are pulmonary inflammations (especially tuberculosis), vasculitis, coagulation disorders, and malignant diseases.

Clinical Aspects

> The D-dimer level is not a useful diagnostic criterion in ICU patients.

Symptoms. Pulmonary embolism presents clinically with respiratory distress of sudden onset in the absence of known lung disease, or an acute exacerbation of respiratory function in known lung disease with abrupt onset of dyspnea or tachycardia. PE may lead to circulatory collapse with systemic hypotension, usually resulting from a massive central pulmonary vascular occlusion, and is believed to be responsible for approximately 15% of "sudden deaths." Pleuritic pain and hemoptysis are manifestations of pulmonary infarction due to peripheral embolism.

> The extent of thromboembolism does not correlate with clinical manifestations, which may even be absent.

PE may also produce no clinical symptoms. The extent of the thromboembolism does not correlate with the severity of clinical manifestations.

Laboratory findings and ECG. Laboratory indicators of PE are an elevation of plasma D-dimer, a fall in the platelet count, nonspecific changes in coagulation markers, and a rise of serum creatine kinase (CK). ECG shows tachycardia along with signs of pulmonary hypertension (incomplete right bundle branch block, right deviation of the QRS axis, a high P-wave, and ST-T changes). Massive PE is associated with arterial hypoxemia, hypocapnia, and respiratory alkalosis. A normal oxygen tension does not exclude PE, however.

Differential Diagnosis

A single clinical symptom such as dyspnea or acute chest pain is nonspecific and would be consistent with many other diseases, which require rapid and effective differentiation from PE (**Table 2.40**).

Diagnostic Strategy

Pretest Probability

Various analytic schemes have been described in the literature for determining clinical pretest probability, but only the simplified Wells score will be referenced here. A score below 2 indicates a low pretest probability, 2–6 indicates a modest probability, and above 6 indicates a high probability (**Table 2.41**).

D-Dimer

D-dimers are fibrin breakdown products that form during the proteolysis of a thrombus by plasmin. While D-dimer is very sensitive for the diagnosis of acute PE, it is nonspecific because it is also elevated in the postoperative state, for example, and in several other medical conditions (**Table 2.42**). As a result, a positive D-dimer level is not a useful diagnostic criterion in ICU patients; *a negative D-dimer, however, is well accepted for excluding PE.*

Radiography

The chest radiograph is the primary imaging study in acute PE because it is rapidly available and can exclude clinical *differential diagnoses* such as a new pneumotho-

Table 2.40 Clinical differential diagnosis of acute pulmonary embolism (PE)

- Pneumonia
- Myocardial infarction
- Aortic dissection
- Pleural effusion, pericardial effusion
- Pneumothorax, pneumomediastinum
- Rib fractures
- Mediastinitis, abscesses
- COPD
- Diaphragmatic hernia

Table 2.41 Modified Wells score for determining the pretest probability of PE

Criteria	Points
Clinical signs and symptoms of lower extremity venous thrombosis	3
Alternative diagnosis less likely than PE	3
Tachycardia > 100 bpm	1.5
Immobilization in previous 4 weeks	1.5
Hemoptysis	1
Malignancy within the last 6 months	1

Table 2.42 Diseases and situations that are associated with elevated D-dimer levels

- Venous thrombosis
- Infection
- Malignancy
- Heart failure
- Acute myocardial infarction
- Renal failure
- Stroke
- Connective-tissue diseases
- Liver diseases
- Pregnancy
- Postoperative state
- Trauma

rax or pneumonia. Chest radiographs cannot exclude PE, however.

Echocardiography

The advantage of echocardiography is that it provides an immediate bedside examination that is particularly useful in bed-confined patients. It can exclude important *differential diagnoses* such as aortic dissection and pericardial tamponade.

The detection of *right-heart overload* by echocardiography (dilatation of the right ventricle and main pulmonary artery trunks, paradoxical septal motion and tricuspid insufficiency) is useful for diagnosing massive PE in patients with no prior history of right ventricular dilatation. Echocardiography has no role in diagnosing acute PE in an unselected population.

Computed Tomography

Today, CT is considered the method of choice for the detection of acute PE. As a general rule, the thinner the slices, the better the ability to evaluate the peripheral segmental and subsegmental vessels.

Multislice CT can scan the entire thorax in submillimeter or 1-mm slices during a single breath-hold.

--- Practical Recommendation ---

The following points should be noted:
- The injected contrast volume depends on the speed of the available scanner.
- The use of a test-bolus injection to evaluate circulation time or automated scan triggering during optimum enhancement of the pulmonary arteries is most essential when using a high-speed scanner with a scan time of just a few seconds. With fast (32- and 64-slice) scanners, an extra scan delay should be added after peak enhancement (10 s at 100 HU, 5 s at 150 HU) to ensure good enhancement throughout the lung.

- An NaCl chaser bolus is routinely recommended to reduce contrast-induced streak artifacts, prolong the plateau phase of maximum intravascular enhancement, and reduce the necessary contrast dose.
- Nonventilated patients should receive good preparation and instruction to avoid a Valsalva maneuver. With a scan time of only 5 s this maneuver can reduce intravascular enhancement to a nondiagnostic level. Patients with significant *dyspnea* should take quiet, shallow breaths during the examination. In ventilated patients, scanning should be performed with breath held at full inspiration.

Imaging

Radiography

The chest radiograph has no role in the diagnosis of PE. Even in non-ICU patients, chest radiographs are false-negative in ca. 40% of cases. Nonspecific chest radiographic findings in PE are summarized in **Table 2.43**.

Computed Tomography

The CT diagnosis of PE is based on direct visualization of the thrombus, which appears as a partial or complete intraluminal filling defect in the pulmonary artery (**Fig. 2.96a**). An abrupt cutoff of the intravascular contrast column and nonopacification of the vessel (in the soft-tissue window) are evidence of complete occlusion (**Fig. 2.96c**). A thrombus-filled vascular segment may be markedly dilated (**Fig. 2.96b**). Oligemia with decreased vascular markings (especially on side-to-side comparison) is also diagnostic (**Fig. 2.97**).

The CT correlate of pulmonary *infarction* is a wedge-shaped or bandlike area of consolidation that directly abuts the pleura. Foci of liquefaction may develop within the consolidated area, even after a period of months (**Fig. 2.97c**).

Mosaic perfusion describes a CT pattern of higher and lower parenchymal attenuation due to variations in perfusion. It is common only in the setting of chronic PE, however (**Fig. 2.98**).

> PE appears as a partial or complete filling defect in the pulmonary artery on postcontrast CT.

> Multislice CT is the method of choice for the diagnosis of pulmonary embolism.

Table 2.43 Frequency and nature of chest radiographic findings in PE

Finding	Frequency (%)
Atelectasis (consolidation)	70
Pleural effusion	35–50
Westermark sign (oligemia)	20
Fleischner sign (dilatation of central vessels)	15
Elevation of the hemidiaphragm	20
Hampton hump (subpleural infarction)	15

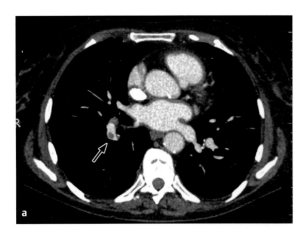

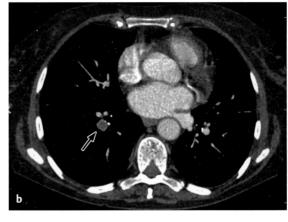

Fig. 2.96 a–c **Typical signs of pulmonary embolism on CT scans.**
a Sharply circumscribed intravascular filling defect.
b Vascular caliber enlarged by thrombus material.
c Complete arterial occlusion (multiplanar reformation).

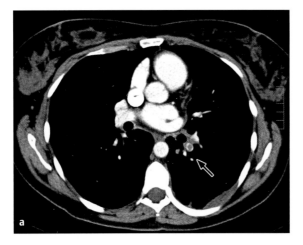

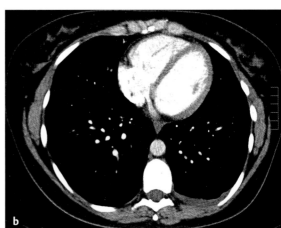

Fig. 2.97 a–c **Central embolism leading to pulmonary infarction.**
The central embolism (a) has caused pronounced, asymmetrical hypoperfusion of the downstream lung (b) and a subpleural infarction (c).

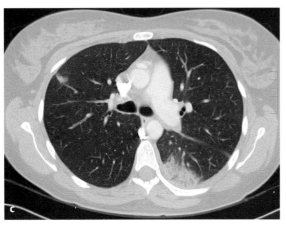

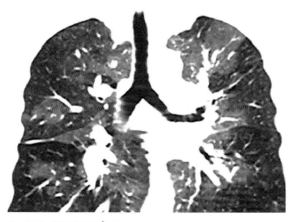

Fig. 2.98 **Mosaic perfusion.**
Mosaic perfusion is a sign of chronic pulmonary embolism (check for pulmonary hypertension).

Obstruction of more than 30% of the pulmonary circulation leads to a significant rise of pulmonary arterial pressure causing an *acute right heart overload* (**Fig. 2.99**). The evaluation of cardiac function, especially in right heart overload, is the domain of echocardiography, although CT may play a greater role in the future. The following, prognostically important signs serve as morphologic CT criteria of right heart overload, even on non-triggered scans:

- dilatation of the right ventricle (ratio of RV to LV transverse diameters > 1.3)
- flattening or convex bulging of the septum toward the left
- dilatation of the pulmonary artery
- dilatation of the coronary sinus

The clinical significance of isolated *subsegmental emboli* is controversial (**Fig. 2.100**). The healthy lung acts as a filter to prevent dissemination of these small emboli into the systemic circulation. Isolated subsegmental thrombi have clinical importance as possible precursors of a severe embolism (lower extremity imaging) and in patients with a limited cardiopulmonary reserve that increases their vulnerability to emboli.

Table 2.44 reviews the typical CT findings of acute and chronic pulmonary emboli.

Table 2.45 lists possible reasons for false-positive and false-negative CT findings in PE. The leading causes of spurious findings, especially in ICU patients, are motion artifacts (respiratory and pulsation artifacts, **Fig. 2.101**)—best detected by correlation with changes in the lung window—and mucus-filled bronchi, which mimic a linear filling defect (also check in lung window) (**Fig. 2.102**).

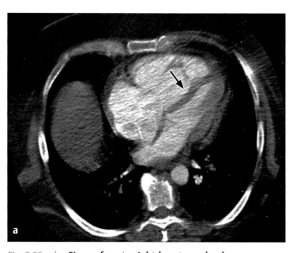

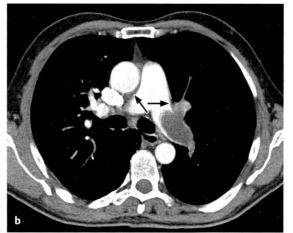

Fig. 2.99 a, b **Signs of acute right heart overload.**
Dilatation of the right ventricle (transverse diameter > left ventricle), bulging of the septum (**a**), and acute dilatation of the pulmonary trunk (**b**) are considered poor prognostic signs in a patient with massive PE.

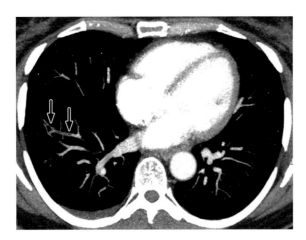

Fig. 2.100 **Subsegmental emboli.**
Fast scanners and submillimeter slice acquisition can detect even the smallest subsegmental emboli (thin-slice MIP, maximum intensity projection).

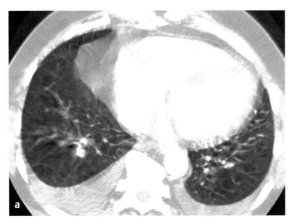

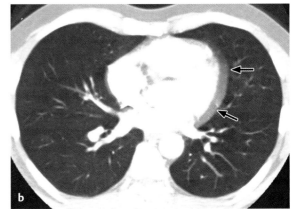

Fig. 2.101 a, b **Respiratory and pulsation artifacts.**
These can mimic intravascular density changes and should not be mistaken for pulmonary emboli.
a Respiratory artifacts (lung window).
b Pulsation artifacts (watch for double contours of the heart and vessels).

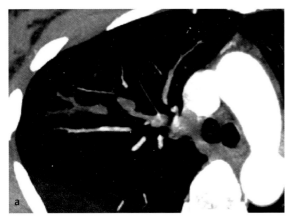

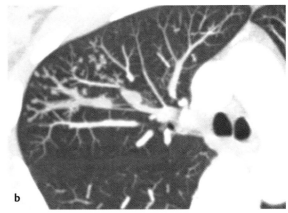

Fig. 2.102 a, b **Typical spurious finding.**
Mucus-filled bronchi form tubular structures that mimic nonopacified vessels (**a**). Always correlate with findings in the lung window (**b**).

Table 2.44 Morphologic criteria for the differentiation of acute and chronic PE

Acute PE	Chronic thromboembolic pulmonary hypertension
Central intravascular thrombus outlined by contrast medium	Mural thrombus Recanalized or calcified thrombus Intraluminal webs
Dilatation of intrapulmonary vessels	Intrapulmonary vessels smaller than normal, irregular vessel margins
Wedge-shaped area of parenchymal consolidation (infarction)	Mosaic perfusion
Right heart enlargement with normal heart wall	Right heart enlargement with thickened heart wall
No dilatation of bronchial arteries	Dilatation of bronchial arteries
Possible pleural effusion, atelectasis	Pericardial effusion, ascites

Table 2.45 Reasons for false-positive and false-negative findings and possible solutions

False-negative	Solution
Poor vascular opacification	Repeat scan
Motion artifacts	Check for artifacts in lung window; streaks transcend the vessel wall
Faulty scan parameters	
Beam-hardening artifacts caused by contrast medium	
Isolated PE in subsegmental vessel	

False-positive	Solution
Hilar lymph nodes	MPR
Partial volume effects	MPR
Incorrect scan delay	Repeat scan
Focal decrease in lung perfusion (e. g., emphysema)	Correlation with lung window
Misinterpretation of nonopacified veins	Trace vessels centrally
Contrast variations due to respiratory or pulsation artifacts	Look for heart wall pulsations and respiratory artifacts in the same scan

MPR, multiplanar reformation.

Summary

Portable chest radiographs are no longer obtained on a routine daily basis owing to concerns about radiation safety and cost. The depth of inspiration is adequate when the hemidiaphragm is displayed at the level of the fifth anterior rib in the midclavicular line.

The **correct interpretation** of portable chest radiographs requires an awareness of previous therapeutic and diagnostic actions.

Intrathoracic **tubes and lines** should be completely visualized on chest radiographs.

- The **central venous catheter** is usually introduced via the subclavian vein or internal jugular vein. The catheter tip should be positioned between the sternal attachments of the first three ribs in the AP radiograph close to the origin of the azygos vein. Pneumothorax is the most frequent complication of subclavian vein catheterization.
- A chest radiograph should always be obtained after the insertion of a **pulmonary artery catheter**.
- AP and lateral radiographs are both necessary for the accurate localization of **cardiac pacemakers and implantable cardioverter defibrillators**.
- Every **endotracheal intubation** should be followed by a chest radiograph to evaluate tube position. With the head in a neutral position, the tip of the endotracheal tube should be 5–7 cm above the carina.

The most reliable signs of **hydrostatic edema** are cardiomegaly and a mediastinal width greater than 7 cm. Interstitial (grade 2) edema and alveolar (grade 3) edema are on a continuum and frequently coexist.

The diagnosis of **adult respiratory distress syndrome** (ARDS) is based on a combination of clinical and imaging findings. The clinical manifestations of ARDS may precede imaging findings by more than 12 hours. Radiographs can demonstrate the successive phases of ARDS, which are marked by increasing opacities that may spread throughout the lung (in extreme cases producing a "white lung" with a positive air bronchogram) and finally show a less compact distribution with focal and patchy opacities. PEEP ventilation can reopen microatelectases, resulting in improvement of compliance, functional residual capacity, and gas exchange. Possible complications include pneumonia and, in ventilated patients, pulmonary interstitial edema, pneumothorax, and pneumomediastinum.

Community-acquired **pneumonia** is an outpatient infection whereas, by definition, nosocomial pneumonia develops at least 72 hours after hospitalization. The radiographic hallmark of pneumonia is opacity of the lung parenchyma. An air bronchogram identifies an opacity as being located in the lung (as opposed to the pleural space) but is not seen in all pneumonias. The radiologic diagnosis of pneumonia is often difficult in ventilated patients. To avoid misinterpretation, the radiologist must be aware of any changes in ventilator settings or patient positioning. Complications of pneumonia are pulmonary abscess formation, pneumatoceles, pleural empyema, and bronchopulmonary fistulas.

Atelectasis is common in ICU patients and most frequently affects the posterobasal region of the left lung. Patients with obstructive atelectasis (no air bronchogram) will often benefit from bronchoscopy, unlike patients with compression atelectasis (positive air bronchogram). Atelectasis generally shows signs of diminished lung volume whereas pneumonia usually shows a volume increase.

A **pneumothorax** may still develop hours or days after a tube thoracostomy. In the supine patient, the air tends to be distributed in the anterior and basal portions of the pleural space. It usually appears as a rounded or oval area of increased radiolucency ("black oval") or as an avascular area. The cardinal signs of a **tension pneumothorax** are a contralateral shift of mediastinal structures (tracheal shift!), herniation of the collapsed or retracted lung toward the mediastinum, and inversion of the diaphragm.

A **pleural effusion** must have a volume greater than 200 mL to cause visible opacity in a portable chest radiograph. Free-flowing effusions may collect in the major and minor fissures, while loculated effusions may assume a globular shape and form a pseudotumor, depending on their volume.

Multislice CT is the method of choice for the diagnosis of **pulmonary embolism**. The thinner the slices, the better the ability to evaluate the peripheral segmental and subsegmental vessels. CT diagnosis is based on direct visualization of the thrombus, which appears as a partial or complete filling defect in the pulmonary artery.

Pneumonectomy 93
Lobectomy 101
Segmental Lung Resection 102
Sleeve Resection 103

Lung Transplantation 103
Cardiovascular Surgery 106
Heart Transplantation 109
Esophageal Surgery 110

Lung resections vary in their extent from wedge resections of peripheral lesions to complete pneumonectomy. The excision may be extended to include portions of the chest wall, pericardium, diaphragm, or great vessels, depending on the extent of disease.

Postoperative chest radiographs or computed tomography (CT) scans usually show pronounced anatomical changes. The radiologist should be aware of previous surgical interventions to understand the changes and interpret them correctly.

M. Fuchsjaeger and C. Schaefer-Prokop

The radiologist should be aware of previous surgical interventions when interpreting postoperative chest radiographs and CT scans.

Pneumonectomy

A pneumonectomy is performed under standard conditions through a posterolateral thoracotomy.

The most common operation is an *intrapleural* pneumonectomy, which includes removal of the lung and visceral pleura. It involves opening the pericardium and dissecting the great vessels.

An *extrapleural* pneumonectomy involves an en-bloc resection of the lung including the parietal and mediastinal pleura, pericardium, and diaphragm.

The mortality rate of pneumonectomy is ca. 5%. Most deaths result from pneumonia, respiratory failure, pulmonary embolism, myocardial infarction, bronchopleural fistula, or pleural empyema.

Normal Postoperative Findings

The volume of the operated hemithorax is reduced after pneumonectomy. The ribs are spaced closer together and are directed at a steeper angle. The contralateral, nonoperated hemithorax often shows increased volume due to compensatory hyperinflation, especially in younger patients, while also showing signs of increased perfusion (**Fig. 3.1**).

Air–fluid level. The pleural space on the operated side fills increasingly with serous fluid, which appears on radiographs as a homogeneous opacity with an air–fluid level (**Fig. 3.2**). The air–fluid level may persist for months. A double air–fluid level is caused by fibrinous septa. Multiple fluid levels occur in up to 25% of patients with a normal postoperative course and require differentiation from pleural empyema (see under Pneumonia in Chapter 2, p. 49). Once fluid has completely filled the pneumonectomy cavity, it is gradually reabsorbed. This is accompanied by a reduction of hemithoracic volume due to organization of the residual fluid and increasing fibrosis.

Ordinarily the pneumonectomy cavity shows a *continuous* decrease in air accompanied by a rising fluid level. Any *sudden* increase in the air volume (sudden fall of the fluid level) is suspicious for a complication such as bronchopleural fistula or a bronchial anastomotic leak.

Mediastinal shift. The mediastinum is shifted from the midline toward the operated side, accompanied by a shift of the trachea. The clamped main bronchus generally does not show a reduction in its diameter.

A continuous decrease of air and increase of fluid is normal after pneumonectomy. A sudden increase in air volume is suspicious for a complication.

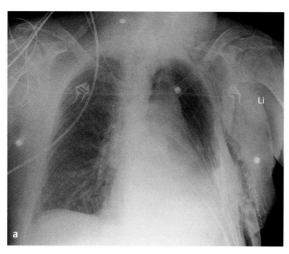

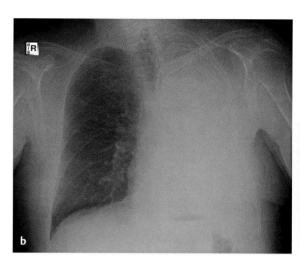

Fig. 3.1 a, b **Increased perfusion of the remaining lung.**
Pneumonectomy is followed initially by increased perfusion of
the remaining lung, which should not be interpreted as "engorgement." Compare the pulmonary vessels on postoperative day 1 (**a**) and postoperative day 7 (**b**).

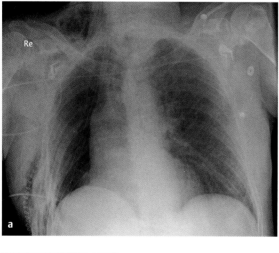

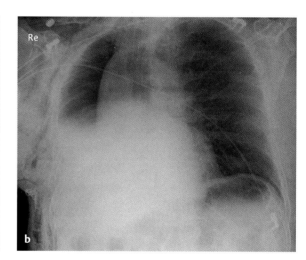

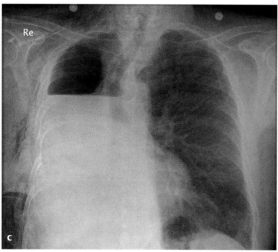

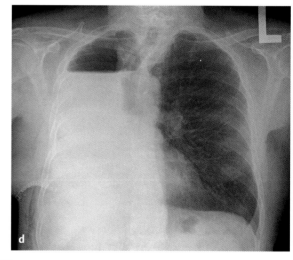

Fig. 3.2 a–d **Normal progression of findings after pneumonectomy.**
The pneumonectomy cavity is increasingly filled with fluid.
a Postoperative day 1.
b Postoperative day 2.
c Postoperative day 5.
d Postoperative day 10.

Following a *left-sided* pneumonectomy, the aortic arch maintains its anteroposterior orientation while the anterior or posterior portion of the right lung may herniate into the pneumonectomy space. The outline of the diaphragm is still defined by negative contrast from the gastric bubble and left colic flexure. Following a *right-sided* pneumonectomy, it is common to find rotation of the mediastinum with a transverse orientation of the aortic arch and anterior herniation of the left lung. In most cases the right hemidiaphragm is no longer defined.

Specific Postoperative Complications

Postpneumonectomy Edema

Postoperative edema has an incidence of up to 5% after pneumonectomy (right > left) and less than 1% after lobectomy, typically occurring ca. 2–3 days after the resection. It is marked *clinically* by rapid progression of dyspnea and hypoxia. The prognosis with treatment is good. The *pathophysiology* of postpneumonectomy edema may relate to a fluid overload in the remaining lung, left heart failure, a disturbance of capillary membrane permeability

Table 3.1 Complications after pneumonectomy

Early complications
- Empyema
- Cardiac herniation
- Pulmonary edema (hydrostatic, permeability edema)
- Chylothorax
- Hemothorax
- Bronchopleural fistula
- Wound infection
- Esophagopleural fistula

Late complications
- Postpneumonectomy syndrome
- Tumor recurrence
- Esophagopleural fistula

due to sepsis or prolonged ventilation, or a surgically induced disruption of lymphatic drainage.

Radiography. Interstitial edema is visible on chest radiographs and may spread to form patchy areas of alveolar consolidation.

Hemothorax

A hemothorax is usually the result of persistent bleeding from a bronchial artery or a vessel in the chest wall. The bleeding rarely originates from a central pulmonary vessel. The mortality rate is less than 0.1%. Hemothorax is diagnosed clinically in patients who have a chest tube in place.

Radiography. Hemothorax appears radiographically as a rapidly increasing pleural effusion (possibly accompanied by typical clinical signs such as tachycardia, hypotension, and a fall of hematocrit) with an associated mass effect based on its size (**Fig. 3.3a, b**).

Computed tomography. CT demonstrates a pleural fluid collection, frequently lobulated (loculated), of variable density. The effusion often has biconvex margins and produces a mass effect based upon its size and typical rapid enlargement.

The *attenuation values* of a hemothorax range from 15 HU to more than 40 HU, depending on the age of the hemorrhage. It is common to find layering effects within the pleural effusion. As the hemorrhage becomes more organized, the effusion may acquire a tumorlike aspect. It is distinguished from a tumor by noting its high attenuation values on plain scans and its lack of enhancement after IV contrast administration.

▸ The attenuation values of a hemothorax range from 15 to 40 HU, depending on the age of the hemorrhage.

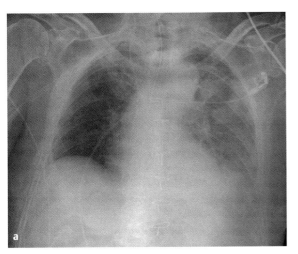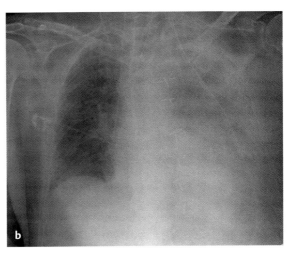

Fig. 3.3 a, b **Hemothorax.**
A rapidly progressive pleural effusion after surgery (12 hours passed between **a** and **b**) is suspicious for a hemothorax in patients with corresponding clinical symptoms.

Chylothorax

A chylothorax results from injury to the thoracic duct or one of its tributaries. Sites of predilection are the left inferior paravertebral hemithorax following extrapulmonary pneumonectomy, the aortopulmonary window region following lymphadenectomy, and the region of the pulmonary ligament on both sides.

Radiography. Like a hemothorax, chylothorax appears radiographically as a rapidly increasing pleural effusion (**Fig. 3.4**).

Computed tomography. Negative, fat-equivalent CT attenuation values confirm the diagnosis of chylothorax. Negative attenuation values are not always present, however, due to the protein content of the collection.

Negative, fat-equivalent CT densities confirm a chylothorax but are not always present.

Pleural Empyema

Extensive infections of the pleural cavity occur in up to 5% of cases, depending on the patient subgroup. A pleural empyema may develop as an early (weeks) or late complication (months to years). The main causative organisms are staphylococci, *Pseudomonas*, streptococci, and *Aerobacter aerogenes*.

An empyema occurring in the *early postoperative period* usually results from the intraoperative spread of infec-

tious organisms or a bronchial leak. The main cause of a *late* infection is bronchopleural fistulation.

The following factors predispose to the development of a (late) postpneumonectomy empyema:
- secondary pneumonectomy after an initial lobectomy
- preoperative radiation
- sepsis
- mediastinal lymphadenectomy
- prolonged mechanical ventilation

The drainage of an empyema is described under Pneumonia in Chapter 2 (complications, empyema, p. 67).

Radiography. The following signs are noted, depending on the timing of the infection:
- Unusually rapid filling of the hemithorax with fluid
- Shift of the mediastinum toward the healthy side (mass effect from the pleural fluid) (**Fig. 3.5**).
- Sudden drop of the air–fluid level in the operated hemithorax via a communication with the main bronchus or a fistula in the pleural wall
- Reappearance of air in a completely opaque hemithorax due to a bronchopleural fistula or gas-forming bacteria
- Appearance of multiple air–fluid levels at various locations (caution: multiple air–fluid levels are a normal finding in up to 25% of patients; they are suspicious when multiple new air–fluid levels appear after initial

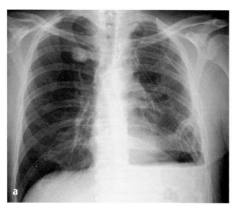
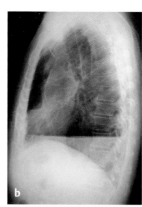

Fig. 3.4 a, b **Basal chylopneumothorax after lobectomy.**
Note extension of the air–fluid level along the full sagittal thoracic diameter (unlike an abscess) (**a**) and the anterior loculated pneumoserothorax, which also contains an air–fluid level (**b**).

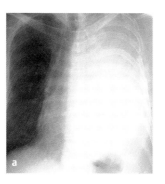
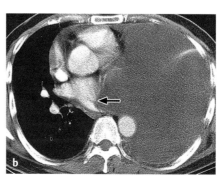

Fig. 3.5 a, b **Pyoserothorax with mass effect.**
The collection has caused a contralateral shift of the mediastinum.

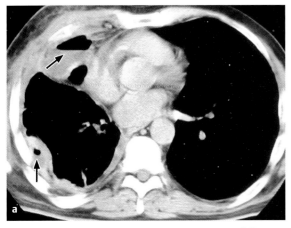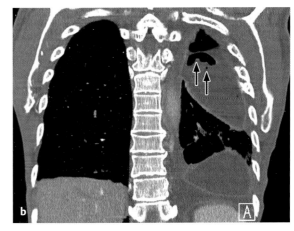

Fig. 3.6 a, b **Postoperative pleural empyema in two different patients.**
The pleura is thickened and shows increased contrast enhancement. Multiple air inclusions are seen at different levels.

homogeneous fluid filling of the hemithorax) (**Fig. 3.6**).

Ultrasonography. Ultrasound scanning can detect septations earlier and with greater clarity than CT. Echogenicity that is increased or variable due to septations and reverberations from air inclusions are typical sonographic features of a "complicated" effusion (see **Fig. 2.91**).

Computed tomography. CT signs of pleural empyema are a thickened pleura showing increased contrast enhancement and dense exudate with attenuation values greater than 20 HU. CT is better than radiographs for revealing associated mass effects (**Fig. 3.6**).

— Practical Recommendation —

A bronchopleural fistula (BPF) should be excluded whenever a pleural empyema is detected. Pleural empyema (pus) or infected pleural fluid (complicated effusion) may be present even in the absence of peripheral rim enhancement, which is why attention should be given to possible mass effects (**Fig. 3.5**) and air inclusions.

Bronchopleural Fistula

Small air leaks in the main bronchus are not uncommon and will generally heal spontaneously with conservative therapy. Large or persistent leaks give rise to bronchopleural fistulas (BPFs). The origin of the fistula is usually located in the bronchial stump. Generally the diagnosis is confirmed by bronchoscopy.

BPFs rarely occur in the early postoperative period. They more commonly develop as a delayed complication after a bronchial stump infection, bronchial ischemia, extensive lymphadenectomy, tumor recurrence, or in cases where the bronchial stump has been ligated at a too-

proximal level. Predisposing factors are preoperative radiation and preoperative pleuropulmonary infection.

BPF is the leading cause of pleural empyema.

Radiography. The following radiographic signs may be noted at varying intervals after a pneumonectomy:
- Persistent or increasing pneumothorax with a chest tube in place
- Increasing subcutaneous or mediastinal emphysema
- More than a 2-cm drop in the air–fluid level with a mediastinal shift toward the healthy side
- Sudden onset of pneumoserothorax with a preexisting serothorax (**Fig. 3.7**)
- Consolidated areas in the contralateral lung caused by fluid overflow from the pneumonectomy cavity or by direct communication through a BPF

Computed tomography. In up to 50% of cases, thin-slice CT can directly visualize a BPF between the airway (bronchial stump) and pleural space, or between the lung parenchyma and pleural space (**Fig. 3.8**).

If the fistula cannot be directly visualized, persistent air and fluid collections in the mediastinum or pleural space may suggest the correct diagnosis.

Esophagopleural Fistula

This rare complication (< 1%) occurs most commonly after a right pneumonectomy (direct contact between the esophagus and right pleura).

An esophagopleural fistula (EPF) of *early onset* (within 2 weeks) may be caused by direct esophageal injury or decreased blood flow to the lower esophagus. *Later* occurrence of the fistula (from 2–6 weeks postoperatively) may result from an empyema, extensive lymphadenectomy, or BPF. An EPF caused by tumor recurrence may develop more than 2 years after the operation.

When the detection of pus confirms a pleural empyema, a bronchopleural fistula should be excluded.

Thin-slice CT can directly visualize a bronchopleural fistula in up to 50% of cases.

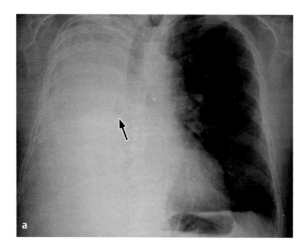

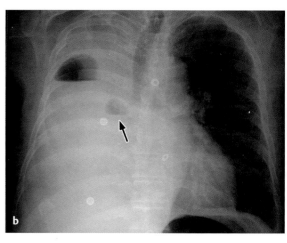

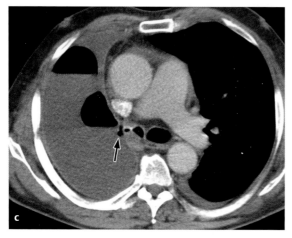

Fig. 3.7 a–c **Anastomotic leak after pneumonectomy.**
The pneumonectomy cavity is completely filled with fluid (**a**). This is followed by secondary air inclusions with air–fluid levels (**b**), which continue to increase during follow-up (**c**).

Patients typically present with fever, chest pain, and significant dysphagia. The presence of food constituents in the drained pleural fluid provides direct evidence of an EPF.

— **Practical Recommendation** —

Every patient who develops dysphagia after pneumonectomy should undergo oral contrast examination of the esophagus with a water-soluble medium to exclude an esophagopleural fistula.

Radiography and CT. Direct visualization of the fistula (e. g., after oral contrast administration) may be difficult. Visualization is aided by moving the patient to a lateral decubitus position with the operated side down (**Fig. 3.9**). Imaging can be done by conventional esophagography or by CT after the oral administration of water-soluble contrast medium.

Cardiac Herniation

The heart may herniate through the pericardial defect created by an intrapericardial pneumonectomy. This complication occurs within the first few hours after an intrapericardial pneumonectomy and is extremely rare in cases where the pericardial defect has been closed. Cardiac herniation may occur through a pericardial defect of any size.

A *right-sided herniation* is manifested clinically by obstructed venous return leading to a rise of central venous pressure (due to counterclockwise rotation of the heart about the superior vena cava). A *left-sided herniation* leads to shock symptoms with hypotension and tachycardia (caused by strangulation of the left ventricle in the pericardial defect).

Radiography. The cardiac silhouette is markedly displaced toward the side of the pneumonectomy, with the cardiac apex touching the lateral chest wall. An empty, air-filled pericardial space may also be seen.

(Right) Pneumonectomy Syndrome

Pneumonectomy syndrome is a delayed complication usually following a right-sided pneumonectomy. Marked compensatory hyperinflation of the left lung shifts the mediastinum toward the right side, obstructing the left main bronchus and promoting intermittent pneumonia

▣ Cardiac herniation toward the left side leads to shock symptoms with tachycardia and hypotension due to strangulation of the left ventricle in the pericardial defect.

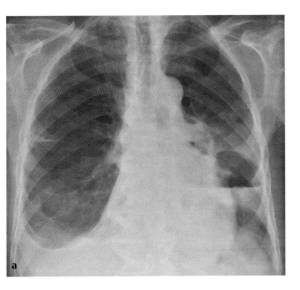

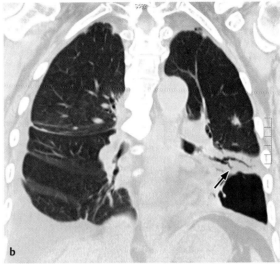

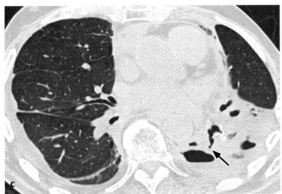

Fig. 3.8 a–c **Bronchopleural fistula.**
This patient has a chronic bronchopleural fistula and persistent pneumothorax caused by a communication between the bronchus and pleura.

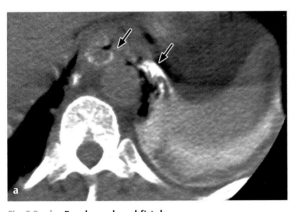

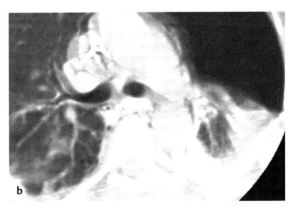

Fig. 3.9 a, b **Esophagopleural fistula.**
CT shows direct contrast extravasation from the esophagus into the left pleural space through an esophagopleural fistula (here, an iatrogenic fistula caused by balloon dilation of the esophagus). Pneumothorax and mediastinal emphysema are also present.

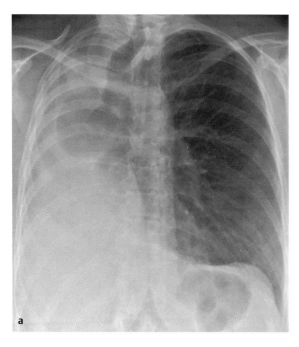

Fig. 3.10 a–c **"Pneumonectomy syndrome" following a right pneumonectomy.**

a, b Chest radiograph and CT show complete displacement of mediastinal structures toward the right side with compression of bronchial or vascular structures (in this case, the left lower lobe bronchus) by the spinal column.

c Postoperative CT. The mediastinum has been repositioned with a prosthesis implanted into the pneumonectomy space.

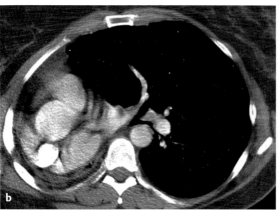

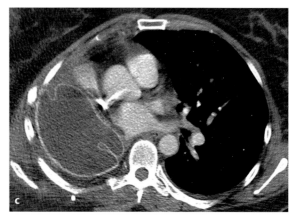

and dyspnea. In rare cases cardiac problems may develop due to compression of the (inferior) left pulmonary vein with damming back of blood into the pulmonary circulation.

Computed tomography. CT demonstrates rotation of the mediastinum with stretching of the left main bronchus and/or inferior pulmonary vein across the spinal column (**Fig. 3.10**). Signs of intrapulmonary congestion may also be found (ground-glass opacity and thickened interlobular septa).

Nonspecific Complications after Pneumonectomy

Besides the specific complications of pneumonectomy described above, patients who have undergone thoracic surgery are highly susceptible to nonspecific complications such as atelectasis and pneumonia.

Atelectasis may result from the retention of secretions, postoperative swelling of the airways, impaired ciliary motility, and partial denervation. Superinfection and/or aspiration are not uncommon. The prevalence of *pneumonia* after pneumonectomy is ca. 20%; prolonged mechanical ventilation is a predisposing factor. Causes include superinfected atelectasis and the aspiration of gastric contents (gram-negative bacteria). The most serious complication is *necrotizing pneumonia*.

Lobectomy

The principal indications for lobectomy are the resection of:

- bronchial carcinoma
- large emphysematous bullae
- centrally located (obstructive) benign tumors
- focal lesions such as fungal infiltrates, pulmonary cysts, bronchopulmonary sequestration, or arteriovenous malformations

Bronchoplastic techniques are used if the tumor involves only one lobe but has infiltrated the main bronchus central to the lobar bronchus. Tumors of this kind are removed by a lobectomy with a sleeve resection of the infiltrated portion of the main bronchus. Bronchial continuity is restored by reanastomosis.

Normal Postoperative Findings

The chest radiograph shows a moderate mediastinal shift toward the side of the lobectomy with a diminished lung volume on the operated side, ipsilateral elevation of the diaphragm, and compensatory hyperinflation of the remaining pulmonary lobes.

A *pneumothorax* or *hydrothorax* may develop, even in patients with a well-positioned chest tube. A mild pneumomediastinum or soft-tissue emphysema may also occur. A small pleural effusion or residual pneumothorax may persist for several days after removal of the chest tube. The mediastinum will later return to its midline position, but the remaining lobes will continue to be hyperinflated.

Arrangement of the pulmonary lobes. The arrangement of the remaining lobes follows a predictable pattern. Since the more anterior lobes are more mobile than the posterior lobes, the middle lobe and lingula tend to leave their anatomical position following an upper or lower lobectomy, occupying and filling the vacant space. On the other hand, resection of the lingula or middle lobe is not followed by a significant displacement of the remaining upper and lower lobes.

Lobectomy is followed by a rotation of the remaining bronchi, which increases the distance between the bronchi and artery. The ipsilateral hilum is generally twisted and appears smaller than the contralateral hilum on projection radiographs.

Specific Postoperative Complications

Generally speaking, the complications described for pneumonectomy, such as bronchopleural fistula and empyema, may also occur after a lobectomy.

Lobar Torsion

True lobar torsion is a rare complication. It is most common to find the middle lobe twisted about the true bronchovascular axis following an upper lobectomy. The central vascular obstruction initially compromises venous blood flow, causing an ischemia that culminates in infarction and lobar gangrene. This condition is marked by rapid clinical deterioration and has a poor prognosis, even when promptly diagnosed.

Fully developed lobar torsion is less common than atelectasis, which may be associated with superinfection and a variable ischemic response caused by *vascular kinking* of the middle lobe bronchus, which is directed sharply upward after the surgery. A typical presentation is "middle lobe syndrome" following right upper lobectomy (**Fig. 3.11**).

Radiography. The chest radiograph initially shows increasing opacity of the twisted lobe. A temporary volume increase due to hyperinflation is followed later by volume loss and complete opacity of the affected lobe.

Computed tomography. Postoperative CT shows increasing consolidation of the affected lobe. Hyperinflation, infection, or atelectasis may increase the lobar volume or, more commonly, may cause a volume decrease. Multiplanar reformatting of 3D-CT data sets can demonstrate the angled, narrowed, or twisted condition of the bronchi and the vessels that supply them.

▶ Upward angulation of the middle lobe bronchus after lobectomy may cause vascular kinking leading to atelectasis and ischemia.

▶ The middle lobe or lingula tends to migrate after an upper or lower lobectomy, occupying and filling the vacant space.

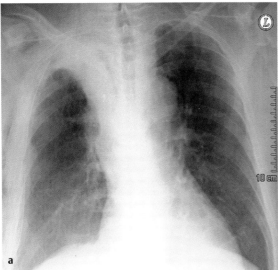

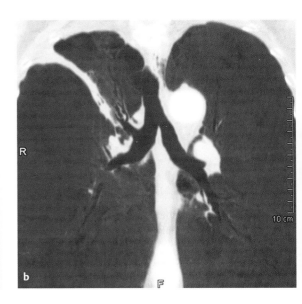

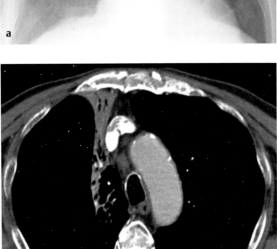

Fig. 3.11 a–c **Postoperative middle lobe syndrome.**
The middle lobe bronchus is angled sharply upward following upper lobectomy. Poor poststenotic ventilation and recurrent infections have led to complete atelectasis (with kind permission of D. Wormanns, Berlin).

Segmental Lung Resection

The indications for segmental pneumonectomy include benign neoplasms, bronchiectasis, pulmonary cysts and abscesses, and metastases.

Patient positioning and surgical approach are the same as for lobectomy. A segmental lung resection is more technically demanding than a lobectomy due to anatomical variations in lung segmentation, but surgical mortality is low at only 0.5%.

Normal Postoperative Findings

The chest radiograph following a segmental lung resection is comparable to that after a lobectomy, except that the effects caused by a reduction in lung volume are less pronounced than after lobectomy.

Specific Postoperative Complications

Since the surgical defects created by a segmental resection are not covered by visceral pleura, postoperative *air leaks* are relatively common. Persistent pneumothorax is another frequent occurrence.

Postoperative intrapulmonary opacities are generally attributable to small *intraparenchymal hemorrhages*. These opacities will resolve in a matter of days or weeks leaving nothing more than focal parenchymal scars.

After the removal of a nodular mass, *fluid may collect* in the operative area and form a "pseudotumor" in place of the excised nodule. This change is usually transitory, although rarely a "permanent nodule" may persist and mimic the appearance of a recurrent tumor.

Sleeve Resection

In this operation, portions of the central respiratory tract are resected and continuity restored by reanastomosis. This is illustrated by the resection of an advanced bronchial carcinoma with tracheobronchial invasion, in which the contralateral main bronchus is reanastomosed to the distal trachea.

Specific Postoperative Complications

A leaky bronchial stump may cause a tension pneumothorax to develop during the early postoperative period. Bronchial anastomotic leak occurring at a later stage usually results in empyema. Anastomotic stricture is the most common late complication, occurring in up to 20% of cases.

Radiography. The appearance of a new air–fluid level on the chest radiograph is suspicious for empyema formation due to an anastomotic leak.

Computed tomography. The most sensitive CT sign is the direct visualization of a wall defect. The detection of extrabronchial air close to the anastomosis is sensitive but not very specific. Bronchial wall irregularities are another nonspecific finding. The diagnosis is confirmed by bronchoscopy. Anastomotic stricture is detected by thin-slice CT with multiplanar reformatting.

Anastomotic stricture occurs at a late complication in up to 20% of sleeve resections.

Lung Transplantation

Single lung transplantation is performed through a posterolateral thoracotomy. Bilateral lung transplantation can be performed as a sequential unilateral transplantation or via a median sternotomy. The bronchial anastomosis is sometimes covered with peribronchial lymphatic tissue to reduce the risk of dehiscence. The pulmonary arteries are joined by end-to-end anastomosis. Postoperative immunosuppression is generally indicated.

Normal Postoperative Findings

The position of the chest tubes is checked immediately after the operation. One tube should be placed near the apex and another near the base.

Pleural effusion. A variable ipsilateral pleural effusion will develop due to impaired lymphatic drainage and should resolve within 2 weeks. If the effusion increases during that period, the possibility of infection should be considered. Effusion may also occur in the setting of a hemothorax or chylothorax.

Reperfusion edema. Noncardiogenic pulmonary edema, known also as reperfusion edema or reimplantation response, consistently develops after lung transplantation. Causal factors are an ischemic increase in capillary permeability (after transient hypoxia), impaired lymphatic drainage, sympathetic denervation, and surgical trauma. Hypertension and consequent increased edema may develop in the first lung of a double-lung transplantation, depending on the sequence of intraoperative implantation.

Radiography. The radiographic features of reperfusion edema are like those of interstitial and alveolar lung edema (**Fig. 3.12**). They invariably appear during the first 2 days after lung transplantation, and one-third of recipients manifest these changes during the first 12 hours. The edema initially increases until the fifth postoperative day and then clears by the 10th postoperative day or the 14th day at the latest.

Computed tomography. CT shows edematous thickening of the bronchial walls and interlobular septa, accompanied by reticular markings and ground-glass opacity or

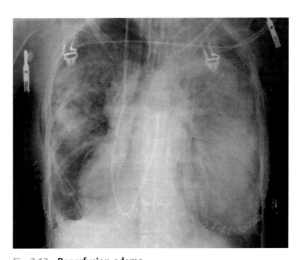

Fig. 3.12 **Reperfusion edema.**
Significant reperfusion edema is found in a 24-year-old woman who received one lobe in each hemithorax (split lung transplantation) because of her small size. Slight mediastinal emphysema and pneumothorax are also noted on the right side.

Reperfusion edema is caused by an ischemic increase in capillary permeability, impaired lymphatic drainage, sympathetic denervation, and surgical trauma.

even consolidations of the lung parenchyma dependant on the amount of intrapulmonary fluid.

Specific Postoperative Complications

Despite its lack of specificity, the routine chest radiograph is important in the detection of complications such as pneumonia and allograft rejection. Clinical or radiographic suspicion of pneumonia or rejection should be investigated by bronchoscopy with bronchoalveolar lavage. Bronchoscopic biopsy may be added if required.

Early complications may consist of pneumothorax, acute allograft rejection, pneumonia, bronchial ischemia or dehiscence, bleeding, or phrenic nerve palsy. Perioperative organ injury, ischemia, or vascular stenosis may lead to initial graft dysfunction.

Possible *late complications* are infection, acute or chronic rejection, bronchial stenosis, and post-transplant lymphoproliferative disease.

Initial Dysfunction

Initial dysfunction describes a condition in which reperfusion edema does not resolve within the first two weeks and the graft shows increasing opacity and functional deterioration.

Radiography and CT. The chest radiograph displays features of DAD/ARDS: diffusely increased density of the lung parenchyma (ranging from ground-glass opacity to consolidation) with superimposed intralobular and interlobular reticular changes (see page 37).

Acute and Chronic Progressive Rejection

An acute rejection response during the first 3 months is manifested clinically by cough, fever, dyspnea, and decreased oxygen saturation.

Radiography. Radiographic changes are subtle or even absent in many cases. Generally speaking, they resemble the radiographic signs of rejection, reperfusion edema, cardiogenic lung edema, or pneumonia. The most common radiographic changes are thickened interlobular septa and increasing pleural effusions.

Computed tomography. CT and especially HRCT may demonstrate a variety of changes, which are ultimately nonspecific (**Table 3.2**, **Fig. 3.13a**). It can be difficult to distinguish between acute rejection and infection (especially with CMV and *Pneumocystis jirovecii*).

The hallmark of (chronic progressive) allograft rejection is bronchiolitis obliterans. Approximately 10% of all lung transplant recipients develop bronchiolitis obliter-

ans during the first year after surgery, and ca. 20% by the second year. Classic bronchiolitis obliterans without other superimposed parenchymal changes produces only a mosaic pattern with air trapping, appreciated more clearly in expiration than in inspiration. This is followed by increasing airway changes with a tree-in-bud pattern, bronchiectasis, bronchiolectasis, bronchial wall thickening, and progressive signs of interstitial fibrosis (**Fig. 3.13b**). Similar changes are also found in pulmonary graft-versus-host disease (GvHD) after bone marrow transplantation.

Airway Complications, Anastomotic Leak

Anastomotic leak is a typical complication during the initial days after lung transplantation. It has an ischemic cause, as the bronchial tissues close to the anastomosis receive only a retrograde blood supply via pulmonary arterioles or by diffusion, since the bronchial arteries are not reanastomosed after the transplantation. Although the incidence of anastomotic leak was still quite high a few years ago, today it has been drastically reduced through improved suturing techniques, better immunosuppression to prevent acute rejection, adjunctive rheologic measures (heparin, prostaglandin 2), and more efficient prophylaxis of infection.

Small defects will generally heal without sequelae. Larger defects lead to necrosis resulting in anastomotic dehiscence. These defects can be managed by bronchoscopic stent insertion if necessary, and a worst-case scenario may necessitate retransplantation. Bronchial strictures may develop as a late complication.

Computed tomography. HRCT with a slice thickness of 1–2 mm will detect even small extraluminal air collections. Small, diverticulum-like peribronchial air collections associated with small wall defects are distinguished from large, pouch-like protrusions with extensive bronchial wall defects, which predispose to bronchial scarring and stenosis (**Fig. 3.14**).

Table 3.2 CT findings in acute and chronic progressive rejection

CT in acute rejection
▪ Thickened bronchial walls
▪ Thickened interlobular septa
▪ Focal or diffuse alveolar opacities (perihilar)
▪ Ground-glass opacities
▪ Pleural effusion

CT in chronic progressive rejection (bronchiolitis obliterans)
▪ Thickened bronchial walls
▪ Thickened interlobular septa
▪ Cylindrical bronchiectasis
▪ Decreased vascularity
▪ Air trapping (expiratory views)
▪ Focal peribronchial opacities
▪ Fibrosis

Chronic progressive rejection after lung transplantation presents as bronchiolitis obliterans.

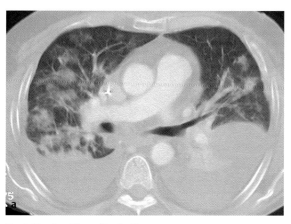
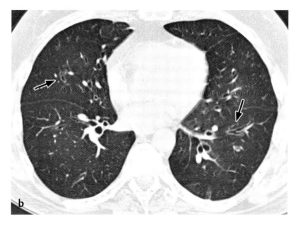

Fig. 3.13 a, b **Allograft rejection.**

a Acute rejection response is marked by extensive, bilateral pleural effusions and focal pulmonary opacities as in DAD/ARDS. These findings are nonspecific, however, and may also result from infection.

b Chronic rejection with bronchitis, bronchiolitis, and fibrotic parenchymal changes (similar to GvHD in the lung after bone marrow transplantation).

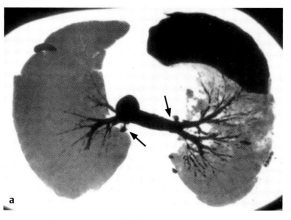
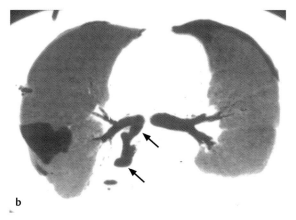

Fig. 3.14 a, b **Anastomotic leak.**

Anastomotic leak is manifested by a small diverticulum-like air collection (**a**) and a larger extrabronchial air collection (**b**). While the former usually resolve without sequelae, the latter predis- pose to infection and subsequent bronchial strictures (stent implantation).

Infection

Infections are the most frequent complication of lung transplantation and are the leading cause of death in lung recipients. The risk of infection is increased not only by immunosuppression but also by transplantation-induced ischemic changes, the disruption of lymphatic pathways, and a diminished cough reflex.

The most frequent causative organisms are bacteria such as *Pseudomonas* and staphylococci, CMV and other viruses, and fungi. Bacterial infections generally occur within the first two months after transplantation. CMV infections occur within the first 4 months (immunosup- pression). Fungal infections are rare but are associated with a high mortality.

Radiography and CT. Bacterial infections cause more or less pronounced areas of consolidation that are difficult to distinguish from an acute rejection response or edema.

CMV infections are characterized by an interstitial pat- tern of reticulonodular opacities, ground-glass opacities, or consolidated areas, often accompanied by small pleu- ral effusions.

Fungal infections most commonly produce multiple nodular or focal opacities.

Infections are the most frequent complication of lung transplanta- tion and the lead- ing cause of death.

Cardiovascular Surgery

Most cardiac operations are performed through a median sternotomy or extrapleural approach. Similar postoperative problems and complications arise, regardless of whether the surgery involved a coronary bypass or the correction of valvular heart disease (**Table 3.3**).

Normal Postoperative Findings

In an accurate anteroposterior projection of the chest, the aortic valve is projected over the spinal column while the mitral valve is displayed lower and to the left of the spinal column. The pulmonary valve is located at a higher level than the aortic valve and slightly to the left of the midline.

Almost all postcardiac surgery patients display atelectatic changes in the left lower lobe. Although cardiac surgery is performed through a median extrapleural sternotomy, the pleural space will have been opened in some patients (postoperative pleural drainage tube). Small amounts of mediastinal or pericardial air are a normal postoperative finding, as are transient pleural effusions.

Specific Postoperative Complications

Mediastinal Hematoma

Small mediastinal fluid collections, hematomas, and air collections are a normal finding up to 3 weeks after cardiac surgery.

Radiography and CT. Postoperative widening of the mediastinum due to hemorrhage or edema is a common finding after sternotomy. Up to 35% widening of the mediastinum (compare mediastinal widths on preoperative PA and postoperative AP chest radiographs) is of no concern if the patient is stable and there is no clinical evidence of hemorrhage.

More than 50% widening relative to the preoperative radiograph (at the same depth of inspiration) is at least suspicious for hemorrhage (**Fig. 3.15**). The indication for reexploration is based on clinical criteria (> 1500 mL drainage of blood, sudden increase in drainage volume, tamponade or hypotension due to blood loss). More than

60% mediastinal widening is considered a critical radiographic finding.

CT scans show diffuse, sometimes patchy or streaky hyperdense infiltration (> 40 HU) of the mediastinal fat. The mass effect of the collection depends on the extravasated blood volume (**Fig. 3.16**).

Rare complications include *vascular lesions* (pseudoaneurysms, **Fig. 3.17**) at the access site for cardiopulmonary bypass as well as hemorrhagic complications.

Mediastinitis

Postoperative mediastinitis has an incidence of 0.4–5% and is usually associated with sternal dehiscence. It may also result from esophageal perforation or the spread of a cervical infectious process. Even today, mediastinitis has a high mortality rate that exceeds 60%. If conservative antibiotic therapy is unsuccessful, surgical debridement may be considered depending on the extent of the process.

Computed tomography. CT shows stranding or complete obliteration of the mediastinal fat by fluid. Circumscribed abscess formation is uncommon (**Fig. 3.18**). Mediastinitis has a high association with bilateral pleural effusions. Sometimes a communicating process is found between the substernal soft tissues and the infiltrated subcutaneous soft tissues. Aspiration cytology is used to confirm the diagnosis and identify the causative organism.

— **Practical Recommendation** —————————

Mediastinitis is a clinical diagnosis! Negative CT scans exclude mediastinitis, but false-positive findings may be encountered, especially in the immediate postoperative period. More than 75% of patients show fluid infiltration of the mediastinum after surgery. This may persist for ca. 20 days postoperatively in the absence of infection, and rarely it may be detectable for up to 7 weeks. Therefore the CT findings should always be interpreted in relation to the clinical findings and time course. Skin redness does not always signify mediastinitis and may be nothing more than a superficial skin reaction. Other nonspecific findings are retrosternal hematoma, fluid retention, and air inclusions during the initial days after surgery.

Progression of fluid retention combined with bilateral pleural effusions and more than 3 mm of sternal dehiscence later than 2 weeks after surgery are suspicious for an infectious process.

> ▣ Postoperative mediastinal widening by 60% is suspicious for hemorrhage.

> ▣ Increasing fluid retention with bilateral pleural effusions and more than 3 mm sternal dehiscence later than 2 weeks after surgery are suspicious for infection.

Table 3.3 **Early complications of cardiac surgery**

- Perioperative myocardial infarction, cardiac arrhythmia
- Decreased cardiac output (myocardial ischemia, arrhythmia, tamponade, hypervolemia, prosthetic valve dysfunction, etc.)
- Postoperative bleeding
- Mediastinal tamponade
- Thromboembolism
- Infection
- Renal, gastrointestinal, or neurologic complications

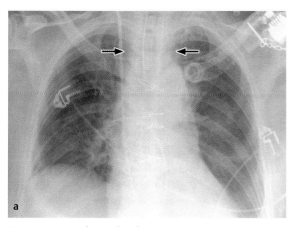
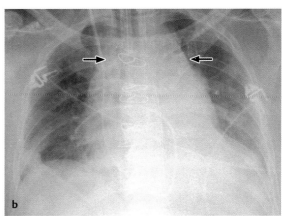

Fig. 3.15 a, b **Mediastinal widening.**
Some degree of mediastinal widening is always present after cardiac surgery. More than 50% widening relative to the preoperative width or a marked increase in mediastinal widening over time is suggestive of a complication (here, mediastinal hematoma after bypass surgery).

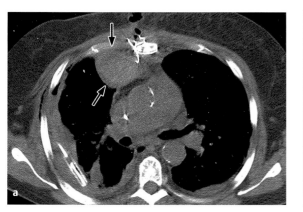

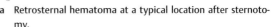
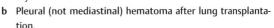
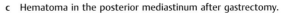

Fig. 3.16 a–c **Hematomas.**
a Retrosternal hematoma at a typical location after sternotomy.
b Pleural (not mediastinal) hematoma after lung transplantation.
c Hematoma in the posterior mediastinum after gastrectomy.

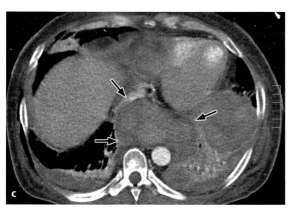

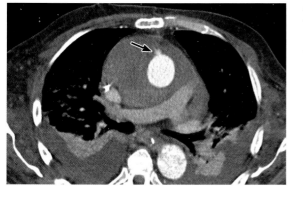

Fig. 3.17 **Small aortic pseudoaneurysm at the cannulation site for cardiopulmonary bypass.**
Note the large pleural effusions and the (hemorrhagic) pericardial effusion.

Sternal Dehiscence and Osteomyelitis

Sternal dehiscence and osteomyelitis are a rare (1–2%) but serious complication of sternotomy. The diagnosis is generally based on clinical findings. Normal postoperative radiographs should show no more than a slight dis-

placement of the fragments and should not show an actual osteotomy gap. A gap larger than 3 mm has been cited in the literature as a criterion for sternal dehiscence, but this finding has proven nonspecific in routine practice (**Fig. 3.19**). Discontinuity and displacement of the

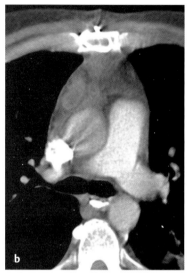

Fig. 3.18 a, b **Mediastinitis.**
Mediastinitis is a clinical rather than CT diagnosis. Multiple air inclusions (a) are strongly suspicious for infection. Densities alone (b) may be a normal postoperative finding (up to 20 days or more) and do not always signify infection.

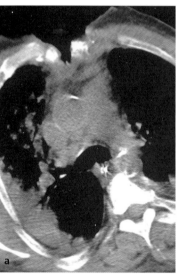

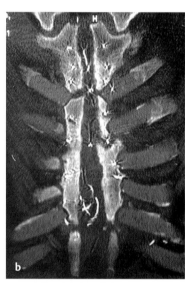

Fig. 3.19 a–c **Sternal dehiscence and osteomyelitis.**
a, b Wide sternal dehiscence (a) and loose suture wires (b) in secondary osteomyelitis.
c Rarely, a fistula may communicate with the pericardium, demonstrated here by contrast instillation.

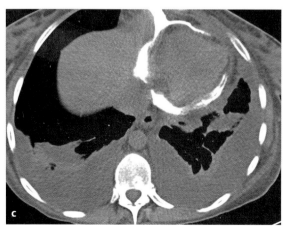

sternal suture wires are a more common and sensitive indicator of sternal dehiscence.

Predisposing factors are diabetes, obesity, osteoporosis, COPD, reoperation for hemorrhage, external cardiac massage, tracheotomy, prolonged mechanical ventilation, and deficient surgical closure.

Fractured sternal suture wires can be identified on chest radiographs. Sternal and chondral infections present in the second or third postoperative week with fever, pain, and purulent discharge. Infections are often associated with sternal dehiscence but rarely spread to involve the mediastinum.

Computed tomography. CT is much more sensitive than conventional radiography and tomography but may be negative in the early stage. Sternal dehiscence is best appreciated on multiplanar reformatted scans, which show decreased structural density and bone destruction along with inflammatory soft-tissue infiltration. The posterior sternal border is often ill-defined and irregular on postoperative scans even in the absence of inflammation, so this is considered a nonspecific sign. CT fistulography can detect bony fistula formation after instillation of a 1 : 10 mL dilution of contrast medium.

Postpericardiotomy Syndrome

Postpericardiotomy syndrome is characterized by fever, pericarditis, pleurisy, and pneumonitis. It develops in up to 25% of patients 2–4 weeks after cardiac surgery but may also occur a few days or even months after the operation.

The chest radiograph shows widening of the cardiac silhouette, a left-sided pleural effusion, and basilar infiltrates. Generally the disease is self-limiting and does not affect the long-term prognosis. Treatment consists of anti-inflammatory medications. Rare complications (1–2%) are pericardial tamponade and constrictive pericarditis.

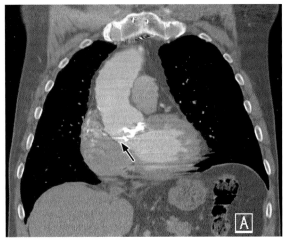

Fig. 3.20 **Periprosthetic leak in a patient who underwent aortic valve replacement.**
This diagnosis was actually confirmed by echocardiography and is more of an "incidental finding" on multidetector CT.

Complications after Valvular Surgery

Infection is a potentially life-threatening complication that may occur during both the early and late postoperative periods. Infections occur at a rate of 1% per year and have a high mortality. The main causative organisms are staphylococci, gram-negative bacteria, and Candida. Infected valves may shed septic emboli into the pulmonary or systemic circulation. Infection leads to valvular dehiscence with periprosthetic leakage (**Fig. 3.20**) and may spread to the lung.

Computed tomography. CT angiography can very accurately define pseudoaneurysmal dilatations, which most commonly occur in the supravalvular ascending aorta at the access site for cardiopulmonary bypass. Paravalvular leaks can be confirmed by CT angiography but are diagnosed primarily by echocardiography.

> Infection is a serious complication of valvular heart surgery and may lead to septic embolism and/or valvular dehiscence.

Heart Transplantation

In an orthotopic heart transplantation, the recipient heart is removed through a median sternotomy, leaving the atria in place along with the distal ends of the ascending aorta and pulmonary trunk. The donor heart is introduced and anastomosed at the level of the atria, aorta, and pulmonary artery.

Normal Postoperative Findings

The postoperative chest radiograph typically shows an *enlarged cardiac silhouette* caused by dilatation of the recipient pericardial sac. The cardiac silhouette dwindles in size during subsequent months. The superimposed donor and recipient atria may cause the right atrium to present a double outline.

CT may demonstrate a *notch* at the anastomosis of the ascending aorta and right atrium (**Fig. 3.21**). The inferior vena cava is frequently dilated. The distance between the superior vena cava (recipient) or pulmonary artery (recipient) and the ascending aorta (donor) may be increased.

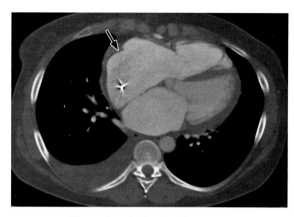

Fig. 3.21 **Visible notch in the border of the markedly dilated right atrium after cardiac transplantation.**

A *pericardial effusion*, often loculated, may persist for weeks or months. Steroid medication may lead to mediastinal lipomatosis.

Specific Postoperative Complications

The main sites of predilection for anastomotic hemorrhage are the aortic anastomosis and the anastomotic site

Acute allograft rejection after heart transplantation is diagnosed by myocardial biopsy of the right ventricular septum.

Esophageal Surgery

Antireflux operations can be performed through a thoracic or abdominal approach. Minimally invasive laparoscopic techniques are most widely used (see Chapter 5, p. 169). The Heller technique of modified esophageal myotomy, performed through a left posterolateral thoracotomy, is the method of choice for the treatment of achalasia.

Various surgical techniques are employed:

- Complete resection of the esophagus with a gastric pull-up reconstruction (Akiyama procedure). The anastomosis is placed at the cervical (extrathoracic) or intrathoracic level.
- Esophageal reconstruction with interposed small bowel or colon. In this case the cervical anastomosis is accompanied by multiple intra-abdominal anastomoses.

Anastomotic leak after esophageal surgery is detected by oral contrast administration.

Specific Postoperative Complications

The complication rate after esophageal surgery is higher than after other gastrointestinal surgery because it is more difficult for the esophagus to retain sutures and staples, due partly to the absence of a serosal layer, and because the gastric pull-up or interposed bowel segment may compromise blood flow.

of the right ventricle. An aortic dissection or aortic pseudoaneurysm develops in less than 1% of cases.

Infection

Infections are responsible for 40% of all deaths following cardiac transplantation. The most frequent causative organisms are *Aspergillus*, CMV, and *Pseudomonas*. Most lung infections occur within the first 3–4 months after heart transplantation. When associated with empyema or mediastinitis, they are an extremely poor prognostic sign. Bacterial pneumonia may develop during the first 2–3 weeks after transplantation.

Acute Allograft Rejection

Acute allograft rejection occurs within 2 weeks to 3 months after transplantation. The risk of allograft rejection declines markedly after the sixth postoperative month. Cardiomegaly is neither sensitive nor specific for rejection.

Acute graft rejection is diagnosed by myocardial biopsy. Possible complications of myocardial biopsy, in which myocardial tissue is taken from the right ventricular septum, are pneumothorax and hemothorax.

Anastomotic Leak

The principal complication, known as the "Achilles heel" of esophageal surgery, is anastomotic leak, which occurs in up to 20% of cases even at experienced centers. The cervical anastomosis is more commonly affected than the mediastinal anastomosis, although a leaky thoracic anastomosis is associated with greater morbidity (**Fig. 3.22**).

Radiography and CT. The leak itself is diagnosed by oral (intraluminal) contrast administration. CT is best for evaluating the degree of mediastinal infiltration, abscess formation, and involvement of the pleural space (empyema). In most cases a direct communication exists between the mediastinum and pleural space, resulting in empyema (more common on the left side than the right). The detection of contrast medium in the pleural space after oral contrast administration confirms an esophageal perforation. Mediastinal emphysema is frequently present.

Treatment. While leaks accessible to external drainage can sometimes be successfully managed by conservative therapy, large leaks with associated mediastinitis require reoperation. Oversewing the leak or revising the esophagogastrostomy is appropriate only if the esophagus and

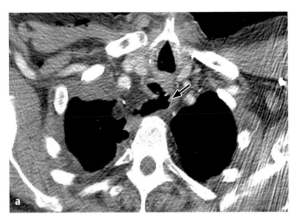

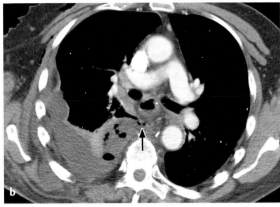

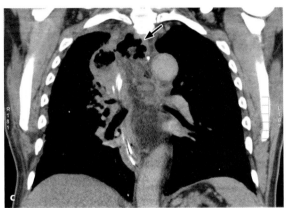

Fig. 3.22 a–c **Anastomotic leaks.**
Anastomotic leaks at the cervical level (**a**, **c**) and thoracic level (**b**) after esophageal resection usually result from ischemic complications. They may lead to sizable leaks with mediastinitis and pleural empyema.

gastric tube have an adequate blood supply. Otherwise the only option is resection of the gastric tube, blind closure of the stomach, and the creation of a cervical esophagostomy. A catheter jejunostomy is constructed for enteral feeding. Alimentary continuity is restored secondarily with an interposed colon segment.

Pulmonary and Tracheal Complications

Postoperative pulmonary complications such as atelectasis, pneumonia, and respiratory failure are common (up to 30%), regardless of the specific operative technique, and may have serious consequences.

There is an ca. 5% incidence of circumscribed *tracheal necrosis*, usually involving the membranous part, following an extensive lymphadenectomy in the upper mediastinum. Tracheal necrosis is a very serious complication with a high mortality rate. Less frequent complications are chylothorax and recurrent laryngeal nerve palsy.

Summary

Following **pneumonectomy**, the pleural space on the operated side initially fills continuously with serous fluid, which is gradually reabsorbed. The mediastinum is shifted toward the operated side. The principal complications are postpneumonectomy edema, hemothorax and chylothorax, and pleural empyema, which always requires the exclusion of a bronchopleural fistula. Rare complications are esophagopleural fistula, cardiac herniation, and (right-sided) pneumonectomy syndrome.

Lobectomy is occasionally complicated by postoperative atelectasis and a variable ischemic response caused by vascular kinking of the middle lobe bronchus, which is directed sharply upward after the surgery. Anastomotic stricture develops as a late complication in up to 20% of sleeve resections.

Lung transplantation is usually followed by the development of a pronounced ipsilateral pleural effusion, which should clear within 2 weeks, and by reperfusion edema. Initial graft dysfunction presents the radiographic features of DAD/ARDS, whereas chronic progressive rejection after lung transplantation presents as bronchiolitis obliterans. Infections are the most frequent early complication of lung transplantation and are the leading cause of death

The principal **complication of cardiovascular surgery** is mediastinal hematoma. Postoperative widening of the mediastinum by 50% is suspicious for hemorrhage. Mediastinitis is a clinical diagnosis. It is marked by increasing fluid retention with bilateral pleural effusions and more than 3 mm of sternal dehiscence noted later than 2 weeks after surgery.

The principal **complication of esophageal surgery** is anastomotic leak. With an incidence of up to 20% even at experienced centers, this complication is detected by oral contrast administration. CT is best for evaluating the degree of mediastinal infiltration, abscess formation, and involvement of the pleural space (empyema).

Acute Abdomen in Intensive Care Patients

4

Acute Pancreatitis 113
Acute Cholezystitis and Cholangitis 120
Acute (Pyelo)nephritis (Urosepsis) 123
Acute Renal Failure 127

Acute Gastrointestinal Bleeding 129
Inflammatory Bowel Diseases 135
Acute Intestinal Ischemia 140

This chapter reviews the causes and radiologic features of the acute abdomen in intensive care patients. Particular attention is given to the pathologic conditions that may lead to an acute abdomen in the intensive care setting and must be considered in the differential diagnosis of sudden clinical deterioration in intensive care unit (ICU) patients, even if the patient does not or cannot complain of abdominal pain. They include conditions such as (se-vere) pancreatitis and (acalculous) cholecystitis, acute gastrointestinal bleeding, acute intestinal ischemia, inflammatory bowel diseases with risk of perforation, and pyelonephritis.

These complications may arise in both medical and surgical ICU patients. The complications associated with abdominal surgery are discussed in Chapter 5.

Acute Pancreatitis

M. Uffmann

Acute pancreatitis is characterized by the leakage of pancreatic enzymes from the acinar cells into the adjacent parenchyma and, since the pancreas lacks a capsule, into extrapancreatic tissues. Even today, severe necrotizing pancreatitis has a high mortality rate and requires intensive medical care.

The most important imaging modality for evaluating acute pancreatitis is computed tomography (CT). The primary imaging goal is *not* to make a diagnosis but to assess the severity of the disease and detect complications.

Pathogenesis

The causes of pancreatitis are diverse and range from intrinsic, usually chronic sources of irritation such as alcohol abuse, hypercalcemia, hyperlipidemia, and hepatobiliary stones (biliary pancreatitis) to acute extrinsic causes such as trauma or stress (postoperative), medications, or previous ERCP (endoscopic retrograde cholan-giopancreatography). Patients with pancreas divisum are at increased risk for pancreatitis.

Clinical Aspects

Various clinical scores have been devised to evaluate the severity and prognosis of pancreatitis (**Table 4.1**). Severe pancreatitis is indicated by the presence of at least three Ranson criteria identified at the start of the disease or during its course. The mortality rate ranges from 1% (0–2 criteria) to 100% (7 or 8 criteria).

Possible *associated clinical findings* in severe pancreatitis are paralytic ileus (see Chapter 5, p. 164), acute renal failure, or circulatory impairment with tachycardia and hypotension ranging to shock.

Diagnostic Strategy

Plain abdominal radiographs (supine, left lateral decubitus) are useful for excluding "free air" due to a perfora-

> The main goals of imaging in acute pancreatitis are the assessment of severity and the detection of complications.

Table 4.1 Ranson criteria for evaluating the severity and prognosis of pancreatitis

Criteria at admission		Criteria at 48 hours	
Age	> 55 years	Hematocrit	Fall by > 10 %
White blood cell count	> 16 000/µL	Urea	Increase by > 5 mg/dL
Blood glucose	> 200 mg %	arterial pO$_2$	< 60 mmHg
Base excess	> 4 mEq/L	Calcium	< 8 mg/dL
Serum LDH	> 350 IU/L	Sequestration of fluids	> 6 L
Serum AST	> 250 IU/L		

tion and for detecting associated signs (paralytic ileus), although they are of limited value in supine ICU patients.

Pancreatic changes are demonstrated more clearly by *abdominal ultrasonography*, but the results are often compromised by gaseous distension of the bowel.

The most important imaging modality for the evaluation of acute pancreatitis is *computed tomography* (**Tables 4.2**, **4.3**). The goals of CT imaging are to assess the severity of the disease and detect possible complications. CT is not essential for the diagnosis of acute pancreatitis.

> ▣ CT is the principal imaging study for acute pancreatitis.

Imaging

Plain Abdominal Radiograph

The plain abdominal radiograph will sometimes show an isolated, gas-distended small bowel loop in the left upper quadrant of the abdomen (sentinel loop sign) or a distended transverse colon segment that terminates abruptly near the inflamed and enlarged pancreas (colon cutoff sign). Isolated distension of the duodenum may

also signify an inflammatory process of the pancreatic head (**Fig. 4.1a**). These signs are neither sensitive nor specific for acute pancreatitis, however. It is more rewarding to look for complications of other diseases in the abdominal cavity (e. g., a perforated duodenal ulcer) or check for associated signs such as paralytic ileus and pleural effusions.

Ultrasonography

Under favorable conditions, abdominal ultrasound scanning can evaluate the parenchymal echogenicity, homogeneity, margins, and size of the pancreas. Acute edematous pancreatitis may be associated with an inhomogeneous, predominantly hypoechoic parenchyma (**Fig. 4.1b**) accompanied by enlargement of the gland (pancreatic head > 3 cm, rest of pancreas > 2 cm).

Computed Tomography

Classification of the severity of acute pancreatitis is based on morphologic CT changes, clinical findings, and laboratory markers. The goal of CT scanning is to detect parenchymal and extraparenchymal areas of necrosis (**Table 4.4**).

Acute pancreatitis is basically classified into simple and severe forms. Severe acute pancreatitis is characterized by extensive changes in the peripancreatic fat and hemorrhagic fluid collections in the retroperitoneum.

Serous exudative form. CT scans in the serous exudative form of acute pancreatitis show hypodense, nonenhancing exudates with inflammatory spread along preexisting fascial spaces (anterior pararenal space along the Gerota fascia, along the mesenteric root, along the gastrohepatic, gastrosplenic and gastrocolic ligaments; **Fig. 4.2**). Enzymatically active exudates may also produce fluid collections in the lesser sac, perirenal spaces, and mediastinum. These exudative fluid collections are sometimes difficult to distinguish from areas of fat necrosis. The latter have less well-defined margins, however, and usually show higher CT attenuation (> 25 HU).

Table 4.2 Recommendations for the timing of initial CT in patients with acute pancreatitis

Clinical findings	Time after onset of signs and symptoms
Lack of clinical responseto conservative therapy	≥ 72 h
Suspicion of necrotizing pancreatitis	≥ 72 h
Equivocal clinical diagnosis	≥ 48 h
Sudden deterioration after initial improvement with suspected complications	Immediate
Clinically severe pancreatitis (Ranson score > 3)	Immediate

> ▣ The CT Severity Index is used to evaluate and quantify the inflammatory process and the degree of pancreatic necrosis.

Table 4.3 Recommended indications for CT follow-up in patients with acute pancreatitis

CTSI	Clinical findings
3–0	Lack of improvement or deterioration in response to therapy
3–0	At 7–10 days or before discharge to exclude clinically latent complications
0–2	CT indicated only if complications are suspected

CTSI = CT Severity Index (see **Table 4.4**).

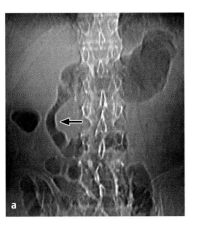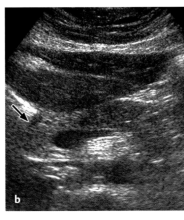

Fig. 4.1 a, b **Acute pancreatitis.**
a Abdominal radiograph (CT scout view) shows the air-filled duodenal loop splayed open by the enlarged, edematous head of the pancreas (sentinel loop sign).
b Ultrasound image shows a thickened, hypoechoic pancreatic head.

Table 4.4 CT Severity Index (after Balthasar et al. 1990) for the quantification of parenchymal and extrapancreatic necrosis

Evaluation of the acute inflammatory process		
Grade A	Points = 0	Normal pancreas
Grade B	Points = 1	Intrinsic pancreatic changes, focal or diffuse pancreatic enlargement, slightly heterogeneous parenchyma, small intrapancreatic fluid collections (< 3 cm)
Grade C	Points = 2	Same as grade B, but with mild inflammatory changes in peripancreatic tissue
Grade D	Points = 3	Peripancreatic inflammatory changes greater than in grade B but limited to fluid collections
Grade E	Points = 4	Multiple or widespread extrapancreatic fluid collections or abscess formation
Degree of pancreatic necrosis		
Normal	Points = 0	No necrosis, normal contrast enhancement of the parenchyma
Slight	Points = 2	Necrosis involving < 30 % of the pancreas
Moderate	Points = 4	Necrosis involving 30–50 % of the pancreas
Extensive	Points = 6	Necrosis involving > 50 % of the pancreas

Hemorrhagic necrotizing form. The hemorrhagic necrotizing form is characterized by focal, sometimes confluent, areas of pancreatic necrosis. The gland is markedly enlarged, inhomogeneous, and poorly demarcated from peripancreatic tissue. The necrotic areas are hypodense. Parenchymal sequestra may appear isodense, while hemorrhagic portions of the pancreas may be hyperdense (**Figs. 4.3, 4.4, 4.5**).

The extent of the necrotic areas in the pancreas is best appreciated after contrast administration, as necrosis does not enhance with the rest of the gland.

Bacterial contamination of necrotic areas is common and requires immediate surgical or interventional treatment. Drainage is unnecessary if the necrotic material is solid, but liquefied material can be drained. Proper management requires close cooperation between the radiologist and surgeon, close-interval CT follow-ups, and frequent catheter changes in most patients.

Complications and Intervention

Acute pancreatitis may be complicated by superinfection (suppurative pancreatitis or pancreatic abscess), pseudocyst formation, and vascular complications.

Suppurative form. This is a serious complication characterized by superinfection (usually with intestinal bacteria) and abscess formation (**Fig. 4.6**) occurring ca. 4 weeks after the onset of inflammation. CT-guided fine-needle biopsy to detect bacterial infection is a valuable aid to further treatment planning (surgery versus CT-guided abscess drainage or possible surgical intervention at a later, less critical time). The suppurative form of pancreatitis generally has a poor prognosis with a high mortality rate.

Pancreatic abscess. Pancreatic abscess cannot always be positively distinguished from an (uninfected) pseudocyst by CT. Both lesions appear as well-defined fluid collections (10–30 HU) with an enhancing wall. The detection

Viable pancreatic tissue enhances on CT while necrotic parenchyma does not.

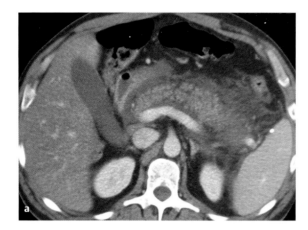
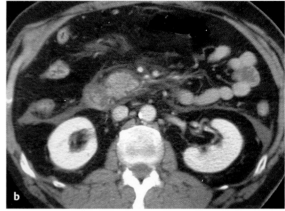

Fig. 4.2 a–c **Acute exudative pancreatitis (three different patients).**

a Infiltration of peripancreatic fat.

b Bilateral tracking of exudate along the Gerota fasciae.

c The inflamed pancreas has a spongy edematous structure but still shows homogeneous perfusion. Other findings are ascites and infiltration of the peripancreatic fat.

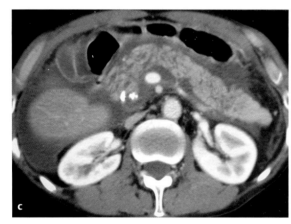

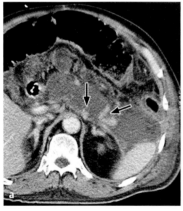
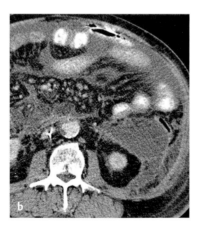
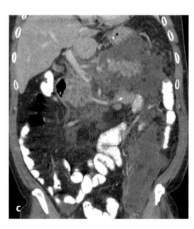

Fig. 4.3 a–c **Necrotizing pancreatitis.**

a CT shows extensive necrosis in the pancreatic bed with only fragmentary areas of perfused pancreatic tissue (CT Severity Index 6, see Table 4.4).

b Ascites and extensive spreading of necrosis along the Gerota fascia (grade E).

c Spread of necrosis into the lesser pelvis (CT Severity Index 4, grade E).

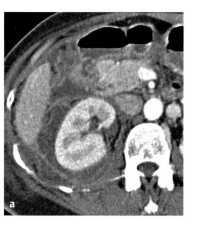
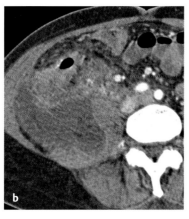

Fig. 4.4 a, b   **Necrotizing pancreatitis.**
a   With involvement of the perirenal space.
b   With abscess formation due to super-infection.

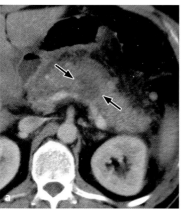
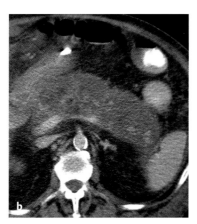
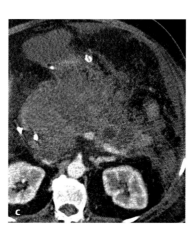

Fig. 4.5 a–c   **Necrotizing pancreatitis (three different patients, see Table 4.4).**
a   With focal necrosis (grade B).
b   With diffuse necrosis and mild perifocal reaction (CT Severity Index 6, grade B).
c   With diffuse necrosis and extrapancreatic spread (CT Severity Index 6, grade D).

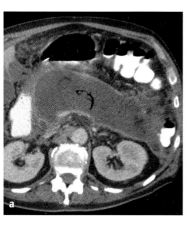
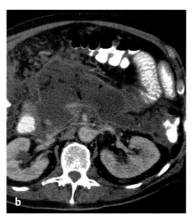

Fig. 4.6 a, b   **Infected necrotizing pancreatitis.**
CT shows extensive abscess formation, air inclusions, and rim enhancement.

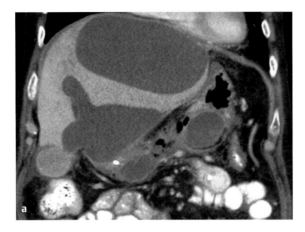

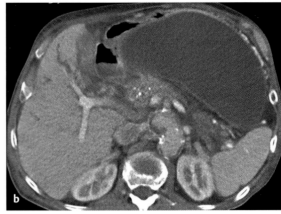

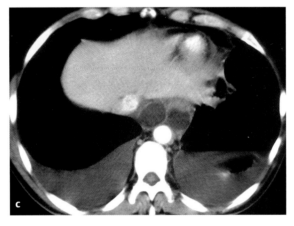

Fig. 4.7 a–c **Pseudocysts.**
a   Perihepatic pseudocyst accompanied by a pseudocyst in the pancreatic bed.
b   Giant pseudocyst in the lesser sac.
c   Mediastinal spread.

of gas inclusions is considered a reliable CT sign of bacterial superinfection when other causes (gastrointestinal fistula, previous percutaneous aspiration) have been excluded.

> Pancreatic abscess and pseudocyst are not always distinguishable by CT. Gas inclusions of unknown cause signify bacterial superinfection.

— **Practical Recommendation** ————————

The drainage catheter should have a large lumen (14–18F) and multiple sideholes. A lateral (retroperitoneal) approach is favored over the anterior approach, passing through the right or left perirenal space to the region of the pancreatic head or tail. Anterior transgastric or transhepatic approaches are an option, in principle, but they are more complex and require fluid drainage against the natural force of gravity. Alternatively a transgastric drainage can be performed endoscopically.

Pseudocysts. Pseudocysts (**Fig. 4.7**) are a noninfectious complication that may develop approximately 4–6 weeks after the onset of pancreatitis. They are often larger than 6 cm and, when untreated, persist for several weeks. Many (but not all!) pseudocysts do not resolve sponta-

neously and are drained to prevent complications. The indications for drainage are pain, infection, compression of adjacent organs, diameter greater than 5 cm, and recurrence following aspiration or surgery. Aspiration alone is often insufficient and most pseudocysts require drainage, possibly over a period of months.

Vascular complications. Vascular complications include pseudoaneurysms of the visceral arteries, which develop in ca. 10% of cases. The splenic artery is most commonly affected, followed by the pancreaticoduodenal artery and the gastroduodenal artery. Another vascular complication is stricture formation with associated ischemic effects in dependent organs. Pseudoaneurysms may cause acute, life-threatening hemorrhage (**Fig. 4.8**). Diffuse hemorrhage may also be encountered (**Fig. 4.9**). In patients with diffuse thickening of the bowel wall, the differential diagnosis has to include ischemic disease in addition to inflammatory disease (**Fig. 4.10**).

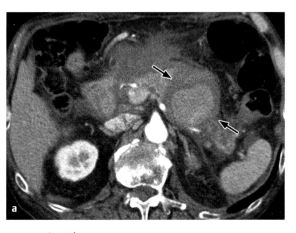 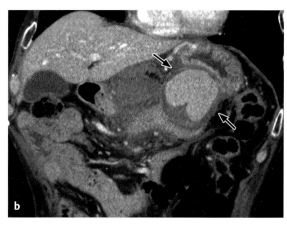

Fig. 4.8 a, b **Splenic artery aneurysm.**

a   Slight perfusion is noted during the arterial phase.

b   Perfusion is increased during the venous phase.

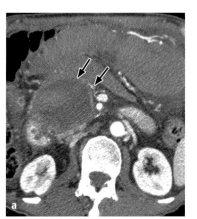 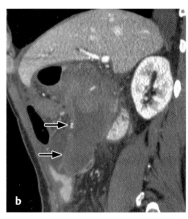

Fig. 4.9 a, b **Extensive hemorrhage.**

a   The hemorrhage probably originates from a branch of the mesenteric vein.

b   Layering of sediment in the supine patient.

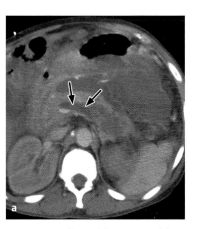 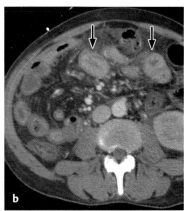 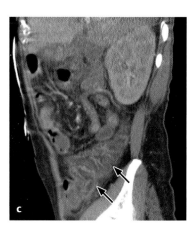

Fig. 4.10 a–c **Necrotizing pancreatitis.**

a   Extensive extrapancreatic exudation, thrombosis of the splenic vein, and partial thrombosis of the portal vein.

b, c   Reactive wall thickening of the small bowel (b) and colon (c).

Acute Cholecystitis and Cholangitis

M. Uffmann

Pathogenesis

Acute cholecystitis. Inflammation of the gallbladder is caused by lithiasis in more than 90% of cases. Cholestasis and bacterial superinfection give rise to a purulent or suppurative cholangitis, which may culminate in a highly acute septic–toxic state with high mortality.

Even in the absence of lithiasis, ICU patients on parenteral nutrition may develop a gallbladder inflammation (acalculous cholecystitis) that may also lead to sepsis.

Cholangitis. The etiology of acute cholangitis is analogous to that of acute cholecystitis and is based on an acute obstruction of the bile duct, rather than the cystic duct, by a stone or other process. The obstructed drainage leads to biliary colic and incites an ascending bacterial cholangitis. The development of rapidly progressive sepsis and shock is among the most serious complications. Multiple biliary, pyogenic liver abscesses may develop as a result of acute suppurative cholangitis.

Imaging

Ultrasonography

Although the detection of gallstones is suggestive of acute cholecystitis, the stones may also be an incidental finding. The most reliable sign of acute cholecystitis is *thickening of the gallbladder wall* to more than 3 mm, with an average thickness of 9 mm (**Fig. 4.11**). Ultrasound scanning may demonstrate *stratification* of the gallbladder wall. Perfusion of the gallbladder fundus on color duplex scans is another sign but is less reliable because color-flow signals may also appear in the normal gallbladder wall. Echogenic areas in the omentum and pericholecystic fat are suggestive signs of inflammation but are rarely detectable.

It should be noted that other diseases are also associated with thickening and stratification of the gallbladder wall and with intraluminal membranes in the absence of acute cholecystitis. They include:

- acute hepatitis
- hypalbuminemia in the setting of portal hypertension with ascites
- HIV cholangiopathy
- heart failure
- renal failure

Complicated acute cholecystitis. Definitive signs of complicated acute cholecystitis are gas collections in the gallbladder wall (emphysematous cholecystitis) and focal hypoechoic areas in the gallbladder wall or bed (pericholecystic abscess).

Acute acalculous cholecystitis. Acute acalculous cholecystitis is frequently difficult to diagnose and is often recognized only by noting the development of complications. Ultrasound scanning shows thickening of the gallbladder wall, which may increase on serial scans. Color duplex examination shows increased mural flow signals indicating hyperemia of the gallbladder wall. A hypoechoic rim in the precholecystic fat and gallbladder bed may signify inflammatory edema.

Acalculous cholecystitis is often associated with *gallbladder hydrops* (gallbladder transverse diameter > 4 cm, longitudinal diameter > 10 cm), and this may be the only diagnostic clue (**Fig. 4.12a**). Thus, acalculous cholecystitis

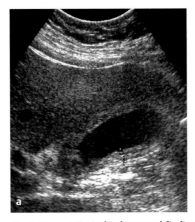
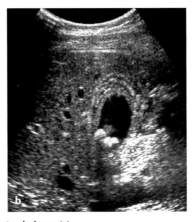
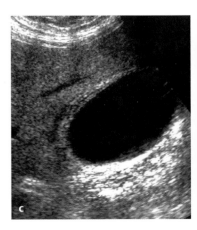

Fig. 4.11 a–c **"Typical" ultrasound findings in cholecystitis.**

a Inflammatory wall thickening (> 3 mm).

b Stones and wall thickening.

c Three wall layers.

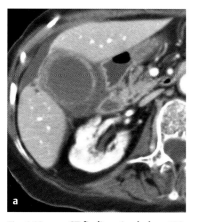 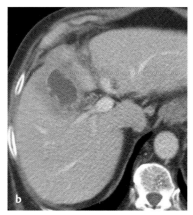 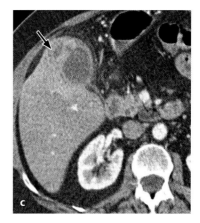

Fig. 4.12 a–c **CT findings in cholecystitis.**

a Thickened, intensely enhancing gallbladder wall with perihepatic fluid and fluid in the gallbladder bed.

b Incipient pericholecystic abscess formation.

c Confined gallbladder perforation with a frank pericholecystic abscess.

should be considered whenever gallbladder hydrops is found in an ICU patient with sepsis.

Computed Tomography

CT is generally used in cases where complications are suspected in the setting of cholecystitis (see below). As in ultrasonography, the gallbladder *wall* is thickened and shows increased contrast enhancement (**Fig. 4.12**). Usually the adjacent *fat* is infiltrated owing to pericholecystic inflammation, or fluid may be detected in the gallbladder bed.

Wall thickening and enhancement in the *bile ducts* (see **Fig. 4.14b**) is suggestive of cholangitis. Suppuration cannot be detected by analyzing the attenuation values of the biliary fluid.

Complications

The complications of acute cholecystitis include gangrenous or empyematous cholecystitis, gallbladder perforation with the development of a pericholecystic abscess, and gallstone ileus.

Gangrenous Cholecystitis

Gangrenous cholecystitis may develop as a result of gallbladder distension secondary to an obstruction. This condition will not have serious sequelae if early cholecystectomy is performed.

Sonographic hallmarks of gangrenous cholecystitis are *stratification* of the gallbladder wall and intraluminal membranes formed by sloughed layers of mucosa. The sonographic Murphy sign (tenderness over the gallbladder) is often negative in these patients.

Pericholecystic Abscess

Untreated, the ischemic wall changes may lead to perforation of the gallbladder followed by the development of a mural or pericholecystic abscess (**Fig. 4.12a, b**). This may occur even in acalculous cholecystitis. Although a perforation does carry a risk of generalized peritonitis, inflammatory spread at the perforation site is usually contained by omental tissues, resulting in the formation of a circumscribed abscess cavity. Gallbladder perforation may occur, even in the setting of acalculous cholecystitis.

Hypoechoic pericholecystic areas on ultrasound scan are suspicious for abscess formation. With CT the diagnosis of pericholecystic abscess can securely be established by infiltration, possibly accompanied by air inclusions. Neither ultrasonography nor CT can always detect the wall perforation that precedes abscess formation, however.

Emphysematous Cholecystitis

Emphysematous cholecystitis has a relatively high mortality rate (15%). Patients with diabetes mellitus are predisposed. Males predominate by a 5 : 1 ratio. Emphysematous cholecystitis is caused by infection with gas-forming bacteria (Clostridium). Intramural air can typically be detected 24–48 hours after the onset of symptoms. A possible complication is gallbladder perforation with peritonitis.

Diagnosis is based on *gas detection* in the gallbladder wall by ultrasonography (echogenic foci with acoustic shadowing), CT, and even conventional radiographs in pronounced cases (air–fluid level, **Fig. 4.13**).

Gallbladder hydrops in an ICU patient with sepsis should raise suspicion of acalculous cholecystitis, even in the absence of wall thickening and perifocal fluid.

Gallbladder perforation may occur, even in ICU patients with acalculous cholecystitis.

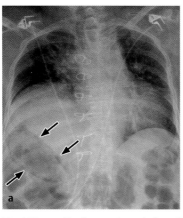
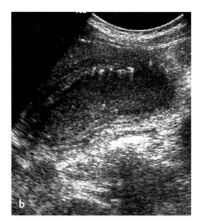
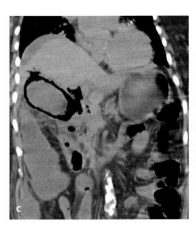

Fig. 4.13 a–c **Emphysematous cholecystitis.**

a An abnormal elliptical infradiaphragmatic air collection is visible on the portable chest radiograph.

b Ultrasound scan demonstrates echogenic air bubbles in the gallbladder wall.

c CT shows extensive intramural air inclusions, air in the common bile duct, and perihepatic ascites.

Gallstone Ileus

In rare cases the inflamed gallbladder may perforate into the duodenum, resulting in gallstone ileus. Stones larger than 3 cm may become impacted, usually at the ileocecal valve, causing a mechanical bowel obstruction (see Chapter 5, p. 164).

Hepatic Abscess

Hepatic abscess is a potential complication of ascending bacterial cholangitis (**Fig. 4.14**). Other causes of hepatic abscess are as follows:

- hematogenous spread via the portal vein in intra-abdominal sepsis (appendicitis, diverticulitis), pyelophlebitic abscess
- hematogenous spread via the hepatic artery in sepsis or bacteremia
- spread by local extension (**Fig. 4.15**)

> As it takes 2–4 weeks for an abscess to form a membrane, the absence of typical rim enhancement does not exclude a liver abscess.

Regardless of the etiology, there are three *stages of abscess formation* (**Table 4.5**), which are distinguishable by their morphologic features. Differential diagnosis is often difficult with ultrasonography, and CT can provide a more accurate classification.

Hepatic abscess appears on CT scans as a rounded or irregular area of low attenuation (0–45 HU). The center of the mass does not enhance after contrast administration. The abscess may appear initially as a cluster of small cystic lesions that coalesce over time.

Typical *rim enhancement* is seen only after a mature abscess membrane has formed. But granulation tissue takes 2–4 weeks to develop, so the absence of typical peripheral enhancement does not exclude an hepatic abscess (**Fig. 4.15c**).

Contrast enhancement of the granulation tissue may be masked during the portal venous phase by enhancement of the normal liver parenchyma, or the granulation tissue may appear hypodense. The ill-defined appearance of the abscess margins before and after contrast administration is an important differentiating feature.

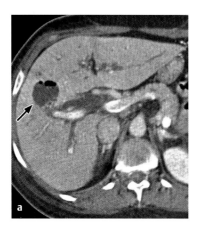
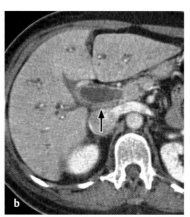

Fig. 4.14 a, b **Biliary liver abscess.** CT reveals an intrahepatic abscess with air inclusions (**a**) in cholangitis (**b**) with dilated intra- and extrahepatic bile ducts and increased enhancement of the duct walls.

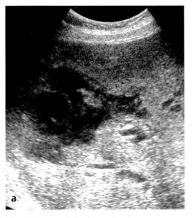 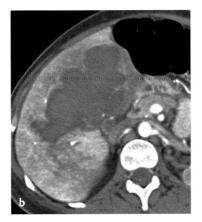 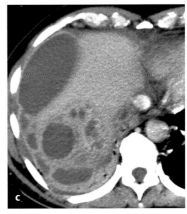

Fig. 4.15 a–c **Intrahepatic abscesses.**

a   On ultrasound scans intrahepatic abscesses are often hypoechoic.

b, c   On CT the abscesses may be multilobular with increased peripheral enhancement (**b**) or may have a cystlike appearance (**c**).

Table 4.5   Stages in the development of hepatic abscess

Stage	Time	Features
Necrosis	0–10 days	Incipient parenchymal necrosis, small fluid areas
Reabsorption	10–15 days	Reabsorption of the necrosis with liquefaction
Mature abscess	> 15 days	Abscess encapsulated by a fibrous wall

Besides enhancement of the abscess membrane, IV contrast administration may also produce a ring pattern of contrast enhancement in the adjacent healthy liver parenchyma. This *"double-target sign"* is caused by increased capillary permeability. Gas collections within an abscess are specific for infection with gas-forming bacteria, but they are very rarely observed.

Acute (Pyelo)nephritis (Urosepsis)

G. Heinz-Peer

Acute pyelonephritis is an infectious nephritis that involves the renal pelvis. In ICU patients with sepsis, pyelonephritis is one possible focus (urosepsis, see section on Sepsis in Chapter 5, p. 154). A diffuse interstitial form is distinguished from a focal form (acute focal bacterial nephritis).

Emphysematous pyelonephritis. Emphysematous pyelonephritis is a particularly severe form of bacterial pyelonephritis caused by gas-forming bacteria. It is common in diabetics (90% of all cases) and is an indication for immediate surgery.

Pyonephrosis. Pyonephrosis results from the infection of a hydronephrotic kidney, and is often associated with an obstructing stone and renal function impairment.

Renal abscess. An intrarenal or perirenal abscess is a complication of infectious nephritis, pyelonephritis, or septicemia. It may result from an ascending infection (gram-negative bacteria) or hematogenous dissemination (*Staphylococcus aureus*).

The hematogenous spread of infection (usually in staphylococcal sepsis) incites the formation of multiple small renal abscesses. In contrast to ascending pyelonephritis, they are located predominantly in the well-perfused renal cortex. These cortical foci facilitate the spread of infection to the perirenal space.

Diagnostic Strategy

The diagnosis of nephritis and pyelonephritis is based on laboratory serology and clinical findings. Ultrasonography can be helpful in evaluating the degree of obstruction. CT is used to investigate suspected complications (intrarenal or perirenal abscess) and to determine pathogenesis. The possibility of urosepsis with inflammatory renal changes should always be considered when looking for an infectious focus in ICU patients with sepsis.

CT is also used acutely in pyonephrosis to determine the location of the causal obstruction.

CT is used acutely in pyelonephritis to investigate suspected complications and is used electively to determine the cause. Always consider the possibility of urosepsis in ICU patients with sepsis!

Imaging

Sonography

Acute pyelonephritis. Acute pyelonephritis is a clinical and serologic diagnosis. Ultrasonographic findings are usually normal. Rarely, the ultrasound scan may show an enlarged kidney with a bulky, hypoechoic parenchyma and effacement of the sinus echo complex.

Pyonephrosis. Pyonephrosis, unlike hydronephrosis, has no pathognomonic sonographic findings. The fluid collection may show increased echogenicity due to echogenic aggregates of cells (pus), but this is not consistently seen. The echogenicity may be so high that it creates a tumorlike appearance with complete obliteration of the central echo complex. As in CT, ultrasonography may show marked thickening of the renal pelvic wall in some cases (**Fig. 4.16**; see also **Fig. 4.18**). Abscesses and areas of liquefaction may also have a cystlike appearance. Ultrasonically or CT-guided fine-needle aspiration should confirm the diagnosis prior to drainage.

Computed Tomography

Acute pyelonephritis. Acute pyelonephritis leads to focal or diffuse enlargement of the kidney. Focal or wedge-shaped areas of increased attenuation on unenhanced CT may signify hemorrhage, while areas of decreased attenuation indicate edema or necrosis.

Affected areas of the renal parenchyma show decreased contrast enhancement during the parenchymal phase, sometimes forming a radial pattern that extends past the corticomedullary junction. The walls of the renal pelvis and ureter may be thickened and show increased enhancement (see **Fig. 4.18**).

Focal bacterial nephritis. Focal bacterial nephritis (focal pyelonephritis, **Fig. 4.17a**) has a tumorlike appearance with a focal, ill-defined zone of decreased contrast enhancement. Again, a radial pattern may be seen in the late phase of enhancement, and lack of enhancement indicates necrosis or abscess formation. A focal abscess (**Fig. 4.17b**) requires differentiation from an infected cyst (**Fig. 4.17c**).

Renal abscess. A renal abscess appears on CT as a mass with a hypodense center and enhancing rim (**Figs. 4.18, 4.19**). Its attenuation values (10–30 HU) are higher than an uncomplicated cyst, and peripheral enhancement is not invariably present. Fungal infections tend to cause microabscesses, obstruction, and calcifications. Renal abscess cannot always be distinguished from a tumor with central necrosis.

Emphysematous pyelonephritis. Emphysematous pyelonephritis is characterized by the presence of gas in the renal parenchyma and collecting system as well as at parapelvic, subcapsular, and retroperitoneal sites (**Fig. 4.20**).

Pyonephrosis. The wall of the renal pelvis in pyonephrosis is thickened and shows increased contrast enhancement. Layering of (opacified) urine and pus is found in the dilated renal pelvis, the intrapelvic fluid showing attenuation values > 20 HU (pus). Rare cases show retroperitoneal or even intraperitoneal spread of infection with the development of peritonitis (**Fig. 4.21**).

The CT changes may persist for months despite appropriate and successful treatment.

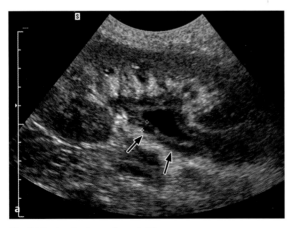 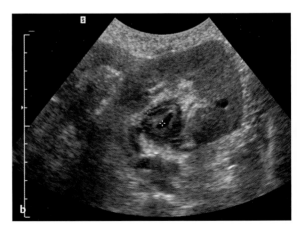

Fig. 4.16 a, b **Acute pyelonephritis.**
The walls of the renal pelvis and ureter are thickened in a patient with acute pyelonephritis (see also **Fig. 4.18**).

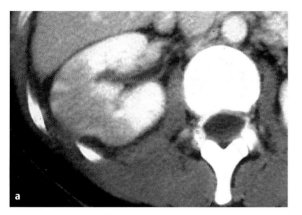
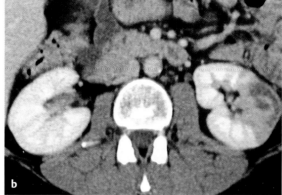
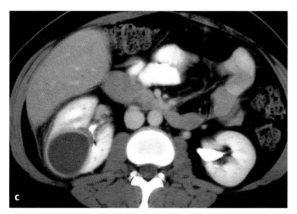

Fig. 4.17 a–c **Complications.**

a, b Focal hypodensities in the renal parenchyma are consistent with focal nephritis (**a**) or frank abscess formation (**b**) as a complication of infection.

c A cyst with a thickened, enhancing wall is typical in infections.

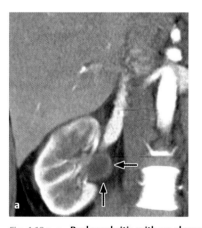
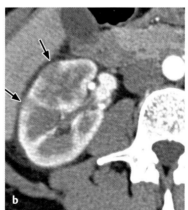
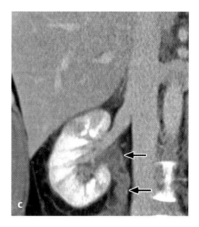

Fig. 4.18 a–c **Pyelonephritis with an abscess.**
Postcontrast CT shows a thickened, enhancing renal pelvic wall in pyelonephritis (**a**) with a parenchymal abscess (**b**) and a dilated ureter with a thickened wall (**c**). Note also the increased density of the urine.

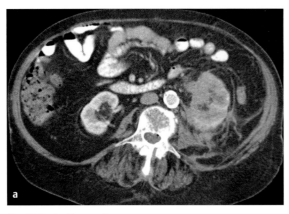
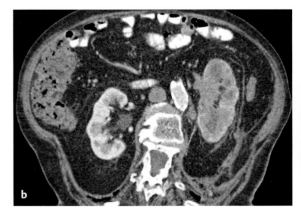

Fig. 4.19 a, b **Urosepsis.**
CT demonstrates multiple abscesses in the left kidney, general swelling of the organ, and a perifocal reaction.

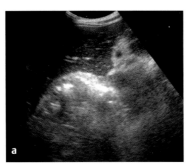
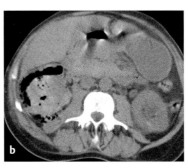
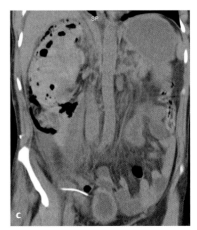

Fig. 4.20 a–c **Emphysematous pyelonephritis in a diabetic patient.**
The kidney shows extensive inflammatory changes with intrarenal and perirenal air inclusions.

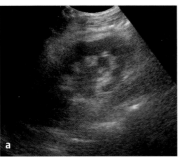
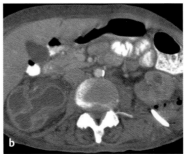
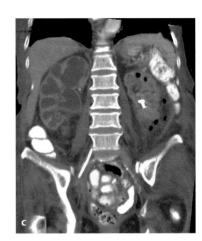

Fig. 4.21 a–c **Pyonephrosis in a woman with metastatic cervical cancer.**
A tube has already been inserted on the left side for drainage of pyonephrosis.

Acute Renal Failure

G. Heinz-Peer

Pathogenesis

Acute renal failure is classified by its pathogenesis as prerenal, renal ("intrinsic"), or postrenal ("urologic"). Prerenal renal failure is based on impairment of renal blood flow (shock). The renal form is based on tubular necrosis or inflammatory renal dysfunction, and the postrenal form has an obstructive cause (**Table 4.6**).

Renal cortical necrosis. Renal cortical necrosis is a rare cause of acute renal failure based on microcirculatory impairment due to intravascular coagulation (in the setting of shock or sepsis, or as a complication of pregnancy).

Crush kidney. "Crush kidney" is caused by a sudden obstruction of the renal tubules by hemoglobin and myoglobin leading to tubular necrosis. Hemoglobin and myoglobin may be released after crushing-type injuries to muscle or after major burns.

Postoperative. *Transient postoperative renal failure* is usually the result of an intra- or postoperative fall in blood pressure sufficient to cause temporary renal ischemia.

Acute renal failure following transurethral resection of the prostate (TUR), known as *TUR syndrome*, also has a prerenal cause. TUR syndrome is characterized by a severe disturbance of the water and electrolyte balance caused by perforation of the prostatic capsule and entry into the venous plexus, allowing irrigation fluid to enter the circulation during the prostatic resection.

Diagnostic Strategy

Ultrasonography is the imaging modality of choice in acute situations. It aids in distinguishing between obstructive uropathy, irreversible chronic renal failure, and acute renal failure and can help to direct therapeutic actions in acute cases.

As with the liver, however, both ultrasonography and CT have only a relatively small role in differentiating the causes of diffuse parenchymatous renal diseases. This is because the sectional image of the kidney in various forms of acute and chronic nephritis and nephrosis may appear *normal* or may show only nonspecific changes.

Imaging

Sonography

Important differentiating sonographic criteria are the size of the kidneys, the echogenicity of the renal parenchyma relative to the liver and spleen, and visualization of the corticomedullary junction (**Table 4.7**).

The ultrasonographic appearance of acute renal failure changes over time and often shows no abnormalities. Hypoechoic expansion of the renal parenchyma with narrowing of the central echo complex is sometimes seen due to edematous swelling of the organ (**Fig. 4.22**). As renal failure continues to progress during protracted shock with increasing tubular injury, necrosis, and diminished blood flow, the renal parenchyma becomes more echogenic with prominent medullary pyramids and a narrow sinus echo.

Hydronephrosis is recognized by a fluid-filled collecting system in the normally high-level echoes of the central complex. Hydronephrosis in a normal-sized kidney is

▶ Ultrasound scanning is helpful in acute situations for distinguishing treatable obstructive uropathy from a renal or prerenal cause of renal failure.

▶ Key differentiating sonographic criteria are renal size, renal parenchymal echogenicity, and corticomedullary differentiation.

Table 4.6 Causes of acute renal failure

Prerenal
Ischemic:
- Renal vascular occlusion, embolism, renal vein thrombosis, or traumatic avulsion of the renal pedicle
Hypovolemic:
- Shock (trauma, endotoxins, anaphylaxis)
- Profuse diarrhea, prolonged vomiting
- Severe heart failure

Renal
Glomerulonephritis, polycystic kidneys, and systemic diseases with renal involvement

Postrenal
Acute, bilateral urinary tract obstruction (ureter, bladder, urethra)

Table 4.7 Differential diagnosis of underlying renal diseases correlated with different sonographic patterns

Large kidneys, hypoechoic parenchyma
- Acute renal failure
- Acute nephritis
- Right heart failure
- Renal vein thrombosis
- Acute urinary retention

Large kidneys, hyperechoic parenchyma
- Shock kidney
- Acute glomerulonephritis
- Septic toxic
- Acute pyelonephritis
- Amyloidosis
- Graft rejection
- AIDS- or heroin-induced nephropathy
- Diffuse lymphomatous infiltration

Small kidneys
- Hypoplasia
- Renal artery stenosis
- Atherosclerosis
- Chronic pyelonephritis
- Analgesic nephropathy
- Chronic glomerulonephritis
- Diabetic nephropathy

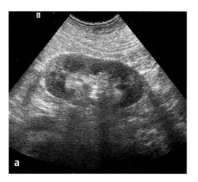
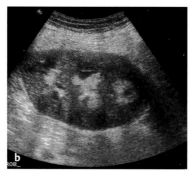
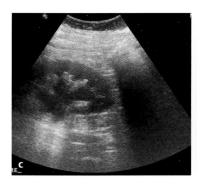

Fig. 4.22 a–c **Acute renal failure.**
a Ultrasonographic findings in acute renal failure are usually normal.
b Ultrasound scans in some cases will show a swollen organ with hypoechoic parenchyma.
c The goal of ultrasonography is to exclude postrenal failure.

suggestive of acute obstruction whereas hydronephrosis in a small-sized kidney is more consistent with chronic obstruction.

Computed Tomography

CT reveals a swollen kidney with absent or diminished corticomedullary differentiation after IV contrast administration (**Fig. 4.23**).

Patchy inhomogeneous enhancement during the parenchymal phase after contrast administration is a sign of advanced parenchymal damage and functional impairment.

In the acute phase of renal cortical necrosis, contrast enhancement is limited to the renal medulla. The nonenhancing cortex is bordered by a thin, hyperdense "cortical rim." The further course is marked by the appearance of cortical calcifications and increasing atrophy.

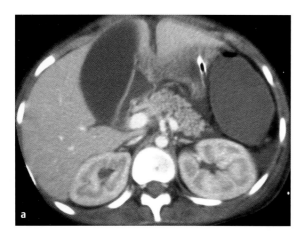

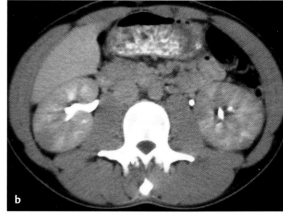

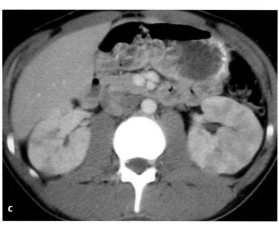

Fig. 4.23 a–c **CT findings in acute renal failure.**
Intravenous contrast administration should be avoided whenever possible in patients with acute renal failure. If a contrast study is considered vital, it will show ill-defined (**a**) or markedly decreased (**b**) cortical enhancement, with delayed scans showing slight, inhomogeneous parenchymal enhancement (**c**).

Acute Gastrointestinal Bleeding

C. Loewe,
E. Schober, and
M. Ceijna

Acute gastrointestinal (GI) bleeding is still associated with a high morbidity and mortality (from 20 to 40%, depending on the severity of the bleeding and hemodynamic instability).

The radiologic detection of GI bleeding (by selective angiography or CT angiography) requires continuous, active bleeding at a rate greater than 0.5 mL/min. It should be noted, however, that bleedings are often intermittent rather than continuous. This explains the frequent paradox of negative CT or angiographic findings in a patient with impressive clinical signs of active or prior hemorrhage (melena, etc.).

Pathogenesis

Upper GI bleeding. By definition, upper GI bleeding originates proximal to the ligament of Treitz, that is, in the esophagus, stomach, or duodenum. Upper GI bleeding is approximately twice as common as bleeding in the lower GI tract and occurs predominantly in younger patients.

The most frequent causes of upper GI bleeding are ulcer hemorrhage and bleeding esophageal varices (up to 50% mortality) (**Table 4.8**). Symptoms of acute upper GI bleeding in ICU patients should always raise suspicion of an acute ulcer hemorrhage, even in patients on medication for ulcer prophylaxis.

Endoscopy is the primary tool for the diagnosis of upper GI bleeding, although it cannot identify a bleeding source in up to 20% of cases, even with massive bleeding (> 1 mL/min). Peritonitis and sepsis due to an untreated perforated ulcer develop within 6 hours in 5% of cases, within 24 hours in 40% of cases, and have a high mortality.

Lower GI bleeding. Lower GI bleeding may originate in the small bowel, colon, or rectum. It is less common than upper GI bleeding and occurs predominantly in older patients. The most frequent causes are diverticulitis and angiodysplasia (**Table 4.9**). There is controversy as to whether invasive angiography or CT angiography is better for evaluating lower GI bleeding. The method of choice will depend on individual patient status and the severity of the bleeding.

Intramural small bowel bleeding. These bleeds most commonly result from coagulation disorders. Besides anticoagulant therapy, significant causes include coagulopathies secondary to liver disease, lytic therapy, hemophilia, and thrombocytopenia.

Bowel ischemia increases intestinal permeability, leading also to submucous hemorrhage and edema. The cause may be a complicated obstruction (strangulation, incarceration) or mesenteric ischemia (arterial or venous).

Diagnostic Strategy

Endoscopy

Endoscopy is the method of choice for the diagnosis of upper GI bleeding in most cases. It plays a minor role in the acute evaluation of lower GI bleeding, although it is not uncommon for physicians to order endoscopy as the initial examination.

Computed Tomography

Multislice scanners have revolutionized the role of CT angiography in the primary localization of bleeding in both the upper and lower GI tract. One reason for this is that CT appears to be more sensitive than angiography for detecting bleeding at rates below the angiographic threshold of 0.5 mL/min (as low as 0.3 mL/min based on published data).

Another reason for the superiority of CT is its ability to discriminate the cause of the bleeding (tumor vs. diverticulum vs. angiodysplasia) and detect complications that may require immediate surgical intervention (e.g., perforation or large hematoma). Interventionalists value the ability of CT to demonstrate possible anomalies of vascular anatomy and localize the bleeding site, so that the interventional procedure can be planned and performed more efficiently.

▶ Symptoms of acute GI bleeding in ICU patients are suspicious for an ulcer hemorrhage, even in postoperative patients and patients on acid-suppressive medication.

▶ CT can detect bleeding at less than 0.5 mL/min. It can also supply information on causes and complications.

Table 4.8 Causes of upper gastrointestinal bleeding

Cause	Frequency
Gastroduodenal ulcer	50–70%
Bleeding gastroesophageal varices	15%
Mallory–Weiss tears	7%
Gastric carcinoma	3%
Paraesophageal hernia, reflux esophagitis	10%

Table 4.9 Causes of lower gastrointestinal bleeding

Cause	Frequency
Diverticulitis	Up to 50%
Angiodysplasia	Up to 40%
Neoplasm	26%
Colitis	20%
Anorectal lesions, hemorrhoids	10%

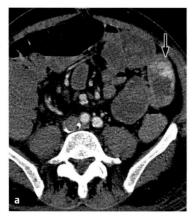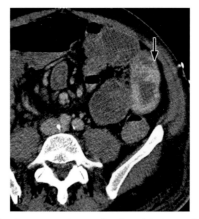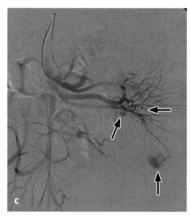

Fig. 4.24 a–c **Recurrent gastrointestinal bleeding in a patient with Schoenlein–Henoch purpura.**

a Arterial enhancement.

b Venous pooling.

c Extravasation in arterial angiography. Note also the multiple microaneurysms detected by mesenteric arteriography.

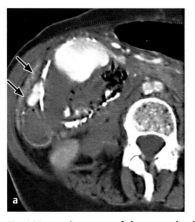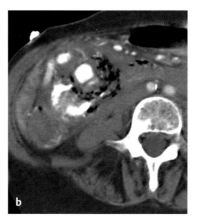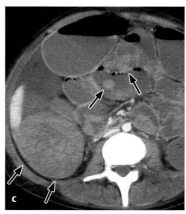

Fig. 4.25 a–c **Aneurysm of the gastroduodenal artery.**

CT demonstrates a large, perforated aneurysm of the gastroduodenal artery (air inclusions suggest possible infection) with contrast extravasation into the free peritoneal cavity and thrombi in the large and small bowel. Blood had been present in the stool for several weeks, and the patient died in acute shock.

Technique. When intra-abdominal bleeding is suspected, an initial noncontrast series should be obtained to distinguish a fresh extravasation from intraintestinal thrombi or hyperdense structures due to other causes (e. g., oral contrast residues) and enhancing lesions. The subsequent contrast series (120–140 mL at 3.5–4 mL/s, 370–400 mg iodine/mL) can be acquired during the arterial perfusion phase (ca. 10-s delay after the aortic peak of 150 HU) or the late arterial phase (25 s after the aortic peak). The advantage of scanning in the late arterial phase is that it is more sensitive to slower bleeds and provides good visualization of even the small peripheral mesenteric branches. A second scan performed during the portal venous phase (70–75 s) can detect venous extravasation, aid in defining possible neoplastic causes of hemorrhage, and assess bleeding activity by measuring the density and increasing size of the extravasate (pooling or arterial blush) (**Fig. 4.24**, see also **Fig. 4.28**). Sometimes the source is easily identified based on obvious vascular pathology

(e. g., postinflammatory aneurysm or pseudoaneurysm) (**Fig. 4.25**). Attention should also be given to indirect signs such as bowel wall thickening due to intramural hemorrhage, extraintestinal hematoma formation, and intraluminal thrombi (**Fig. 4.26**).

— Practical Recommendation

Comparison of precontrast and postcontrast CT scans has proven to be a more sensitive technique than looking for a focus with > 90 HU attenuation, as some authors have recommended. It is important to distinguish between extravasation and mucosal enhancement; this can be particularly difficult in collapsed bowel (**Fig. 4.27**). It is helpful in these cases to take an additional scan after the arterial phase and check for increased enhancement (blush) on the delayed scan (see **Fig. 4.24**). Significant bleeding is almost always detectable, however, by comparing the plain and contrast-enhanced series and by evaluating enhancement dynamics (increasing enhancement) between the arterial and portal venous phases.

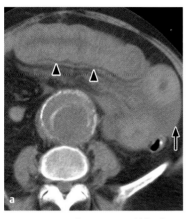 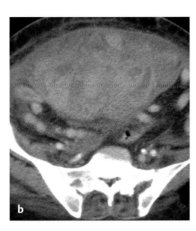 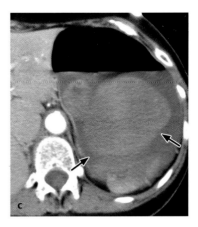

Fig. 4.26 a–c **Indirect signs of bleeding.**
Blood may spread freely within the peritoneal cavity (**a**, arrow). It may also spread in the bowel wall (**a**, arrowheads), form a circumscribed hematoma (**b**), or form a thrombus within the stomach (**c**). It should be interpreted as evidence of previous gastrointestinal bleeding or rebleeding.

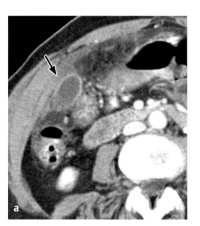 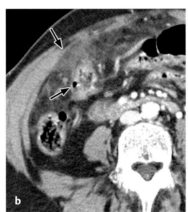

Fig. 4.27 a, b **Bleeding duodenal ulcer.**
Bleeding in the upper gastrointestinal tract is diagnosed (and treated) by endoscopy. CT may rarely or incidentally show findings that warrant further investigation. In the case illustrated, the wall of the duodenal bulb is thickened and shows increased enhancement with hyperdense perifocal infiltration. Gastroscopy confirmed a bleeding duodenal ulcer.

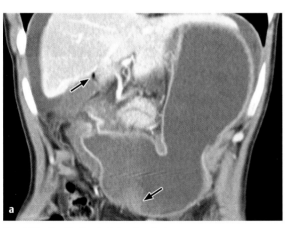 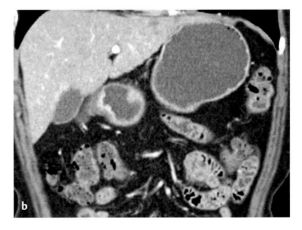

Fig. 4.28 a, b **Perforated duodenal ulcer.**
As in **Fig. 4.27**, the wall of the duodenal bulb is thickened and shows increased enhancement in a patient with a perforated duodenal ulcer. Findings include a small, free subhepatic air-bubble and blood in the stomach.

Complications. CT can reliably confirm or exclude complications (such as minimal free gas, massive damage to the gastric or duodenal wall, coexisting ischemia or obstruction, etc.) and can therefore aid in directing further management (i.e., angiography vs. acute surgery). Thus it is important to detect even minute amounts of free air (**Fig. 4.28**), and it may be necessary to acquire at least one series with a lung window setting.

Comments. Today it is widely acknowledged that CT should be the initial imaging study in all hemodynamically stable patients with GI bleeding at an unknown site. CT is used for:

- localization of the bleeding
- detecting vascular anatomic variants
- detecting or excluding other causes of acute abdomen (e.g., perforation)

Angiography should be the initial imaging study in hemodynamically unstable patients.

Angiography

Angiography should be ordered promptly in patients with significant upper GI bleeding that does not stop spontaneously, after CT has excluded complications that would definitely require surgical treatment. Published reports indicate that angiography can successfully detect a source that is actively bleeding at a rate of at least 0.5 mL/min. Angiodysplasia is the only lesion that can be detected angiographically during the interval between bleeds.

Advantages. Two important advantages of angiography are its capability for the superselective visualization of bleeding sites and the option for immediate therapy (em-

bolization, vasopressin administration) (**Fig. 4.29**, see also **Fig. 4.31**).

Other advantages of angiography besides accurate localization are its ability to detect additional changes in vasculature that are not actively bleeding, such as vascular malformations and pseudoaneurysms, which may also be accessible to immediate interventional treatment.

— Practical Recommendation

The bladder should be catheterized before angiography to ensure that findings are not obscured by a contrast-filled bladder. Sedation and close surveillance of the patient by a clinician (critical care physician) are essential.
Caution: Endoscopy immediately before angiography (or before CT) may lead to false-positive findings due to mucosal irritation or iatrogenic lesions and may hamper the detection of small hemorrhages.
Glucagon can be administered intra-arterially (via the angiographic catheter) or buscopan intravenously for relief of bowel distension.

Technique. The study should employ high contrast volumes and flow rates—keeping in mind that even high flow rates cannot replace superselective angiography using a microcatheter and coaxial technique.

CT will often provide key information on whether the *superior mesenteric artery* should be evaluated before the *inferior mesenteric artery*, as is normally the case. If a bladder catheter has not been inserted, this sequence is generally reversed with initial visualization of the inferior mesenteric artery (otherwise the contrast-filled bladder would be superimposed over the rectum), followed by the superior mesenteric artery and celiac trunk.

If selective mesenteric angiograms are negative, they should be followed by *selective celiac angiography*. If this is negative as well, it is appropriate to repeat the entire study due to the possibility of intermittent bleeding

> It is widely agreed that CT should be the initial imaging study in hemodynamically stable patients, whereas angiography should be the first choice in hemodynamically unstable patients.

> Normally the superior mesenteric artery is evaluated before the inferior mesenteric artery, but this sequence should be reversed if the bladder has not been catheterized.

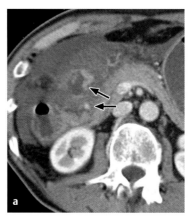 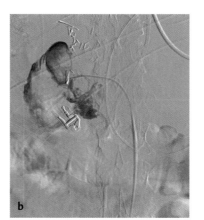 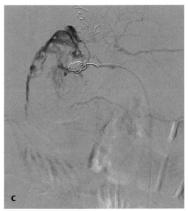

Fig. 4.29 a–c **Angiography with coil occlusion.**
CT demonstrates a bleeding duodenal ulcer with intraluminal and extraenteric contrast extravasation (**a**) and free intraperitoneal fluid. Corresponding angiograms before (**b**) and after (**c**) coil occlusion of the gastroduodenal artery (with kind permission of O. von Delden, AMC, Amsterdam).

(vasospasm). Contrast flow rates should be higher than 6–8 mL/min. If necessary, a vasodilator (papaverine or nitroglycerine) can be administered intravenously to improve opacification, even in hemodynamically compromised patients with severe vascular narrowing. Either the subtracted or precontrast phase may be easier to evaluate, depending on the quality of the angiography and bowel immobilization.

The *provocation of bleeding* with a vasodilator, heparin, or a fibrinolytic agent is a controversial tactic that may be considered after negative superselective angiography and should be used only in a highly controlled setting (see above).

Imaging

Computed Tomography

With a sensitivity, specificity, accuracy, positive predictive value (PPV), and negative predictive value (NPV) of 91%, 99%, 98%, 95%, and 98%, respectively, CT can accurately localize the source of the bleeding by detecting pooling or a plume configuration of contrast medium (**Fig. 4.30**, see also **Fig. 4.24**).

Extravasation. Extravasated blood may assume an oval, ellipsoidal, or linear shape. Significant intraluminal blood volumes in the stomach or bowel can also be reliably detected, as a fresh bleed will significantly increase the fluid-equivalent attenuation values of the stomach or bowel contents. Increased attenuation of the bowel content is more easily recognized by comparison with other bowel loops. CT can also reliably detect any fresh intraintestinal blood clots, which appear as well-circumscribed or cloudy intraluminal masses with average attenuation values of 50 HU (28–82 HU).

Contrast extravasation, on the other hand, has an average attenuation of 150 HU (90–270 HU). When the examination is done in two perfusion phases (e.g., arterial and portal venous), active bleeding will show an increase in attenuation (in one publication averaging approx. 75 HU to 120 HU) and in size (blush) (see also **Fig. 4.24**).

Causes of bleeding. The most frequent cause of upper GI bleeding, gastroduodenal ulcer, is the most difficult to detect by CT. Most spurious findings in published reports of CT angiography have been located in the duodenum. Rarely, CT may show definite local wall thickening with increased enhancement and perifocal infiltration (see **Fig. 4.28**). Perforations of the stomach and duodenal bulb lead to free intraperitoneal air, while perforations of the duodenal loop lead to air collections in the portal vein or retroperitoneum (anterior pararenal space), since all but the first part of the duodenum is retroperitoneal.

In assessing the prognosis of lower GI bleeding, it is important to distinguish between diverticular bleeding and angiodysplasia, because the risk of rebleeding from angiodysplasia, at over 70%, is much higher than the risk of diverticular rebleeding (ca. 20%). Angiodysplasia is frequently associated with multiple bleeding sites (**Fig. 4.31**).

Intramural bleeding. Intramural bleeding requires differentiation from active bleeding with contrast extravasation. A small bowel hematoma appears on CT as a relatively homogeneous thickening of the bowel wall that is fairly dense on unenhanced scans. Unlike tumors, the hematoma does not show significant contrast enhancement. The antimesenteric outer wall presents smooth, well-defined margins, as on ultrasound scans. Because the intestinal lumen may be narrowed, it is also common to find prestenotic dilatation of bowel segments.

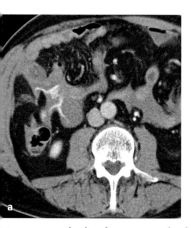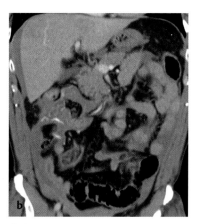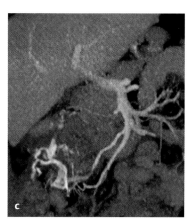

Fig. 4.30 a–c **Bleeding from a gastroduodenal ulcer.**
Contrast extravasation in the area of the hepatic flexure during the venous perfusion phase (**a, b**) with CT angiography (MIP, **c**) in a patient with vascular dysplasia. Note the dilated draining veins.

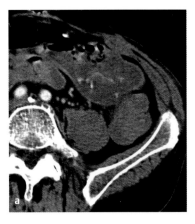 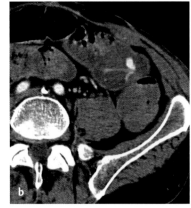

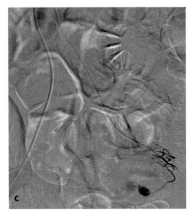 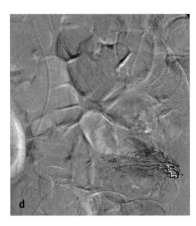

Fig. 4.31 a–d **Lower gastrointestinal bleeding.**
CT angiography shows focal lower gastrointestinal bleeding with arterial contrast extravasation into the bowel lumen (**a, b**). Corresponding arterial angiograms before (**c**) and after (**d**) coil placement (with kind permission of O. von Delden, AMC, Amsterdam).

The main prognostic task of CT is to detect or exclude a mesenteric infarction or mesenteric vein thrombosis! Except for hematomas with an ischemic cause, small bowel hemorrhages have a good prognosis and should resolve by spontaneous reabsorption within a few weeks.

Angiography and Interventional Procedures

Angiodysplasia. The angiography of angiodysplasia typically shows vascular clusters during the arterial phase, an intense blush during the capillary phase, and early venous opacification. The draining veins may have relatively large calibers or may show more prolonged enhancement.

Vasopressin. When angiography is positive for bleeding, subsequent (super)selective vasopressin infusion will at least control the bleeding in up to 90% of cases and create optimum conditions for any surgical treatment that may be needed. Vasopressin is particularly effective in controlling lower GI bleeding (60–90% success rates in the literature), yielding better results for the large bowel than for the small bowel (83% vs. 71%). Vasopressin has the highest success rates for diverticular hemorrhage (92–100%). The differences are due mainly to variations in the size and number of the feeding arteries and the degree of collateralization. These factors also explain the low success rates (15–30%) for pyloroduodenal bleeding. Intravenous nitro-

glycerine should additionally be given to minimize the adverse cardiac side effects of vasopressin (i.e., improve the coronary flow reserve and cardiac output).

Embolization therapy. Transcatheter embolization is accomplished by superselective catheterization of the lesion or leak with a microcatheter followed by embolization using microcoils or particles (**Fig. 4.31c, d**). Liquid embolic agents (*N*-butyl cyanacrylate) are not used for this indication because they are more difficult to control (danger of unwanted distal embolization causing bowel necrosis).

— Practical Recommendation

Transcatheter embolization is not generally recommended owing to potential complications such as bowel ischemia and stricture formation. But it is a good treatment option in cases where the bleeding vessel is easily accessible with a microcatheter by an experienced interventionalist using coils of the appropriate size. Particles should be used only in highly selected cases (see below).

Coils are placed as selectively as possible to occlude large feeding branches (e.g., ulcer hemorrhage from the gastroduodenal artery or left gastric artery) or may be placed in smaller feeding branches for angiodysplasia. Coils cause a flow reduction that produces hemostasis.

Selective vasopressin infusion will at least control bleeding in up to 90% of cases, helping to create optimum conditions for any surgery that may be needed.

Pseudoaneurysms. Bleeding from a pseudoaneurysm can be occluded by the "sandwich technique," which involves embolization of the draining branch(es) (= back door) followed by the feeding branch (= front door). Another option is to pack the aneurysm with coils. The latter method is often combined with the sandwich technique owing to poor visualization of the pseudoaneurysm in three dimensions.

Liquid embolic agents may be used to treat bleeding from a pseudoaneurysm in the upper gastrointestinal tract (e. g., in pancreatitis with vascular erosion and subsequent bowel erosion), provided they can be adminis-tered with good control. Percutaneous thrombin injections have been described in isolated cases.

Diffuse hemorrhagic areas. Diffuse hemorrhagic areas associated with tumors or certain types of angiodysplasia are embolized with particles designed for a specific occlusion level (PVA particles or Embospheres). The smaller the particles, the greater the potential risk of bowel necrosis. Particles in the size range of 500–900 µm will usually cause a massive reduction of perfusion and stop the bleeding.

Inflammatory Bowel Diseases

E. Schober and
C. Schaefer-Prokop

The radiologic findings of enterocolitis are nonspecific in themselves, and similar findings may be noted in infectious enterocolitis, pseudomembranous enterocolitis, graft-versus-host disease, and even during certain stages of ischemia (see section Acute Intestinal Ischemia, p. 140) (**Table 4.10**).

Patients with chronic inflammatory bowel diseases such as *Crohn disease* or *ulcerative colitis* are admitted to intensive care only in the setting of acute exacerbations, complications, or following surgery.

Diverticulitis is mainly important in elderly ICU patients as a potential focus of sepsis, a perforation site leading to peritonitis, or as a source of bleeding.

Infectious Enterocolitis

Infectious enterocolitis is a common differential diagnosis for abdominal symptoms in the emergency department but has almost no role in ICU patients on enteral nutrition. It is important to distinguish infections with toxin-forming bacteria (enterococci, *Escherichia coli, Staphylococcus aureus*) from infections with superficial bacterial invasion and an ulcerative mucosal reaction (*Campylobacter,* enterohemorrhagic *Escherichia coli, Yersinia, Salmonella, Shigelia, Entamoeba histolytica*).

> Diverticulitis is important in elderly ICU patients as a potential focus of sepsis, a perforation site leading to peritonitis, or as a source of bleeding.

Table 4.10 CT findings in the differential diagnosis of various inflammatory bowel diseases (modified from Prokop and Galanski 2003)

Disease	Sites of involvement	CT findings
Crohn disease	Most common in terminal ileum but may involve any portion of the gastrointestinal tract	<ul><li>Segmental wall thickening (15 mm, average 11 mm)</li><li>Acute: – Irregular, enhancing outer border – Smooth, hyperdense and nonenhancing inner border</li><li>Chronic: – Irregular, nonenhancing wall – Fibrofatty proliferation in the mesentery, abscess formation</li></ul>
Ulcerative colitis	Colon, rectum	<ul><li>Continuous, circumferential wall thickening (< 10 mm, average 8 mm); abscess formation very rare</li><li>Acute: – Smooth outer borders but irregular mucosa, stratification of the bowel wall, target pattern with hyperdense inner and outer ring</li><li>Chronic: – Smooth inner and outer borders</li></ul>
Yersinia enteritis	Terminal ileum	<ul><li>Segmental wall thickening, no fat infiltration</li></ul>
Pseudo-membranous enterocolitis	Small and large bowel	<ul><li>Diffuse, circumferential wall thickening with intense, homogeneous contrast enhancement of the mucosa, thickened folds</li></ul>
Ischemic colitis	Distal colon (inferior mesenteric artery), may also involve other bowel segments	<ul><li>Symmetrical, lobulated, segmental wall thickening with irregular luminal narrowing</li><li>Intramural and intravascular air</li></ul>
Graft-versus-host disease	Small bowel > large bowel	<ul><li>Diffuse wall thickening with increased mucosal enhancement</li><li>Ascites</li></ul>
Radiation-induced enterocolitis	Ileum > colon, rectum	<ul><li>Homogeneous wall thickening with irregular wall contours, target pattern</li><li>Stranding of pericolic fat, thickened fasciae</li></ul>

Ultrasonography. Ultrasound scanning shows a variable degree of edematous (hypoechoic) bowel wall thickening and brisk hyperperistalsis with a constant alternation between contraction and dilation. These findings may be accompanied by mild ascites and enlarged lymph nodes.

Pseudomembranous Enterocolitis

Pseudomembranous enterocolitis (complication of antibiotic therapy due to infection with *Clostridium difficile*) is characterized clinically by diarrhea and crampy abdominal pains.

Ultrasonography and CT. Ultrasonography shows hypoechoic hypervascular swelling of the bowel wall. CT shows segmental wall thickening of the large or small bowel with very intense, homogeneous contrast enhancement of the mucosa (**Fig. 4.32**).

The *"accordion sign"* is a radiographic or CT sign referring to edematous haustral folds separated by narrow bands of contrast medium between the folds (after bowel opacification with oral contrast medium).

Graft-versus-Host Disease of the Bowel

Graft-versus-host disease (GvHD) of the bowel occurs after allogeneic bone marrow transplantation. The small bowel (ileum) is more commonly affected than the large bowel.

Abdominal radiograph and CT. The plain abdominal radiograph shows the separation of bowel loops and tubular narrowing of the bowel lumen. CT shows diffuse wall thickening and increased contrast enhancement of the mucosa (**Fig. 4.33**). Ascites is a common associated finding, and there is frequent diffuse infiltration of the mesenteric fat.

Toxic Megacolon

Toxic megacolon is the most serious acute complication of colitis. It may occur in the setting of an acute exacerbation or fulminating initial manifestation of ulcerative colitis or Crohn disease, for example, and is characterized by transmural inflammation with damage to the nerve plexus leading to massive bowel dilatation (**Fig. 4.34**).

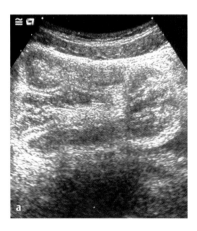
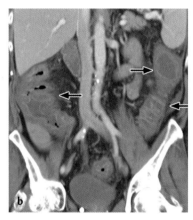

Fig. 4.32 a, b **Pseudomembranous enterocolitis (infection with *Clostridium difficile*).**
Wall thickening in pseudomembranous enterocolitis has caused "thumbprinting" on the ultrasound scan (**a**) and on CT (**b**), which shows marked wall thickening and increased mucosal enhancement throughout the colon.

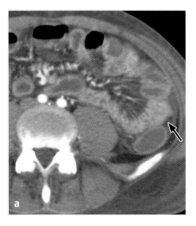
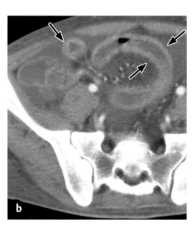

Fig. 4.33 a, b **Graft-versus-host disease (GvHD) of the bowel.**
CT demonstrates wall thickening of the small bowel (**a**) and less pronounced thickening of the large bowel (**a, b**) accompanied by ascites in a patient with acute intestinal GvHD after allogeneic bone marrow transplantation.

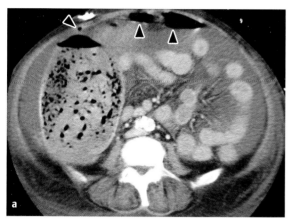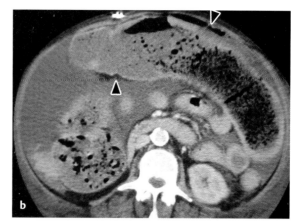

Fig. 4.34 a, b **Toxic megacolon with perforation.**
Free gas is visible along the anterior abdominal wall in a patient with ischemic bowel complications following heart transplantation.

Perforation (usually in the left hemicolon) has a mortality rate as high as 80%, and the risk of perforation is increased when the colon diameter reaches more than 9 cm. Bloody stools are typical but massive intestinal hemorrhage is uncommon.

Toxic megacolon is not specific for ulcerative colitis or Crohn disease and may develop in any form of colitis, including pseudomembranous enterocolitis, ischemic colitis (see section Acute Intestinal Ischemia, p. 140), infectious colitis, diverticulitis, and massive dilatation due to mechanical bowel obstruction.

Radiography. Contrast enemas are strictly contraindicated in toxic megacolon, regardless of the agent used! Daily follow-ups should be scheduled, giving particular attention to signs of perforation and wall ischemia with pneumatosis intestinalis.

Diverticulitis

Approximately 5% of the general population, and 50% of persons over 70 years of age, are affected by diverticulosis. Approximately 25% of all diverticulosis patients develop diverticulitis; this incidence rises with advancing age. The principal complications are a confined perforation with paracolic abscess and/or fistula formation and a free perforation with generalized peritonitis. The imaging modality of choice is CT.

Computed Tomography

CT can accurately detect even small diverticula. Typical signs of diverticulitis are listed below:

- Segmental wall thickening (> 4 mm) (**Fig. 4.35**)
- Signs of peridiverticulitis, that is, linear or (inhomogeneous) patchy densities in the paracolic fat (**Fig. 4.35**)

- Small extraluminal gas collections, often caused by a confined perforation (paracolic gas bubbles) or rarely by a free perforation (pneumoperitoneum) (**Fig. 4.36**)
- Free intraperitoneal fluid (in ca. 30% of cases). It is not always possible to distinguish between loculated ascites and an abscess.
- Circumscribed pericolic abscesses, which may have a hypodense center due to necrosis and liquefaction or may contain gas. They may communicate via inflammatory tracks in the paracolic fat or may coalesce to form larger abscesses (**Fig. 4.36b**).
- The most serious complication is diffuse (fecal) peritonitis with septic shock (**Figs. 4.37**, **4.38**).

It should be noted that the signs of diverticulitis may be very subtle but merit close attention when the focus is sought (**Fig. 4.39**). Signs of perforation may also be very subtle.

> Toxic megacolon is not specific for chronic inflammatory bowel diseases. Contrast enemas are contraindicated!

> Diverticulitis and perforation may have very subtle CT signs.

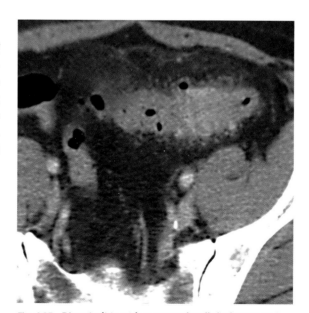

Fig. 4.35 **Diverticulitis with segmental wall thickening and increased density of the paracolic fat.**

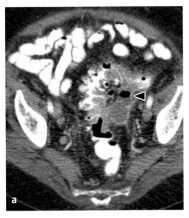
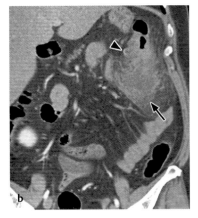
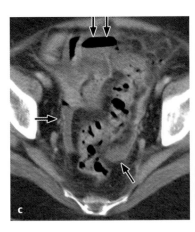

Fig. 4.36 a–c **Complications of diverticulitis.**
a   Confined perforation and peridiverticular abscess.
b   Extensive paracolic abscess formation.

c   Focal peritonitis with ascites and abscess formation between other loops indicating that inflammatory spread has already occurred.

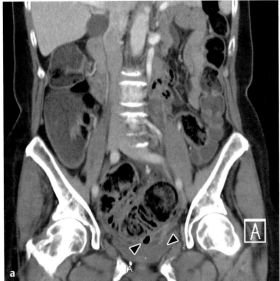

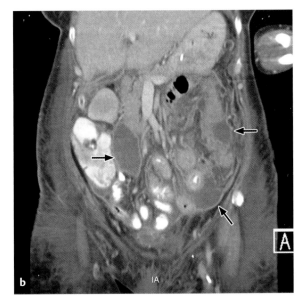

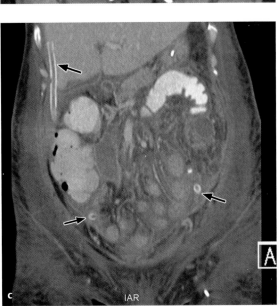

Fig. 4.37 a–c **Diffuse peritonitis after perforated diverticulitis.**
a   Image on the day of admission shows a small abscess and gas collection following the (apparently confined) perforation of diverticulitis.
b   Image 14 days later shows a deep septic pattern with diffuse peritonitis and multiple loop abscesses.
c   Image 5 days later, following the insertion of multiple drains.

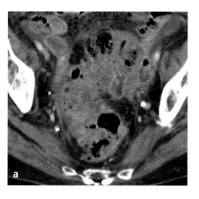
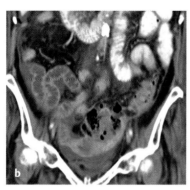

Fig. 4.38 a, b **Perforated diverticulitis with abscesses and peritonitis.**
It can be difficult to distinguish among free air, gas in an abscess, and gas in diverticula.

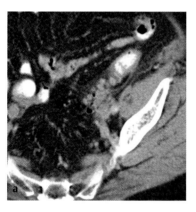
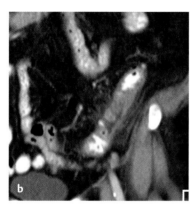

Fig. 4.39 a, b **Mild Diverticulitis.**
The findings may be subtle: mild perifocal reaction and wall-thickened diverticula in uncomplicated diverticulitis (**b**, same patient as in **Fig. 4.40**).

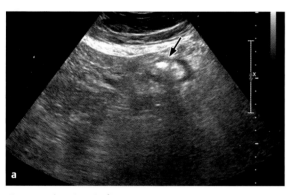
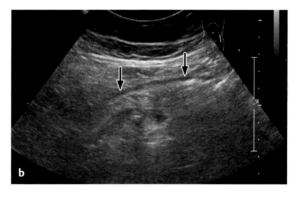

Fig. 4.40 a, b **Diverticulitis.**
Ultrasound scans show wall thickening (**a**) and a gas echo in the diverticulum without a peridiverticular abscess but with a marked perifocal reaction (panniculitis, **b**).

Ultrasonography

Simple diverticulosis. Even simple diverticulosis is usually characterized sonographically by prominent wall thickening of the affected segment, usually with diminished peristalsis, due to hyperplasia of the muscularis propria. Direct ultrasonographic visualization of the diverticula is not always possible. They typically appear as rounded masses adjoining the bowel wall that contain gas echoes with posterior acoustic shadowing. A fluid-filled diverticulum appears hypoechoic, and a stool-filled sac appears hyperechoic.

Diverticulitis. Diverticulitis is characterized by an even greater degree of wall thickening (> 4 mm), generally associated with signs of peridiverticulitis. The inflamed segment is rimmed by a hyperechoic halo (panniculitis) that may have hypoechoic inclusions caused by inflammatory spread (**Fig. 4.40**).

Pericolic abscesses. Pericolic abscesses form hypoechoic masses that may contain gas (reverberations) and fluid. Abscesses are easily mistaken for simple diverticula or hypoechoic lymph nodes due to their similar sonographic features.

Acute Intestinal Ischemia

W. Schima and
M. Prokop

Intestinal ischemia secondary to thromboembolic vascular occlusion without strangulation is among the most serious postoperative complications that may arise.

Pathogenesis

Acute mesenteric ischemia may have several causes:
- arterial vascular occlusion (60–70 %; see also section Strangulated Bowel Obstruction, Chapter 5, p. 165)
- nonocclusive mesenteric insufficiency (NOMI, 20–30 %)
- venous occlusion (5–10 %)

While an arterial vascular occlusion secondary to embolism or thromboembolism is most common in patients with preexisting plaques, nonocclusive mesenteric insufficiency is a very serious complication in ICU patients. Possible causes include hypovolemic shock (maximal intestinal vasoconstriction), sepsis, and heart failure (**Tables 4.11**, **4.12**). Mesenteric venous thrombosis most commonly results from *surgical procedures* or portal hypertension, abdominal inflammatory processes (e. g., diverticulitis, appendicitis, etc.), trauma, paraneoplastic syndrome, coagulopathy, or mass lesions.

▌▶ The most frequent cause of acute mesenteric ischemia is a thromboembolic process.

Clinical Aspects

Patients with intestinal ischemia present with diffuse abdominal pain, constipation or diarrhea, nausea, and dehydration. The abdomen is distended and peristalsis is diminished. Laboratory tests show leukocytosis and elevated values for lactate, LDH, CK/CK-MB ratio, and hematocrit.

Diagnostic Strategy

(Multidetector) CT angiography is the diagnostic study of choice but requires the prospective planning of a suitable imaging protocol.

Compared with the detection of bowel ischemia due to strangulation, CT has the advantage of higher specificity (up to 95 %) but lower sensitivity for detecting ischemia due to vascular occlusion. Thus, while CT can establish the diagnosis by detecting a mesenteric vascular thrombus, the inability to detect a thrombus does not exclude thromboembolism in peripheral vascular branches. In this case the diagnosis is based on indirect (and less specific) findings that are suggestive of ischemia.

Table 4.11 Blood supply of the gastrointestinal tract

Celiac trunk
- Supplies the distal esophagus as far as the descending duodenum
- Anastomosis between the celiac trunk and superior mesenteric artery via the gastroduodenal artery

Superior mesenteric artery
- Supplies the horizontal part of the duodenum, the entire small intestine, and the colon as far as the left flexure

Inferior mesenteric artery
- Supplies the colon from the left flexure to the rectum
- Anastomosis between the superior mesenteric artery and inferior mesenteric artery (Riolan anastomosis)

Arcades
- Four arcades connected in series and in parallel for supplying the muscularis propria, submucosa, and mucosa

Veins
- The inferior mesenteric vein usually drains directly into the splenic vein
- The splenic vein and superior mesenteric vein form the venous confluence, which drains into the portal vein
- Collaterals between the mesenteric veins and the perigastric, paraesophageal, renal, lumbar, and iliac veins

Table 4.12 Causes of arterial or venous occlusions in the gastrointestinal tract

Arterial occlusion
- Thromboembolism (mitral valve disease, ventricular aneurysm)
- Cholesterol emboli
- Thrombosis
- Dissection
- Prior implantation of bifurcated aortic prosthesis (mainly affects the inferior mesenteric artery)
- Antiphospholipid antibody syndrome
- Vasculitis (younger patients, atypical sites of involvement)
- Diabetic microangiopathy
- Amyloidosis
- Hyperoxaluria
- Fibromuscular dysplasia (in children)

Venous occlusion
- Thrombophlebitis
- Tumor infiltration
- Sepsis
- Portal hypertension
- Polycythemia vera
- Thrombocytosis
- Coagulopathies
- Pregnancy
- Contraceptive use
- Strangulation
- Secondary to appendicitis, diverticulitis
- Pancreatitis (direct infiltration or indirect due to vasospasms)

Nonocclusive ischemia
- Hemorrhagic, septic or cardiogenic shock
- Familial dysautonomia syndrome
- Pheochromocytoma
- High-performance athlete

Other causes
- Trauma
- Radiation
- Immunosuppression
- Chemotherapy
- Intoxication:
  - Digitalis, vasopressin, epinephrine, ergotamine, diuretics
  - Neuroleptics, antidepressants, indomethacin
  - Cocaine, crack, heroin

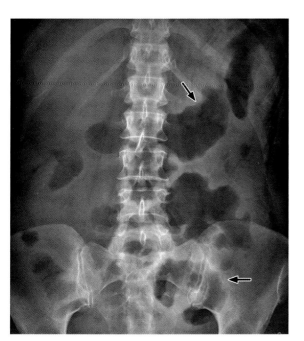

Fig. 4.41 **Thumbprinting.**
"Thumb prints" are a sign of bowel wall thickening due to ischemia.

Imaging

Radiography

The plain abdominal radiograph shows nonspecific signs in the early stage:

- dilated small bowel loops with thickened valvulae conniventes
- separation of bowel loops and thumbprinting due to wall edema (**Fig. 4.41**)

The detection of pneumatosis intestinalis is a sign that irreversible intestinal necrosis has already occurred.

Acute intestinal ischemia is characterized by increasing fluid exudation into the bowel lumen over time, which may eventually create the appearance of a "gasless abdomen." This contrasts with mechanical bowel obstruction and paralytic ileus, which are characterized by increasing amounts of intraluminal air.

Computed Tomography

The CT findings of acute bowel ischemia are variable in accordance with the diverse causes of decreased intestinal blood flow. The ischemia may involve the large or small bowel, typical (left colon) or atypical sites (duodenum, rectum), and may have a diffuse, segmental, or focal distribution.

Early signs of ischemia are distinguished from late signs indicating that (transmural) bowel necrosis has already occurred (**Table 4.13**).

- Arterial embolic and thrombotic occlusions appear on CT angiography as an abrupt cutoff of intravascular contrast, most commonly found in the main trunk of the superior mesenteric artery (**Fig. 4.42**).
- Lack of enhancement after contrast administration is considered the most specific sign of arterial intestinal ischemia. It is not always present, however, and when present it is sometimes difficult to see (**Fig. 4.43**).
- Venous thrombosis with stasis leads to hyperemia, edematous thickening, and subserosal hemorrhage (hemorrhagic infarction). This condition almost always involves the superior mesenteric vein, which normally drains the entire small bowel and the right side of the colon (**Fig. 4.44**). Noncontrast CT shows increased wall density in the affected bowel loops (due to subserosal hemorrhage) and massive wall thickening with submucous edema (halo sign).

Progressive fluid accumulation in the bowel lumen occurs in acute intestinal ischemia, while increasing intraluminal air is characteristic of ileus and mechanical bowel obstruction.

Table 4.13 Early and late signs of mesenteric ischemia

Cause of ischemia	Findings in early stage	Findings in late stage
Arterio-occlusive and nonocclusive small bowel ischemia	- Dilatation or spastic bowel contractions - Little or no wall thickening - No pneumatosis intestinalis	- Exudation into the bowel lumen, thinning of the bowel wall - Possible pneumatosis - Perifocal edema after transmural necrosis - Small bowel feces sign
Arterio-occlusive and nonocclusive large bowel ischemia	- Moderate wall thickening - Paracolic edema - Possible intramural hemorrhages - Pneumatosis (rare)	- Massive wall thickening due to superinfection - Increasing perifocal reaction - Possible intramural hemorrhages - Pneumatosis
Veno-occlusive ischemia of the small and/or large bowel	- Marked wall thickening due to stasis, congested mesenteric vessels and mesenteric edema - Possible intramural hemorrhages - Pneumatosis (rare)	- Progressive wall thickening - Mesenteric edema - Local ascites - Pneumatosis (rare)
Distension ischemia	- Dilatation - Moderate wall thickening - Possible pneumatosis	- Dilatation - Inflammatory perifocal reaction - Increasing pneumatosis
Peripheral vasculitic and postactinic ischemia	- Segmental wall thickening - Spastic contractions - Little or no perifocal reaction	- Increasing wall thickening - Spastic contractions - Increasing perifocal reaction

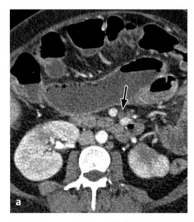 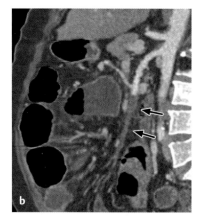 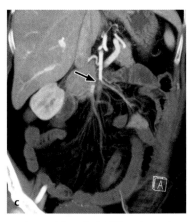

Fig. 4.42 a–c **Acute embolic stenosis of the main trunk of the superior mesenteric artery as imaged by arterial CT angiography.**
a Axial scan.
b Sagittal scan.
c Maximum intensity projection (MIP).

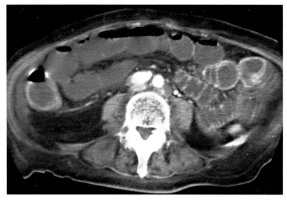

Fig. 4.43 **Lack of enhancement.**
The lack of enhancement of individual bowel loops provides an indirect sign of decreased blood flow.

- Bowel wall thickening is the most common sign of intestinal ischemia. The degree of wall thickening depends on the cause and on the timing of diagnostic imaging.
- The colon shows more pronounced wall thickening than the small bowel due to obligate bacterial super-infection (**Fig. 4.45**). Superficial small bowel ischemia (e.g., in the setting of shock) is more apt to cause contractions or more subtle and diffuse wall thickening, while transmural ischemia leads to atonic, dilated, thinned loops of small bowel.
- Small bowel infarction due to arterial occlusion is associated with dilatation but not with bowel wall thickening and is easily mistaken for a mechanical bowel obstruction or (in the absence of an apparent cause)

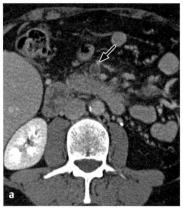 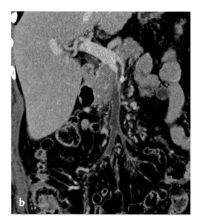 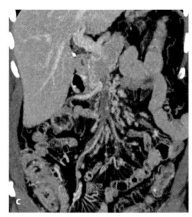

Fig. 4.44 a–c **Thrombosis of the superior mesenteric vein by venous CT angiography.**
a Axial scan.
b Sagittal scan.
c Maximum intensity projection (MIP).

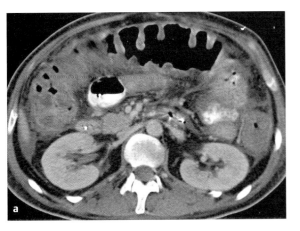

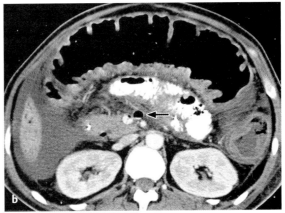

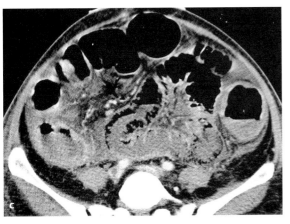

Fig. 4.45 a–c **Bowel wall thickening due to ischemia.**
a Axial CT before contrast administration shows marked ischemic thickening of the colon wall.
b Appearance after IV contrast administration.
c This scan shows extensive pneumatosis intestinalis along with gas in the mesenteric venous vessels.

paralytic ileus (**Fig. 4.46a, b**). A complicated small bowel obstruction (with ischemia) is evidenced by decreased blood flow in the bowel wall, the presence of a small bowel feces sign, ascites, and diffuse infiltration of mesenteric fat (**Fig. 4.46c**).

■ The thickness of the bowel wall does *not* correlate with the severity of ischemia. Whereas strangulation ischemia of the small bowel is associated with massive wall thickening and mesenteric edema as a result of venous congestion, segmental small bowel ischemia due to arterial embolism causes little or no wall thickening, and transmural involvement may even cause thinning of the bowel wall.

■ When hyperdense thickening of the bowel wall is found, it must be determined whether the hyperdensity was present on precontrast scans as a result of submucosal hemorrhage (usually due to venous occlusion and stasis) or whether postcontrast scans show increased enhancement consistent with mucosal hyperemia. The latter condition may result from:
 – reflex hyperperfusion after arterial nonocclusive ischemia (**Fig. 4.47**),
 – venous hyperemia secondary to venous occlusion, or
 – delayed venous drainage in a shock bowel.

■ *Shock bowel* refers to the prolonged and increased enhancement of the small bowel wall that follows hypovolemic shock and is caused by splanchnic vasoconstriction with a slowing of perfusion (**Fig. 4.48**). Shock bowel typically involves only the small bowel, which is dilated and filled with gas or fluid. The large bowel appears normal.

■ *Pneumatosis* and portal venous gas are more specific signs than bowel wall thickening, for example, but they are not pathognomonic. Pneumatosis may consist of very small linear or bubble-like submucous/intramural air collections. The more pronounced the findings, the greater the likelihood of transmural necrosis. A nontransmural infarction may also be associated with subtle findings, however (**Fig. 4.49**).

■ *Bandlike* pneumatosis and the coexistence of pneumatosis intestinalis with portal venous gas are strongly suggestive of irreversible bowel ischemia with infarction. *Vesicular* pneumatosis or an isolated collection of portal venous air was observed in one-third of patients with nontransmural ischemia (**Fig. 4.50**).

■ Pneumatosis intestinalis does *not* always signify bowel ischemia, however. It is also found in nonischemic conditions such as severe bowel distension, trauma, inflammatory or infectious intestinal processes, and neoplasia.

Strangulation ischemia of the small bowel leads to massive thickening of the bowel wall, whereas segmental ischemia due to arterial embolism causes little or no wall thickening.

Pneumatosis intestinalis does not occur exclusively in bowel ischemia; it is also found in nonischemic conditions.

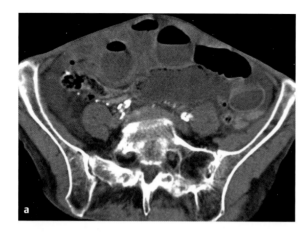

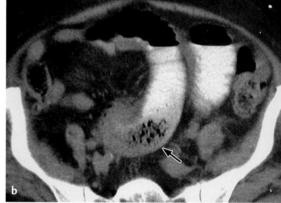

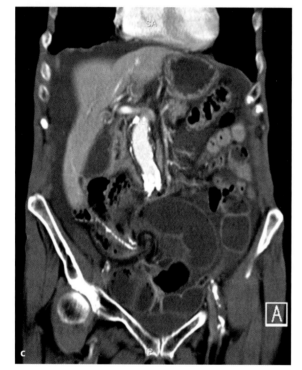

Fig. 4.46 a–c **Ischemic small bowel infarction.**
Ischemic infarction of the small bowel is characterized by marked dilatation, a small bowel feces sign (**b**), massive ascites (**c**), but considerably less wall thickening than in the large bowel (compare with **Fig. 4.45**).

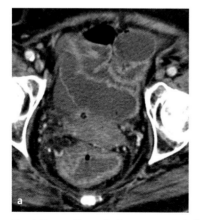

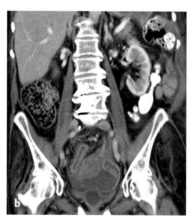

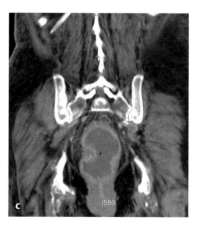

Fig. 4.47 a–c **Nonocclusive mesenteric ischemia.**
In this condition (NOMI) a period of ischemia (e. g., during transient hypotension) is followed by "reactive" hyperemia of the bowel wall.

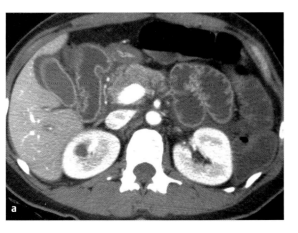

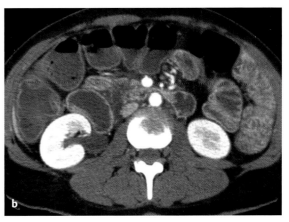

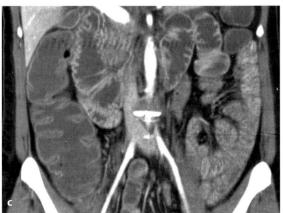

Fig. 4.48 a–c   **Shock bowel.**
Changes similar to NOMI are observed after hypovolemic shock, seen here in a young male who sustained multiple injuries. The reactive hyperemia typically involves the small bowel and is absent or less pronounced in the large bowel.

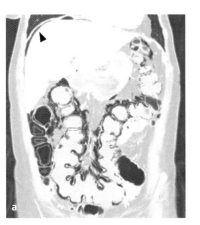

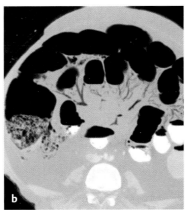

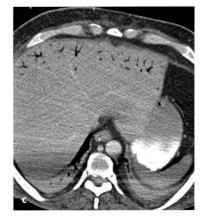

Fig. 4.49 a–c   **Pneumatosis intestinalis.**
a   Pronounced pneumatosis intestinalis.
b   Pneumatosis intestinalis with gas in the mesenteric venous vessels.
c   Gas is also visible in portal vein branches, usually in the periphery of the liver.

Angiography

Angiography in nonocclusive mesenteric ischemia shows a diffuse caliber reduction in the main trunk of the superior mesenteric artery and larger segmental branches with nonvisualization of the small intramural vessels ("leafless tree" pattern). Angiograms in other cases may show a series of spastic, narrowed vascular segments forming a "string-of-beads" pattern. Even large amounts of contrast medium produce little or no parenchymal enhancement, and there is no opacification of the mesenteric vein or portal vein.

Successful treatment has been reported with intra-arterial vasodilators such as alprostadil (Prostavasin) administered as a 20 µg bolus followed by 60 µg/24 h for 2–3 days.

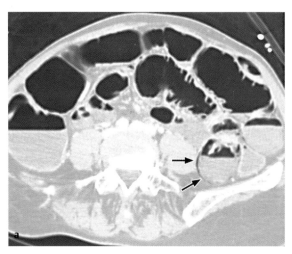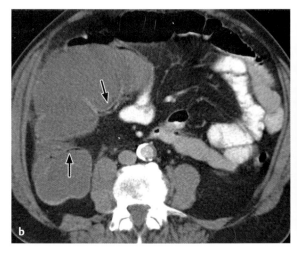

Fig. 4.50 a, b **Vesicular pneumatosis.**
The detection of pneumatosis intestinalis does not always signify irreversible ischemia. Small, bubblelike (vesicular) gas collections are also found in association with infectious changes (**a** in an HIV patient) or massive distension (**b** in a patient with mechanical bowel obstruction).

Summary

Computed tomography (CT) is the most effective imaging modality for classifying the severity of **acute pancreatitis** and detecting parenchymal and extraparenchymal necrosis. CT is also useful for detecting complications of acute pancreatitis (pancreatic abscess, pseudocysts, vascular complications) and directing interventional procedures.

Acute cholecystitis is usually a result of cholelithiasis, but acalculous cholecystitis should also be considered in ICU patients. The principal sonographic signs are thickening of the gallbladder wall to more than 3 mm and the visualization of multiple wall layers. Acalculous cholecystitis is often associated with gallbladder hydrops, which occasionally provides the only diagnostic clue. CT is used in patients with suspected complications such as pericholecystic abscess following gallbladder perforation or an hepatic abscess.

Acute pyelonephritis should be considered as a potential focus for sepsis in ICU patients. Ultrasonography can assess the severity of the obstruction, while CT can detect or exclude suspected complications such as renal abscess or pyonephrosis.

Ultrasonography is used during the initial workup of **acute renal failure** to detect or exclude a potentially reversible and treatable obstructive uropathy. Renal size, renal parenchymal echogenicity, and corticomedullary differentiation are important differentiating criteria in cases with a renal or prerenal cause.

Today it is widely agreed that CT should be the initial imaging study in hemodynamically stable patients with **gastrointestinal bleeding** at an unknown site. Angiography should be the initial study in hemodynamically unstable patients. CT localization of the bleeding site has a sensitivity of 91% and a specificity of 99%. Advantages of invasive angiography are the capability for superselective angiography and the option for immediate treatment (vasopressin infusion, embolization with coils or particles).

In the category of **inflammatory bowel diseases**, diverticulitis is important as a potential focus for sepsis, a site for perforation and peritonitis, or a source of gastrointestinal bleeding, especially in elderly ICU patients. It is imperative to look for CT signs, which may be quite subtle even with a perforation. Toxic megacolon is a serious acute complication that may arise in any type of colitis. Contrast enemas are absolutely contraindicated in this condition.

(Multidetector) CT angiography is the method of choice for the diagnosis of **intestinal ischemia**. Lack of enhancement after contrast administration, bowel wall thickening, pneumatosis and portal venous gas are signs of arterial intestinal ischemia, but they are not always present concurrently and may occur in the setting of other, nonischemic conditions.

Imaging of Intensive Care Patients after Abdominal Surgery

5

Abdominal Drainage 147
Normal Postoperative Findings 150
Postoperative Complications 151
Complications of Specific Operations 169

Abdominal Drainage

*B. Partik and
P. Pokieser*

Several different abdominal drainage systems are used postoperatively or in the setting of interventional procedures. Besides carrying out interventional procedures, the tasks of the radiologist include checking the position of drainage systems and detecting possible complications (e. g., perforation).

Types of Abdominal Drains and their Applications

Classification by Drain Type

The two main types of drain are used: overflow drains and suction drains (**Table 5.1**).

Overflow Drains

In an "open" system, secretions drain into the wound dressing or into a collection bag. This type is illustrated by the *Easy-Flow drain* (a soft silicone tube with a capillary action) and the *Penrose drain* (contains a gauze wick that also drains by capillary action).

In a "closed" system, fluids drain into a collection bag equipped with a valve and stopcock. Examples are the *Robinson drain* (silicone drain with a round cross-section and sideholes) and *Honig drain* (similar design made of soft latex material).

Suction Drains

A *Redon drain* (suction drain) employs a vacuum to draw fluid from the body. A *Jackson-Pratt drain* (bulb drain) is a suction drainage device used primarily in neurosurgery.

Suction–irrigation drains are used in patients with a body cavity infection (e. g., peritonitis or empyema of the knee joint). Typically, two separate lines are used for suction and irrigation.

Special Drains

The *Völcker drain* is a biliary drain that is advanced percutaneously through the bowel following hepaticojejunostomy. The *Tenckhoff catheter* is a drainage device used in chronic abdominal peritoneal dialysis (CAPD).

Overflow drains consist of open and closed systems. Suction drains employ a vacuum to draw fluid from the body.

Table 5.1 Classification and possible applications of various types of drain

Type of drain	Examples	Application
Overflow drain		
▪ Open systems	Penrose drain, Easy-Flow drain	Drainage of anastomoses
▪ Closed systems	Robinson drain Honig drain	Bloody drainage Septic surgery
Suction drains	Redon drain Suction–irrigation drains	Subcutaneous wound drainage Peritonitis
Special drains	Völcker drain Tenckhoff catheter	Percutaneous biliary drainage Chronic abdominal peritoneal dialysis

Classification by Function

Bloody Drainage

Some drains are placed to allow the prompt detection of bleeding and provide for drainage of blood and lymph. The *Robinson drain* and *Honig drain* are most commonly used. These drains are usually removed on the second postoperative day.

Drainage of Anastomoses

Drains are placed close to surgical anastomoses to allow for prompt drainage of anastomotic leaks. The absence of drainage confirms that the anastomosis is secure. These drains are generally removed on the sixth postoperative day. Not all anastomoses are drained. For example, the mobility of a small bowel anastomosis would limit the options for tube placement, whereas a deeply placed rectal anastomosis would be amenable to drainage. Most anastomotic drains are made of soft material (Penrose, Easy-Flow).

Drainage in Septic Surgery

Honig and Robinson drains are preferred for the drainage of abscesses.

Dwell Time

▶ The timing of drain removal depends on the volume and quality of the output.

The timing of drain removal depends on the volume and quality of the drainage. With a pancreatic anastomosis, for example, the drain should be removed when the output falls below 50 mL/day. In the case of an infection, the drain should be left in situ for a longer time.

Feeding Tubes

▶ A water-soluble, nonionic, iodinated contrast medium is instilled for the radiographic localization of a PEG tube or catheter jejunostomy tube.

Small-bore feeding tubes for enteral nutrition have a diameter of 6–8F (1F = 0.3 mm) while large-bore tubes may be as large as 18F. Larger tubes are marked with radiopaque stripes to aid localization. Enteral feeding in intensive care unit (ICU) patients can be done through a nasoenteral tube (gastric, duodenal, or jejunal), percutaneous gastrostomy, or catheter jejunostomy.

Stomach Tube

A correctly placed stomach tube descends through the left upper quadrant of the abdomen. Possible complications are perforation and malposition (e.g., intratracheal or intrapulmonary insertion, placed too high in the esophagus; see also Catheters and Monitoring Devices in Chapter 2). The risk of reflux and aspiration is increased in ventilated, elderly, or unconscious patients. Note that sideholes are often located up to 10 cm from the distal end of the tube.

Duodenal Tube

The tip of the duodenal tube is typically located to the right of the midline in the epigastrium. Positioning is often aided by gastroscopy. A duodenal tube significantly reduces the risk of aspiration compared with a nasogastric tube.

Percutaneous Endoscopic Gastronomy Tube

The percutaneous endoscopic gastronomy (PEG) tube is introduced by percutaneous endoscopy or interventional radiology. Possible complications are clogging of the tube, dislodgement, intraperitoneal malposition, or infection at the incision site.

Catheter Jejunostomy

A jejunostomy tube is placed surgically, usually as part of a larger abdominal operation (gastrectomy, esophageal surgery). The tube may remain in place for up to 3 months. Possible complications are catheter obstruction, accidental removal, intra-abdominal displacement, mechanical bowel obstruction, or local wound infection.

Imaging

Often only a conventional radiograph is taken to assess the position of a stomach tube or duodenal tube. In doubtful cases an additional view is obtained after the instillation of a water-soluble, nonionic, iodinated contrast medium. This material is routinely instilled for the radiographic localization of a PEG tube or catheter jejunostomy. Feeding may commence immediately, once correct placement has been confirmed. If a complication is suspected, further evaluation by CT is indicated.

Biliary Drainage

There is controversy as to the need for biliary drainage in cases where the common bile duct has been opened. Most authors advocate drainage because the rate of complications is higher without it.

The Kehr T-drain is widely used for biliary drainage. Straight, single-lumen tubes with side openings can also be used. The drain is removed between 2 and 3 weeks postoperatively.

The common duct can be stented with a tube to maintain biliary drainage as a palliative measure for stricture or stenosis. A biliary stent can be placed by percutaneous transhepatic cholangiography, the endoscopic retrograde technique, or by nasobiliary catheterization.

Examination Technique

T-tube cholangiography is usually performed on the sixth or seventh postoperative day. A plain radiograph is taken, and then contrast medium is instilled by manual retrograde injection through the T-tube to opacify the biliary tract including the intrahepatic ducts. Approximately 10 mL of undiluted, water-soluble, nonionic, iodinated contrast medium should be used for the detection of peripheral leaks.

— Practical Recommendation —

Special care is taken to avoid injecting small air bubbles into the drain, as they create filling defects in the common bile duct that can mimic stones. Air bubbles are distinguished by their greater mobility in response to position changes.

Complications

Possible complications are residual stones in the common duct, obstruction of the T-drain by inspissated biliary fluid, and blood clots or strictures of the bile duct at the insertion site of the T-drain, which may necessitate reoperation.

Patients occasionally develop postoperative external fistulas through the skin or internal fistulas that communicate with the duodenum, colon, or stomach. Most of these fistulas will close spontaneously and without sequelae in the absence of a distal biliary tract obstruction or biliary tract injury.

Perforation during stenting of the common duct or papilla may lead to cholascos (escape of bile into the peritoneal cavity) with subsequent biliary peritonitis.

Other complications of biliary tract surgery include hemorrhage, suture-line leak, and subhepatic fluid collections including abscess or empyema formation, which are investigated by CT (see sections below on Biliary Tract Surgery and Cholecystectomy).

Urinary Tract Drainage

Percutaneous Nephrostomy and Ureteral Stenting

Percutaneous nephrostomy (PCN) is the procedure of choice for the decompression of hydronephrosis or for establishment of access for nephroscopy, lithotripsy, or antegrade ureteral stenting. Various techniques employ a fine percutaneous needle to catheterize the renal pelvis through a calyx under local anesthesia (using sonographic and/or fluoroscopic guidance). The tract is dilated, and a drainage catheter (12–16F) or ureteral stent is introduced.

Complications. Potential complications are a bleeding arteriovenous (AV) fistula and the development of a false aneurysm or urinoma. Suspected complications should be investigated by ultrasonography (duplex if necessary) and by CT.

Bladder Catheterization

Catheters can be introduced into the bladder by the suprapubic or transurethral route. Bladder catheterization is essential for monitoring and adjusting the fluid balance in ICU patients.

Transurethral catheterization is technically easy to perform but carries a higher risk of infection and late sequelae (strictures, epididymitis) than suprapubic bladder aspiration. The latter procedure is done on a distended bladder under ultrasound guidance using a special disposable instrument set.

Correct catheter placement can be confirmed by fluoroscopically guided contrast instillation. Imaging should be done in two planes (supine and lateral oblique projections).

Complications. Any suspected complications should be investigated by a CT study that includes a delayed series 10 min after IV contrast administration, or by ultrasound scanning of the well-distended bladder. Contrast medium should be diluted 1:20 for intravesical instillation.

Avoid injecting air bubbles into the T-drain, as they may be mistaken for stones.

Transurethral catheterization is easy to perform but carries a higher risk of infection than suprapubic bladder aspiration.

149

S. Kreuzer and C. Schaefer-Prokop

Normal Postoperative Findings

Consistently occurring postoperative findings require differentiation from actual complications. This distinction is aided by noting the typical timeline of specific complications and the types of complication that are most likely to arise after certain operations (**Table 5.2**):

- The most frequent complication during the *early postoperative period* (days 1–2) is bleeding.
- Infections are most common during the *late postoperative period* (days 3–10). The causative dehiscence of a bowel anastomosis typically occurs on day 6 or 7. Other causes of infection or sepsis are retention (abscess), infected hematomas, and the leakage of bile.
- Postoperative mechanical bowel obstruction most commonly occurs on day 4. Intestinal peristalsis will generally resume spontaneously by the third postoperative day.

Resumption of peristalsis generally occurs spontaneously by the third postoperative day.

Postoperative (Physiologic) Fluid Collections

Postoperative intra-abdominal fluid collections are not necessarily an abscess or hemorrhage.

Postoperative intra-abdominal fluid collections do not always signify an abscess or hemorrhage. Fluid retention lasts until postoperative day 4 in ca. 20% of patients, day 8 in 6%, and day 12 in ca. 2%. Typically these (physiologic) fluid collections are crescent-shaped, their shape conforms to surrounding structures, and they occur in preexisting spaces or recesses, where they become spontaneously reabsorbed by the peritoneum.

Postoperative (Physiologic) Intestinal Atony

Reflex or pharmacologically induced gastrointestinal atony (functional or adynamic ileus) consistently occurs during the first two postoperative days, especially after operations that involve the bowel. The paralysis results from premedication and general anesthesia and from the surgical procedure itself (intraoperative therapy, autonomic response).

Usually, peristalsis does not resume until the third postoperative day. The resumption of peristalsis usually occurs spontaneously. Thus, bowel distention is consistently encountered during the immediate postoperative period. It can significantly impede sonographic examination and may increase abdominal circumference in a way that mimics postoperative bleeding.

Imaging

The bowel appears moderately dilated with little or no peristalsis. There is no abrupt cutoff of the gas column, but significant gaseous distention is common. In cases of nonobstructive paralysis, the dilatation involves the small bowel and the ascending colon as far as the hepatic flexure. The rest of the colon has a normal caliber.

Postoperative Pneumoperitoneum

Free intra-abdominal air is a normal finding in the immediate postoperative period. It is highly variable in its duration and extent, depending on patient habitus and the nature of the surgery. The prevalence of postopera-

Table 5.2 Typical timeline for postoperative complications

Postoperative days	Bleeding	Fever, leukocytosis	Ileus
1	Primary bleeding	Postoperative stress response	Physiologic intestinal atony
2	Primary bleeding	Postoperative stress response	Physiologic intestinal atony
3		Anastomotic dehiscence	Physiologic intestinal atony
4		Anastomotic dehiscence	Pathologic ileus
5		Anastomotic dehiscence	Pathologic ileus
6		Anastomotic dehiscence	Pathologic ileus
7	Secondary bleeding	Anastomotic dehiscence	Pathologic ileus
8	Secondary bleeding	Abscess, peritonitis, infected hematoma	Pathologic ileus
9	Secondary bleeding	Abscess, peritonitis, infected hematoma	Pathologic ileus
10	Secondary bleeding	Abscess, peritonitis, infected hematoma	Pathologic ileus

tive free-air decreases with time after surgery, declining from 44% during the first 3 days to 31% by days 4–7.

After 18 days CT no longer demonstrates free intra-peritoneal air, and small amounts of free air before that time do not signify a complication. On the other hand, increasing free air or large amounts of free air are suspicious for an anastomotic leak or perforation.

The quantity of free air is highly variable. Air following a laparoscopy (insufflated CO_2) is absorbed more rapidly than after other types of surgery. Free air has been found with greater frequency and duration in thin patients, male patients, and patients with indwelling drains. Otherwise no correlation has been found between the type of surgery, patient age, and the extent of postoper-ative pneumoperitoneum.

Note that even patients with an anastomotic leak will not necessarily have free air at CT examination, so the exclusion of a pneumoperitoneum does not prove that the gastrointestinal tract is intact.

> Small amounts of post-operative free-air before day 18 do not signify an anastomotic leak or perforation, but increasing or volu-minous free air is suspicious.

Postoperative Complications

*C. Schaefer-Prokop,
S. Kreuzer,
T. Sautner, and
W. Schima*

Diagnostic Strategy and Examination Technique

The imaging strategy will depend upon whether we must evaluate:

- an extubated, mobilized patient who is a good candidate for abdominal radiography and radiographic follow-ups, or
- an ICU patient who is still on mechanical ventilation; radiographs are technically difficult to perform and are rarely diagnostic in this subgroup, and primary sectional imaging studies (ultrasonography and CT) are preferred.

Plain Abdominal Radiograph

A plain abdominal radiograph is indicated in patients with symptoms of ileus and suspicion of a (new) pneu-moperitoneum. It is helpful in identifying residual con-trast medium from prior examinations and differentiat-ing it from contrast extravasation.

Ideally, plain abdominal radiographs should be taken in two planes, although this is usually not practical in the ICU:

- Initial anteroposterior (AP) supine radiograph using a grid cassette (35 × 43 cm) and low kilovoltage (70 kV) demonstrates organs and soft tissues.
- Left lateral decubitus AP radiograph using a grid cas-sette (35 × 43 cm) and high kilovoltage (125 kV) de-tects air–fluid levels, assesses intraluminal gas distri-bution, and detects free air and atypical gas collections (pneumatosis, pneumobilia, etc.). As an alternative, the second view may be a supine cross-table projec-tion with a laterally mounted cassette.

Ultrasonography

Owing to its convenience and availability, ultrasonogra-phy is the primary imaging study for the detection of free fluid or suspected fluid collections.

Even small amounts of intra-abdominal free fluid can be detected with high sensitivity (>90%). Sites of predi-lection for fluid collections are the Morison pouch (hepa-torenal recess) and the lesser pelvis.

As to the limitations of ultrasonography, (small) fluid collections due to leaks *cannot* be distinguished qualita-tively from postoperative reactive or lymphogenous fluid collections that are still within normal limits, or from preexisting ascites. Intraluminal bowel hemorrhages are also difficult to detect on ultrasound scans.

An important *advantage* of ultrasonography (as an ad-junct to CT) is its ability to distinguish an abscess from a fluid-filled bowel loop based on the real-time evaluation of peristalsis.

> Fluid collec-tions in the hepa-torenal recess and lesser pelvis are the earliest post-operative collec-tions that are detectable by ultrasound scan-ning.

Radiography

Radiographic follow-ups after oral contrast administra-tion (water-soluble Gastrografin) for detecting leaks or obstructions are rarely practiced nowadays, especially in ICU patients.

Computed Tomography

CT is the imaging modality of choice for almost all post-operative complications (bleeding, abscess, obstruction, leakage).

Oral contrast administration? The bowel can be opacified in the subacute stage with ca. 1 L of a diluted water-solu-ble contrast medium, administered orally, to distinguish fluid-filled bowel loops from extraintestinal collections. Oral contrast administration is often not possible during the acute stage and will only cause needless delay.

Intravenous contrast administration? Intravenous contrast medium is routinely administered to evaluate the peripheral enhancement of a fluid collection, peritoneal enhancement, as well as vascular and organ perfusion.

In principle, however, an abscess or bowel obstruction can be diagnosed even *without* IV contrast. Thus, a contraindication to contrast medium (renal failure) does *not* justify withholding a CT examination.

CT or ultrasonography? CT is preferred for the diagnosis of intra-abdominal abscess and for locating the focus in postoperative sepsis. Although ultrasound scanning is advantageous in its rapid availability (e. g., in the supine ICU patient), its technical limitations and frequent unfavorable acoustic conditions favor early evaluation by CT. Both modalities can also be used successively and in a complementary fashion.

While intrasplenic, intrahepatic, subhepatic, and subphrenic abscesses can usually be diagnosed with ultrasonography, CT is better for detecting retroperitoneal abscesses and abscesses located between bowel loops or within the lesser pelvis.

Finally, ultrasonography and CT are equally useful in directing diagnostic or therapeutic needle aspiration (and drainage) and for distinguishing an abscess from noninfectious lesions such as pancreatic pseudocyst, hematoma, bilioma, seroma, aseptic necrosis, postoperative fluid collection, or an unexpected tumor.

CT densitometry is better than ultrasonography for differentiating among the fluid components of normal postoperative transudate, proteinaceous exudate, and hemorrhage. Results are compromised, however, by overlaps of measured attenuation values and mixtures of different components (see **Table 5.3**).

Table 5.3 Causes of postoperative bleeding

Intraluminal
- Gastroduodenal ulcer and erosions
- Sloughing of mucosa

Intraperitoneal
- Vascular or organ injury

Nonspecific sites
- Loose or slipped vascular ligature
- Erosion by abscess
- Second or undetected focus
- Hemorrhagic diathesis

During the first 24 hours
- Inadequate hemostasis
- Slipped ligature

Secondary bleeding (days 7–10)
- Abscess
- Anastomotic infection
- Injury by drains
- Granulation tissue

Causes unrelated to the surgical site
- Stress ulcer
- Coagulation disorder
- Occult lesions

Angiography

Angiography or CT? Before fast CT scanners became available, selective angiography was the mainstay for identifying the source and cause of acute bleeding. The advantage of CT is its immediate and high diagnostic accuracy. But most studies require large amounts of contrast medium (up to 150 mL), which may be a limiting factor in acute or postoperative patients with impaired renal function, especially since postcontrast CT is often followed by angiography. This should be a minor handicap in cases where imaging is followed by definitive surgical treatment. The advantage of (super)selective angiography is that it provides access for immediate interventional therapy.

Angiography can detect continuous, active bleeding at rates higher than 0.5 mL/min. It should be noted, however, that not all bleeds are continuous and many sites bleed intermittently. This explains the frequently negative results of CT or angiography in patients with clinical manifestations of gastrointestinal bleeding (melena, etc.; see also the section Acute Gastrointestinal Bleeding in Chapter 4, p. 129).

Sequence of vessel opacification. Often the bleeding site has already been identified, at least with high probability, during previous endoscopy, allowing angiography to be initiated in a specific vascular region (e. g., a bleeding site in the small bowel). The bowel should be effectively immobilized (metoclopramide, glucagon) to create ideal conditions for subtraction views. Otherwise each series should be performed with sufficient contrast medium to allow for satisfactory image interpretation, even in unsubtracted views.

If the source of the hemorrhage cannot be located, all the mesenteric vessels should be selectively visualized in a designated sequence, starting with the inferior mesenteric artery before it is obscured by contrast excretion into the bladder (the imaging sequence does not matter if the bladder has been catheterized). The celiac trunk and superior mesenteric artery are visualized next. Survey angiograms are not sufficient, especially in the celiac trunk and inferior mesenteric artery, and should be supplemented by superselective series of, say, the left gastric artery, gastroduodenal or ileal artery, and jejunal branches, so that the source of the bleeding can be identified with high confidence. Provocation is often done at this stage to locate an intermittent hemorrhage that is still occult. Provocation with intra-arterial heparin or Actilyse is rarely practiced today.

Treatment. Ideally, angiography will demonstrate the extravasation of contrast medium into the bowel lumen. Contrast pooling is another definite sign, and both will document the location of the bleeding site. With both upper and lower gastrointestinal bleeding, the hemorrhagic area is selectively catheterized with a coaxial microcatheter and is embolized with coils as close as possible to the bowel wall.

— Practical Recommendation ——————————

If selective embolization is not possible (vascular caliber, spasms or occlusions upstream), the catheter can be placed as selectively as possible and then used intraoperatively for methylene blue localization of the bowel segment that will be resected. The interval from dye localization to surgery should be as brief as possible to minimize washout of the methylene blue. The microcatheter itself will not actually be palpable during the operation.

Pharmacologic therapy (vasoconstriction by IA vasopressin infusion) is mainly of historical interest but may still be tried in rare cases where a bleeding site cannot be identified.

Scintigraphy

Radionuclide imaging techniques have become much less important owing to the broad and rapid availability of sectional imaging modalities. Only the technetium-labeled red blood cell scan still has a significant role in detecting intraluminal bleeding at rates up to 0.1 mL/min. As with other modalities, intermittent bleeding is frequently occult on radionuclide scans. Unlike conventional and CT angiography, scintigraphy is not useful for acute diagnosis.

Postoperative Bleeding

(Primary) bleeding is classified as an immediate postoperative complication. *Secondary bleeding* is a delayed complication that occurs in the setting of a disorder unrelated to the primary operation, an undetected lesion, or secondary vascular erosion due to inflammation (**Table 5.3**).

Postoperative bleeding may be intraluminal, usually in the bowel, or may spread freely within the intra- or extraperitoneal space.

Pathogenesis

Primary bleeding occurs during the first 24 hours after the operation. It may be caused by the inadequate ligation or cauterization of blood vessels.

Secondary bleeding usually occurs between postoperative days 7 and 10. It may result from infection causing mucosal damage at the anastomotic site, the erosion of large vessels due to abscess formation, vascular injury caused by drains, or bleeding granulation tissue. Secondary bleeding is more common in patients with inflammatory bowel disease (steroid therapy).

Bleeding due to coagulation disorders or anticoagulant medication is rare in patients who have been adequately prepared. The differential diagnosis should include bleeding stress ulcers distant from the primary surgical site and bleeding lesions that were not identified or considered during the operation (e. g., bleeding from angiodysplasia of the ascending colon following a sigmoid colon resection for diverticulosis).

Clinical Aspects

Patients with postoperative bleeding have typical clinical manifestations. Shock symptoms with a fall in blood pressure accompanied by tachycardia, sweating, and a falling hematocrit or low hemoglobin level on blood tests are suggestive of a hemorrhagic complication. Drainage is monitored to check for bleeding from deep drains or direct bleeding from the surgical wound.

The differential diagnosis should always include the possibility of intra-abdominal bleeding, even after operations without a high bleeding risk.

Imaging

Ultrasonography

— Practical Recommendation ——————————

Free intra-abdominal fluid is most easily detected sonographically in the Morison pouch or cul-de-sac. Distinguishing between intraintestinal fluid and extraluminal free fluid requires delineation of the bowel wall and the observation of peristalsis.

The differentiation of "normal" postoperative free-fluid from incipient bleeding or complications may be difficult in any given case. A fluid collection with a spherical or ellipsoidal shape and associated mass effect is suspicious for an abnormal cause (when combined with clinical findings).

Computed Tomography

The CT findings of free intraperitoneal blood depend strongly on the age and extent of the hemorrhage (**Fig. 5.1**). Measured attenuation values are helpful but not definitive (**Table 5.4**).

Mesenteric hematomas. These collections appear on CT as ellipsoidal structures of soft-tissue attenuation (**Fig. 5.2**). Acute, freshly clotted hematomas have attenuation values

Primary bleeding occurs during the first 24 hours after surgery. Secondary bleeding usually occurs between days 7 and 10.

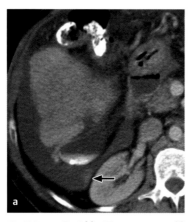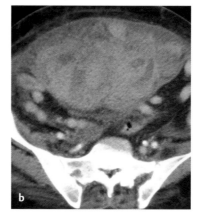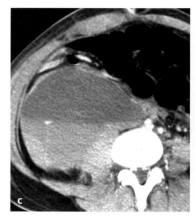

Fig. 5.1 a–c **Variable CT appearance of hematomas.**

a Hematoma appearing as bloody ascites (note the density and sedimentation effect).

b Hematoma appearing as a loculated, inhomogeneous, hyperdense fluid collection following multiple slow bleeds.

c Hematoma appearing as a homogeneous fluid collection with a layer of sedimentation after a single profuse bleed.

Table 5.4 CT attenuation values of various body fluids

Cause	Hounsfield units
Acute hematoma	> 30 HU (caution: > 20 HU in anemia; depends on hematocrit)
Subacute hematoma with clotted blood	40–60 HU. Similar HU values in infection (30–40)
Arterial extravasate	80–130 HU (surrounded by lower-density hematoma); local values up to 170 HU at active bleeding site
Transudate	5–20 HU
Exudate	20–40 HU
Ascites with significant bleeding	> 30 HU
Seroma	10–25 HU
Bilioma	0–10 HU; slightly higher with infection (10–15 HU)
Abscess (pus)	20–35 HU (30–40)

in the range of 20–40 HU, but these values decline over a period of 1–2 weeks due to the breakdown of hemoglobin. The initially homogeneous structure of the hematoma is transformed into an inhomogeneous "mass." This makes it difficult to distinguish a chronic hematoma from an abscess with attenuation values of 15–35 HU. As the hematoma continues to age, however, it becomes progressively smaller and finally assumes the size and density (12–25 HU) of a seroma.

Free hemorrhage. Even with CT, it can be difficult to distinguish free intraperitoneal bleeding from an abscess. CT will sometimes show fine sedimentation in the posterior dependent recesses as evidence of bleeding in preexisting ascites.

Retroperitoneal hematomas. A definite advantage of CT is its ability to evaluate the retroperitoneum and detect retroperitoneal hematomas (e. g., following aortic surgery or due to a coagulation disorder). Retroperitoneal hematomas appear on CT as patchy, relatively hyperdense masses (> 30 HU) that displace normal retroperitoneal structures (**Fig. 5.3**).

Intraparenchymal hematomas. These collections appear as crescent-shaped masses that compress the organ parenchyma (spleen, liver) when subcapsular (**Fig. 5.4**).

Abdominal wall hematomas. Abdominal wall hematomas are not uncommon and are demonstrated equally well by ultrasonography and CT, although ultrasound scanning is often more difficult postoperatively and CT provides a better overview of findings.

Postoperative Sepsis and Focus Identification

Sepsis describes a systemic response to an infectious focus located in the body (not necessarily intra-abdominal). Any monitoring change noted in the postoperative patient may be an initial sign of early sepsis: cardiovascular parameters, blood gas analysis, ventilation, laboratory values, body temperature, or general status.

Common findings in postoperative sepsis are paralytic ileus with distention of the small and large bowel and diffuse subcutaneous edema. The patient is febrile and, when conscious, complains of nausea and vomiting. A precipitous fall in white blood count (e. g., from 13 000 to 3000) is indicative of gram-negative sepsis.

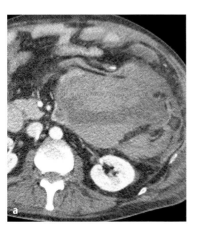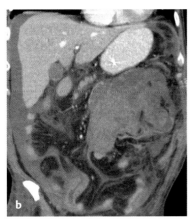

Fig. 5.2 a, b **Extensive intraperitoneal (mesenteric) hematoma.**
Shown here with a sedimentation layer and bloody ascites.

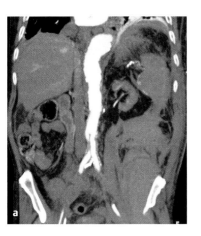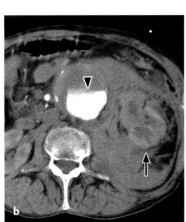

Fig. 5.3 a, b **Extensive retroperitoneal bleeding from the aorta with displacement of the left kidney (arrow).**
Note in **b** the sedimentation of contrast medium in the aneurysmatic aorta (arrowhead) due to impaired left ventricular function.

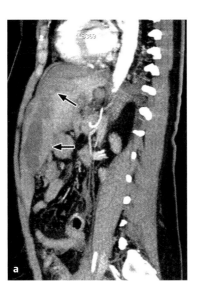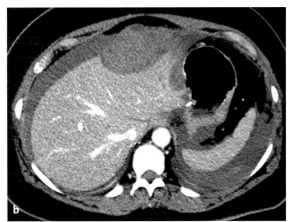

Fig. 5.4 a, b **Subcapsular hematoma in the liver.**
A subcapsular hematoma is impressing on the (soft) liver tissue. Patient presented with a sudden decrease of hemoglobin level 8 days after partial gastrectomy.

Table 5.5 Timeline of postoperative complications in the abdomen

Postoperative days	Abdominal complications
Days 1–2	▪ Postoperative days 1–2 are marked by an inflammatory "stress response" with fever, tachycardia, hyperventilation, and an extravascular and extracellular fluid shift. ▪ Abdominal sepsis is rarely causative; when it is, it is referable to a (major) anastomotic leak with rapid development of peritonitis.
Days 2–3	▪ This period is marked by a physiologic reversal of the extravascular fluid shift with increasing diuresis and potential pulmonary edema formation (especially in patients with preexisting heart and/or renal failure). ▪ Fever may be attributable to pneumonia. ▪ Consider anastomotic leak in patients with poor diuresis and no resumption of peristalsis.
Days 3–6	▪ This is the period in which abdominal sepsis is most common! ▪ Paradoxical diarrhea (do not misinterpret as improvement), intestinal atony, dysuria, cardiopulmonary insufficiency, fever and leukocytosis are symptoms that may be associated with anastomotic leak and peritonitis.
Days 7–14	▪ Most postoperative complications during this period are caused by localized abscess formation, usually secondary to an anastomotic leak.

▦ The "four P's" in the differential diagnosis of sepsis in ICU patients are pneumonia, peritonitis, phlebitis, and pyelitis.

"Four P's" should be considered in the differential diagnosis of sepsis in ICU patients: pneumonia, peritonitis, phlebitis, and pyelitis. The development of septic complications after surgery follows a classic timeline (**Table 5.5**). Awareness of this timeline can be helpful in narrowing the differential diagnosis.

Peritonitis

Peritonitis is defined as an inflammatory reaction of the peritoneum to pathogenic stimuli such as bacteria, viruses, and chemical agents.

Classifications

▦ Primary (spontaneous) peritonitis is distinguished from secondary peritonitis (due to a perforated hollow viscus) and from tertiary (persistent) peritonitis.

Primary peritonitis (hematogenous, lymphogenous, or luminal invasion/contamination) is distinguished from *secondary* peritonitis due to a perforated hollow viscus and from *tertiary* or persistent peritonitis. While secondary peritonitis is treated by surgical eradication of the focus and pharmacologic therapy serves only as an adjunct, the causal treatment for primary peritonitis is antibiotic pharmacotherapy.

Surgical treatment is appropriate for primary peritonitis only in cases that have not responded to antibiotics. Therapeutic options are debridement and copious irrigation of the abdominal cavity to reduce microorganism counts.

For the prevention of persistent "tertiary" peritonitis and intra-abdominal abscess formation (ca. 20 % incidence after secondary peritonitis), it is generally agreed that eradication of the focus should be followed by additional surgical measures based on the principle of "need-oriented relaparotomy" (= reoperation prompted by a deterioration of the patient's general condition).

Postoperative peritonitis, which most commonly results from anastomotic leak, affects a patient that is already traumatized by the previous operation and is subject to an "acute-phase response" (with systemic activation of mediators). Today it is believed that the acute-phase 20 % incidence after secondary peritonitis), it is generally agreed that eradication of the focus should be followed by additional surgical measures based on the principle of "need-oriented relaparotomy" (= reoperation prompted by a deterioration of the patient's general condition). Response combined with the infectious "second hit" may initiate the development of multiorgan dysfunction syndrome (MODS). The mortality rate of this condition, at 50 %, is substantially higher than that of a primary hollow viscus perforation.

The routine clinical description of "(single) quadrant peritonitis" or "multiquadrant peritonitis" is based on a gross subdivision of the abdomen into four quadrants and does *not* follow predefined anatomical boundaries.

Clinical Aspects

The main clinical symptoms of peritonitis are abdominal pain and tenderness, rigidity, aperistalsis (silent abdomen), and systemic disease manifestations. They are accompanied by circulatory symptoms (fever, chills, tachycardia and tachypnea, and eventual signs of shock). The severity of the symptoms correlates with the cause and mortality risk (**Table 5.6**).

The symptoms of peritonitis may be masked in postoperative or immunocompromised patients and in very

Table 5.6 Grades of severity of peritonitis (after Way, modified from Krestin 1994)

Severity	Cause	Mortality
Mild	▪ Appendicitis ▪ Perforated gastroduodenal ulcer ▪ Acute salpingitis	< 10 %
Moderate	▪ Diverticulitis ▪ Nonvascular perforation of the small bowel ▪ Gangrenous cholecystitis ▪ Multiple injuries	< 20 %
Severe	▪ Perforation of the large bowel ▪ Ischemic perforation of the small bowel ▪ Postoperative complications	20–80 %

young or very old patients. The diagnostic challenge is not to diagnose peritonitis but to identify its cause.

Imaging

Plain Abdominal Radiograph

Due to the frequency of perforation-induced peritonitis, a diagnosis of peritonitis should be considered whenever a pneumoperitoneum is found. Abdominal radiographs show generalized intestinal atony and distention with fluid levels in the small and large bowel. Specific signs of peritonitis are not seen. Displacement and obvious asymmetry of bowel loops is suggestive of an abscess.

Ultrasonography

Ultrasound reveals atonic, fluid-filled bowel loops. Free fluid is detected at sites of predilection. Attention is given to the morphology of the gallbladder (caution: cholecystitis) and to any fluid collections that are suspicious for an abscess (see below).

Computed Tomography

Acute peritonitis is characterized by ascites with dilatation of the mesenteric vessels and diffusely increased density of the mesenteric fat. The parietal layer of the peritoneum is diffusely thickened and shows increased contrast enhancement (**Fig. 5.5**).

Peritonitis is classified as single-quadrant or multiquadrant based on the extent of the inflammation. Localized fluid collections, including abscesses, are almost always present in the setting of (diffuse) peritonitis, and their accessibility to percutaneous drainage should be assessed (**Fig. 5.6**, see also the section on Postoperative Bowel Obstruction, p. 163).

— Practical Recommendation ————

The location and distribution of abnormal fluid and air collections are important in making an etiologic diagnosis, just as the anatomical sites of predilection for abscess formation vary with the underlying disease and the nature of the previous operation (**Table 5.8**). The localization of even small inflammatory foci is aided by noting that fluid tends to gravitate toward the posterior recesses, directed there by preexisting and surgically created anatomical compartments (**Table 5.7**).

The differentiation of a "physiologic," noninfectious postoperative peritoneal reaction may be difficult or impossible to distinguish from infection-induced inflammation based on morphologic imaging findings alone.

Spontaneous bacterial peritonitis. Spontaneous bacterial peritonitis is a special form of peritonitis caused by the

The symptoms of peritonitis may be masked in postoperative or immunocompromised patients and in very young or very old patients.

Postoperative, noninfectious peritoneal reactions are not always distinguishable from infection-induced inflammation based purely on morphologic imaging findings.

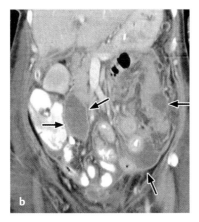

Fig. 5.5 a, b **Diffuse peritonitis.**
Diffuse peritonitis with thickened, enhancing peritoneum, diffuse infiltration of peritoneal fat, and multiple abscesses located between bowel loops (following perforated diverticulitis). Note also the thickening of the small bowel wall and the diffuse subcutaneous edema, which is typical of a patient with sepsis.

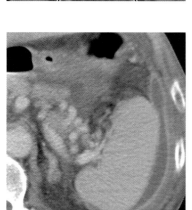
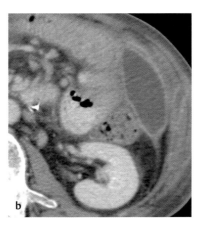

Fig. 5.6 a, b **Focal abscesses are distributed about the spleen and colon and show rim enhancement.**

infection of ascites in the absence of an intestinal lesion. It is a frequent complication in patients with hepatic cirrhosis but also occurs in malignant ascites. Patients present with diffuse abdominal pain and fever. The diagnosis is established by abdominal paracentesis and the detection of granulocytes in the aspirate, or by microbiological findings (usually a monomicrobial infection with gram-negative bacteria).

Abscess

Despite improved surgical techniques and perioperative antibiotic therapy, postoperative abscess formation continues to pose a serious problem and diagnostic challenge. The mortality rate is as high as 30%, depending on the extent of involvement, and rises to more than 80% without treatment. More than 60% of all abdominal abscesses have a postoperative cause. The following operations have the highest association with postoperative abscess formation:

- gangrenous cholecystectomy
- perforated appendectomy or diverticulitis
- gastrointestinal resections for inflammatory or neoplastic disease

Sites of occurrence. Abscesses may form at the primary operative site or may develop distant from the operative field due to the spread of microorganisms along anatomical pathways between communicating intraperitoneal compartments. Synchronous abscesses arising at multiple sites are found in up to 25% of cases.

Sites of predilection for intraperitoneal abscess formation are subphrenic, subhepatic, paracolic, the lesser pel-

vis, between bowel loops, and intraparenchymal (**Tables 5.7, 5.8**). The most common nonintraperitoneal site is the psoas muscle. The Morison pouch (right hepatorenal recess) is the most dependent peritoneal recess in the supine patient, making it a frequent site for abscess formation (**Figs. 5.7, 5.8**). Infected cavities may also develop in the subcutaneous layers of a laparotomy scar.

Pathogenesis

An abscess may form as a result of direct contamination, generalized sepsis, an anastomotic leak or enteric leak, fistulation, or perforation. The causative organisms are gram-negative enterobacteria such as *Escherichia coli*,

Table 5.7 Peritoneal compartments

Upper abdomen, supramesocolic	
Subphrenic	Divided by falciform ligament into left and right subphrenic space
Right subphrenic space	Between the liver and right kidney
Left subphrenic space	Between the liver and stomach
Lesser sac	Between the pancreas and liver, extending to the caudate lobe and splenic hilum
Lower abdomen, inframesocolic	
Right paracolic	Right of the cecum and ascending colon
Left paracolic	Left of the descending colon
Supramesenteric	Cranial to the mesenteric root
Inframesenteric	Caudal to the mesenteric root
Pelvis	
Vesicouterine pouch (females)	Between the bladder and uterus
Douglas pouch = cul-de-sac (females)	Between the uterus and rectum
Rectovesical pouch (males)	Between the bladder and rectum

Table 5.8 Sites of predilection for the intraperitoneal spread of abscesses

Left subphrenic abscess
- Splenic rupture
- Gastric perforation
- Postoperative

Spread
- Left subphrenic
- Caudal spread prevented by phrenicocolic ligament

Right paracolic and subhepatic abscess
- Appendicitis and perforation
- Biliary-tract and gallbladder infection
- Pelvic abscess
- Bowel inflammations
- Intestinal gangrene
- Postoperative

Spread
- Subphrenic
- Down into lesser pelvis

Left paracolic abscess
- Diverticulitis, perforation
- Pelvic abscess
- Bowel inflammation
- Postoperative

Spread
- Left subphrenic
- Down into lesser pelvis

Abscess in the lesser sac
- Gastric perforation
- After pancreatitis, pancreatic rupture
- Postoperative

Spread
- Into free abdominal cavity (only with patent epiploic foramen)

Cul-de-sac abscess
- Intestinal ischemia
- Diverticulitis
- Meckel diverticulum (perforated)
- Pelvic inflammatory disease
- Bladder rupture (iatrogenic, traumatic)
- Postoperative

Spread
- Left and right paracolic
- Left and right inframesocolic
- Subhepatic
- Right subphrenic

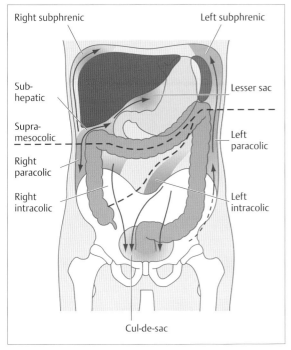

Fig. 5.7 Intra-abdominal abscesses.
Frequent sites of occurrence and routes of spread.

Proteus, Clostridium, Klebsiella, and other enteric organisms.

Clinical Aspects

Leukocytosis that is persistent or resumes after an initially normal white count should raise suspicion of an abscess. Other clinical indicators are an elevated C-reactive protein level, fever, and a delay in the resumption of intestinal peristalsis.

Imaging

Ultrasonography

An abscess often contains internal echoes (debris) on ultrasound scanning, even when its contents show mostly liquid echogenicity. Ultrasonography is much better than CT for defining internal septations and corpuscular debris (**Fig. 5.9**). The abscess margins may be smooth or irregular. Intralesional gas collections are typical of abscesses and appear as areas of increased echogenicity. They may cast an acoustic shadow, depending on their size.

Ultrasound imaging alone cannot distinguish between an abscess and a sterile fluid collection. Even an echo-free structure may be infected, and an infected abscess may contain so much debris that it resembles a solid tumor mass sonographically.

Note that every postoperative fluid collection is not an abscess! Even an enlarging fluid collection is suspicious only when accompanied by suggestive clinical findings. Ultrasound-guided needle aspiration can be used in equivocal cases to help identify the infecting organism and institute antibiotic therapy.

Computed Tomography

Rim enhancement. Most (not all) abscesses display a thin, enhancing peripheral wall. This "ring sign" is most prominent in extraparenchymal abscesses (**Figs. 5.9**, **5.10**). The intensity of the rim enhancement and the thickness of the wall depend on the spatial and temporal development of the abscess. For example, psoas abscesses and abscesses in a setting of Crohn disease or diverticulitis typically present a thick, intensely enhancing wall. This contrasts with postoperative abscesses, which often have a thin wall or may even lack a visible rim. The thickness of the wall increases with the age of the abscess.

> Even an enlarging fluid collection is only suspicious for an abscess within the context of clinical findings.

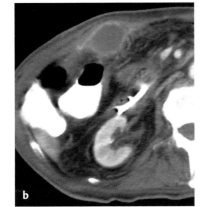
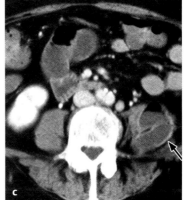

Fig. 5.8 a–c **Abscess sites of occurrence.**

a Abscess in the Morison pouch following a Whipple procedure. The abscess should not be confused with the stomach, which is lateral to it.

b Abscess in the abdominal wall.
c Abscess in the left psoas muscle.

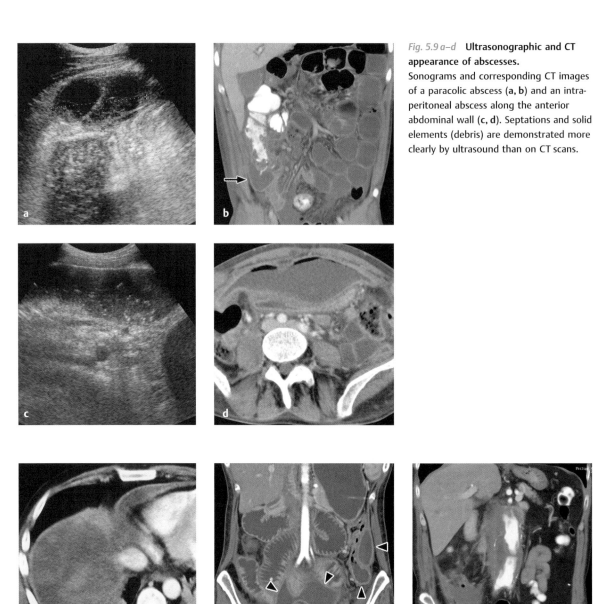

Fig. 5.9 a–d **Ultrasonographic and CT appearance of abscesses.**
Sonograms and corresponding CT images of a paracolic abscess (**a, b**) and an intraperitoneal abscess along the anterior abdominal wall (**c, d**). Septations and solid elements (debris) are demonstrated more clearly by ultrasound than on CT scans.

Fig. 5.10 a–c **CT appearance of abscesses.**
The CT appearance of abscesses varies with their age, cause, and composition (**a**, infected subphrenic hematoma). Some abscesses have a mass appearance with biconvex margins and an enhancing rim (**b**, Crohn disease), while others appear as diffuse infiltration without a visible rim (**c**, status post-appendectomy).

More than 60% of abscesses exhibit a smooth wall, while the remainder present an irregular or "shaggy" wall. Most abscesses exert a mass effect on surrounding tissues.

Density and gas collections. Pyogenic abscesses have attenuation values in the range of 20–35 HU (**Fig. 5.11**). Infected hematomas usually have lower attenuation averaging ca. 15 HU, while infected biliomas average less than 10 HU.

As in ultrasonography, the only pathognomonic CT sign is a gas collection within the abscess cavity (present in up to 40% of cases). This collection may take the form of small, separate air bubbles or may appear as an air–fluid level due to accumulated debris (**Fig. 5.12**).

Intraparenchymal abscesses. Abscesses may form within parenchymal organs like the liver, spleen, or kidneys (**Fig. 5.13**). Intraparenchymal abscesses occur predominantly in the liver and are less common in the spleen.

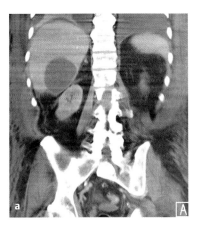
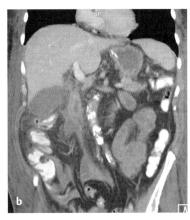

Fig. 5.11 a, b **Uninfected subhepatic hematoma (a) versus abscess (b).** Note the ill-defined margins of the abscess and its higher, less homogeneous density compared with the uninfected hematoma.

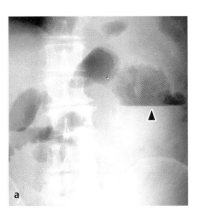
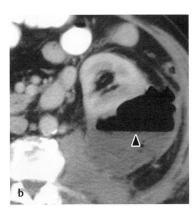

Fig. 5.12 a, b **Extensive retroperitoneal (fecal) abscess with a large air–fluid level.**

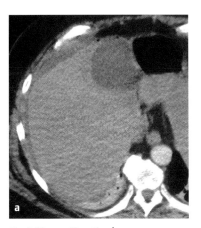
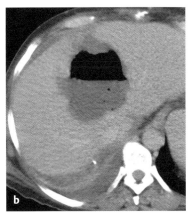
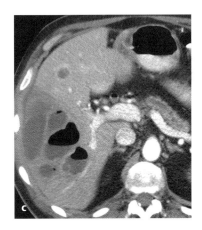

Fig. 5.13 a–c **Hepatic abscesses.**
The abscess in **a** has an almost cystic appearance (note the density) but is associated with a perifocal reaction. Note the air inclusions in **b** and the rim enhancement and air–fluid levels in **c**.

Normally they show very little wall structure but are more clearly demarcated from the surrounding enhancing parenchyma after contrast administration. Even intraparenchymal abscesses are believed to have a thin enhancing wall, but the wall is obscured by surrounding enhancing parenchyma. It is sometimes visible on modern fast scanners during the early arterial phase of enhancement. Gas collections are less commonly found in intrahepatic abscesses than in intra-abdominal abscesses

(< 20%). Both detection and characterization (tumor versus abscess) are facilitated by IV contrast administration.

Differential Diagnosis

Other types of fluid collection such as seromas, hematomas, and biliomas require differentiation from abscesses. Clinical manifestations are of key importance in discriminating these lesions.

A rounded bowel loop may resemble an abscess and should always be excluded (multiplanar imaging in CT, presence of peristalsis in ultrasonography).

An abscess may appear as loculated ascites (without a peripheral rim). Differentiation relies on clinical findings and fine-needle aspiration.

The only pathognomonic sign is the detection of intralesional gas indicating infection by gas-forming bacteria.

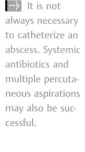 The detection of intralesional gas is pathognomonic for infection by gas-forming bacteria.

Even when massive ascites is present, it is unusual to detect fluid in the lesser sac. When fluid is detected in the lesser sac of a patient who has not had prior surgery, it is suspicious for a lesion in an adjacent organ (e. g., perforated gastric or duodenal ulcer) or a malignant cause. Fluid in the lesser sac is not necessarily abnormal in a patient who has undergone upper abdominal surgery.

Abscess Drainage

The successful interventional therapy of intra-abdominal abscesses requires accurate localization and percutaneous access under sonographic or CT guidance. Interventional therapy may be performed with curative intent or to relieve septic symptoms as a prelude to definitive surgical treatment.

It should be considered that drainage never eliminates the cause. Thus, an interventional procedure is appropriate only if it is reasonable to predict that the underlying cause of the abscess will resolve spontaneously. This rule would apply to postoperative abscesses resulting from a *small* circumscribed suture-line leak and to abscesses following peritonitis that do not communicate with a hollow viscus. It never applies to abscesses that form in a setting of chronic inflammatory bowel disease.

It is not always necessary to catheterize an abscess. Systemic antibiotics and multiple percutaneous aspirations may also be successful.

Approaches

Whenever possible, an approach should be selected that bypasses uninvolved organs (**Fig. 5.14**).

Upper abdomen. Abscesses in the upper abdomen can be accessed via a transhepatic approach. A transpleural approach should definitely be avoided (empyema). The spleen, bowel loops, and stomach should also be avoided. Subphrenic abscesses are an exception and can be drained by a transpleural route in selected cases where a transabdominal approach is not possible (trocar technique).

Pelvis. A transgluteal approach is favored for abscesses in the lesser pelvis. The approach should be as close as possible to the sacrum and above the sacrospinal ligament to avoid irritation of the sciatic nerve and sacral plexus. Deep-seated pelvic abscesses can also be approached transvaginally (with ultrasound guidance) or by the transrectal or transperineal route (with CT guidance or endoscopically).

Catheter Selection and Drainage

It is not always necessary to catheterize an abscess. Systemic antibiotic therapy and multiple percutaneous aspirations may also be successful. The first step is usually to sample material for microbiologic analysis by fine-needle aspiration under local anesthesia.

Pigtail catheters with sideholes are the type most commonly used for abscess drainage. The caliber of the catheter should be appropriate for the abscess fluid (**Table 5.9**). Care is taken to position the sideholes *within* the lesion.

Urokinase or *N*-acetylcysteine can be instilled in an effort to liquefy viscous and solid abscess components, but this is a controversial technique (**Table 5.10**).

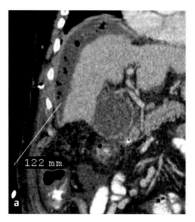
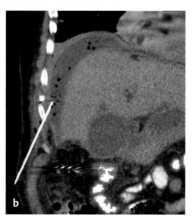
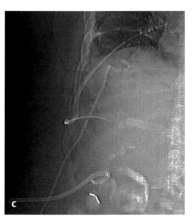

Fig. 5.14 a–c **CT-assisted planning, aspiration, and drainage of a subphrenic abscess.**
Multiplanar reformatted images are helpful in locating and monitoring angled percutaneous approaches to the lesion.

Table 5.9 Catheter calibers recommended for various abscesses

Abscess	Catheter caliber (F)
Low viscosity (bilioma, seroma)	6–8
High viscosity	9–12r
Suction drainage	16
Hematoma	> 9
Pancreatitis	Up to 28 (multiple catheters)

Table 5.10 Urokinase dose recommendations for various abscess sizes

Abscess size	Urokinase units
< 3 cm	12 500 IU
3–5 cm	25 000 IU
5–10 cm	50 000 IU
> 10 cm	100 000 IU
Followed by 10 mL NaCl and 15 min contact time, 3 times daily	

The catheter should be flushed with 10–20 mL NaCl three or four times daily to maintain patency.

Course of Interventional Therapy and Discontinuation

The *duration of catheterization* is determined by the therapeutic effect and drainage activity. The drain may be removed when output falls below 10 mL/day. This is generally the case after 7–10 days. Exceptions are abscesses in pancreatitis, possibly with bowel communication, where the catheter may have to remain indwelling for up to 6 weeks.

The success rates of interventional techniques varies from 30% to 95%. Even complex abscesses are amenable to drainage.

Transient deterioration of the patient's condition may be noted during the first 24 hours of drainage. This is caused by the release of bacteria and bacterial products into the circulation and does not indicate failure of the selected strategy.

Primary surgical treatment is indicated in patients with more than three abscesses, complex abscesses, and situations that cannot be managed by percutaneous drainage alone. This rule does not apply to hepatic abscesses.

Surgical treatment is also indicated in cases where systemic signs of sepsis persist for 3 days despite adequate drainage.

Postoperative Bowel Obstruction

It is important to distinguish physiologic postoperative intestinal atony from the following conditions due to their different clinical significance and treatment implications:

- (prolonged) paralytic ileus
- mechanical bowel obstruction (without vascular involvement)
- ischemic bowel obstruction with hypoperfusion of the bowel, whether due to strangulation or a primary vascular cause (thromboembolism)

Bowel obstruction is a clinical rather than radiologic diagnosis, but imaging is helpful in distinguishing between postoperative paralysis and mechanical obstruction, as CT can reliably detect or exclude a mechanical bowel obstruction.

Paralytic Ileus

Paralytic ileus is caused by the action of toxic substances that paralyze the parasympathetic nervous system. It is usually marked by distention of the small and large bowel and sometimes of the stomach. For example, on CT the small bowel and ascending colon were found to be dilated in more than 80% of cases. The rest of the colon usually has a normal caliber.

It should be noted that gastric or jejunal catheters may decompress the proximal small bowel loops, and this should not be misinterpreted as "improvement" on CT scans.

Mechanical Bowel Obstruction

Postoperative mechanical bowel obstruction is sometimes difficult to distinguish from prolonged paralytic ileus. This distinction is important, however, as a delayed second operation is associated with significantly higher morbidity and mortality. It is difficult to assess the need for relaparotomy based on clinical symptoms, and so imaging studies have assumed a key diagnostic role.

Causes. Approximately 50% of postoperative bowel obstructions occur during the first two weeks after surgery, and 80% of these cases are caused by adhesions (**Table 5.11**). Adhesions are more common in the small bowel than in the large bowel. They are particularly common after small bowel surgery, although small bowel obstruction may also occur after abdominoperineal resections and colon resections.

▸ Decompression of proximal small bowel loops with a gastric or jejunal catheter should not be mistaken for "improvement" on CT.

▸ Surgical treatment is indicated when systemic signs of sepsis persist for 3 days despite adequate drainage.

Table 5.11   Causes of postoperative obstruction

- Adhesion
- Abscess or hematoma at the anastomosis
- Inflammatory stricture
- Edema or technically induced stenosis of the anastomosis
- Volvulus
- Undetected external hernia
- Missed tumor (component)
- Occlusion of mesenteric vessels
- Herniation through a mesenteric or abdominal wall defect
- Intussusception (rare)

The plain abdominal radiograph in mechanical bowel obstruction typically shows dilatation of the small bowel, while paralytic ileus usually shows concomitant dilatation of the stomach and colon.

Symptoms. A simple mechanical bowel obstruction leads to constipation, meteorism, colicky pain, nausea and vomiting. The higher (i.e., the more proximal) the site of the obstruction, the more acute the clinical presentation. A low colonic obstruction causes lengthy prestenotic dilatation of the colon, which delays the onset of obstructive symptoms. As a result, the postoperative presentation of a colon obstruction can mimic the features of postoperative ileus for a period of hours or days.

During clinical evaluation it should be considered that every (primary) mechanical bowel obstruction may progress secondarily to paralytic ileus without treatment.

Plain Abdominal Radiograph

Vertical and cross-table abdominal radiographs are still obtained to investigate acute bowel obstruction and ileus, although their applications and value are limited in immobilized ICU patients (**Fig. 5.15**). Because the dilated small bowel loops assume a radial distribution along the small bowel mesentery, distal loops of ileum may occupy

a higher-than-normal position (e.g., in the right upper quadrant) while loops of jejunum are displaced into the pelvis.

The plain abdominal radiograph in mechanical bowel obstruction typically shows dilatation of the small bowel. Paralytic ileus additionally shows dilatation of the stomach and colon. Fluid levels in the colon may also be a physiologic finding.

Small Bowel Contrast Series

Today the upper gastrointestinal and small bowel series after oral contrast administration has been widely replaced by CT. Occasionally it is still used in the evaluation of "mobile" critical care patients, but it is no longer ordered in postoperative ICU patients.

Ultrasonography

Ultrasonography is an excellent adjunct to radiographs and CT. With its capability for the on-line observation of peristalsis, it can aid in differentiating paralysis from obstruction.

Computed Tomography

CT has become the imaging modality of choice for the investigation of bowel obstruction. Depending on the degree of the obstruction, CT can localize the site of the obstruction, narrow the differential diagnosis, and aid in directing further management. Often it can even define the cause of a mechanical obstruction at the "transition zone" by differentiating a mass lesion from obstruction due to adhesions, incarceration, or inflammation (**Figs. 5.16**, **5.17**).

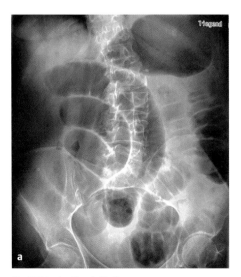
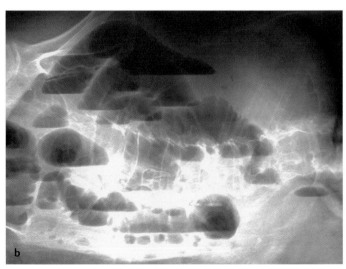

Fig. 5.15 a, b   **Paralytic ileus.**
Radiographs show diffuse dilatation of the small bowel and stomach (**a**) and air–fluid levels in the left lateral decubitus view (**b**).

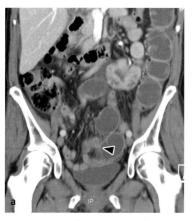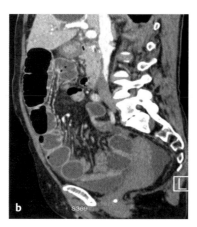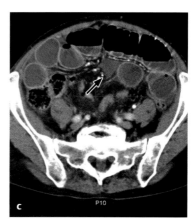

Fig. 5.16 a–c **Adhesive bowel obstruction.**
CT shows an abrupt caliber change (bird-beak sign, arrowhead) in addition to free fluid (arrow).

CT has become an important study for acute, indeterminate cases and for the imaging of ICU patients. The sensitivity of CT in evaluating bowel obstructions depends on the degree of the obstruction. Studies have documented a sensitivity greater than 80% for high-grade stenoses compared with more than 50% for low-grade obstructions, with a specificity of 96%.

The following CT findings are indicative of *mechanical bowel obstruction:*

- *Dilatation of the bowel.* When a bowel segment is obstructed by a pathologic process, it becomes dilated proximal to the site of the obstruction. The following upper cutoff values have been established for the normal diameters of various bowel segments: jejunum 3.5 cm, mid-small bowel 3 cm, ileum 2.5 cm, colon 6 cm.
- *Transition zone.* The transition zone corresponds to the level of the obstruction and denotes the junction between *dilated* bowel loops oral to the obstruction and

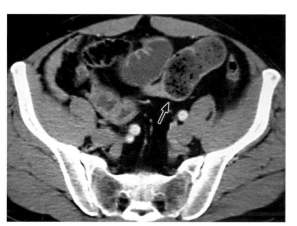

Fig. 5.17 **Small bowel feces sign and abrupt caliber change.**
CT demonstrates multiple small air bubbles in the small bowel (normally seen only in the colon) due to bacterial overgrowth secondary to a long-standing mechanical obstruction.

collapsed bowel loops distal to the obstruction. Direct visualization of the abrupt caliber change at the transition zone is the key criterion for distinguishing between paralysis and obstruction (**Fig. 5.16**). In some cases a "bird beak" configuration of the bowel can be appreciated at the site of an adhesion.

- *Small bowel feces sign.* This is another, less common sign of obstruction based on the identification of gas and stool in a dilated loop of small bowel (air caused by bacterial overgrowth due to prolonged stasis of contents; **Fig. 5.17**).
- *Bowel wall thickening.* Thickening of the bowel wall is a nonspecific but important sign of incipient bowel decompensation with necrosis and risk of perforation.

Bowel distention may be due to obstruction or paralysis. Fluid levels are also easily recognized at CT, although they are not a useful criterion for distinguishing mechanical obstruction from paralysis. A gastric or jejunal tube may mislead the examiner by decompressing the proximal small bowel loops. Direct visualization of the abrupt caliber change at the transition zone is the key criterion for distinguishing between paralysis and obstruction.

Postoperative Strangulated Bowel Obstruction

Adhesions, hernias, or volvulus may give rise to a strangulated bowel obstruction that compromises the mesenteric blood supply with risk of ischemia, gangrene, and eventual perforation (bowel decompensation). Unlike an "ordinary" mechanical obstruction, a strangulated or "closed loop" obstruction occludes the bowel (and associated mesenteric vessels) at two sites (e.g., due to volvulus or incarceration of a bowel loop within a hernial opening). This leads to the more rapid development of

An abrupt caliber change at the transition zone is the key for distinguishing between paralysis and obstruction.

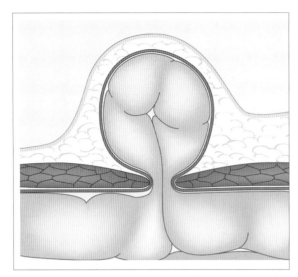

Fig. 5.18 **Diagrammatic representation of vascular strangulation due to herniation, volvulus, etc.**

Causes. The strangulation of a bowel segment may have various causes:

- Bowel may *herniate* through a surgical mesenteric defect, as in cases where the mesentery and peritoneum have not been fully reapproximated during the creation of a stoma.
- Bowel may also herniate through a peritoneal dehiscence in the pelvis, leading to a strangulation that may go undetected for days (**Fig. 5.19**). These *internal hernias* occur when bowel protrudes through a dehiscent suture site in deeper wall layers.
- *Volvulus* may develop secondary to an internal herniation or adhesion. Volvulus should be suspected when markedly dilated bowel loops are found in a setting of postoperative paralysis (**Figs. 5.20, 5.21**).
- Postoperative *intussusception* is rare and occurs predominantly in children (**Fig. 5.22**).
- *Incarceration* occurs when the bowel is narrowed at two or more adjacent sites, usually due to compression, with one or more bowel segments forming a closed loop (**Fig. 5.23**).

intestinal ischemia, necrosis, and peritonitis than an ordinary mechanical obstruction (**Fig. 5.18**). Strangulation is an acute surgical emergency with a mortality rate higher than 40%, compared with less than 10% for an appropriately treated, nonstrangulated obstruction.

Symptoms. Incarceration with strangulation and bowel decompensation is marked by the rapid development of an acute abdomen. Clinical hallmarks are constant ab-

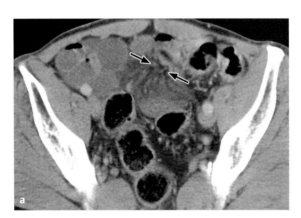

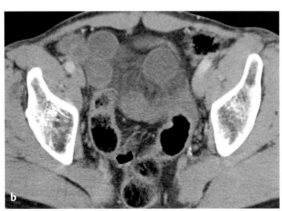

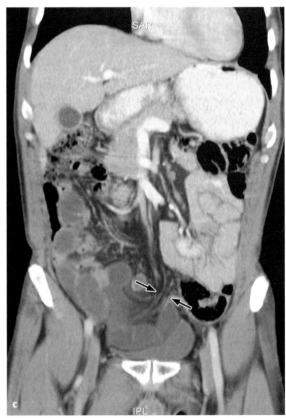

Fig. 5.19 a–c **Strangulated bowel obstruction with twisting of the vascular pedicle.**
Note the slight wall enhancement in the affected bowel segment and the venous dilatation caused by the strangulation.

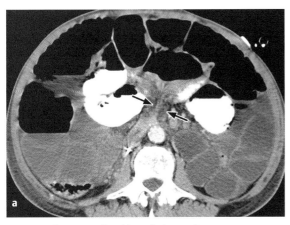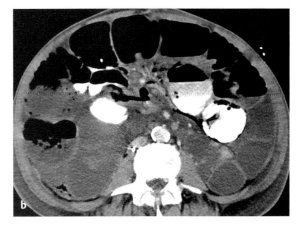

Fig. 5.20 a, b **Strangulated bowel obstruction.**
Torsion of the mesenteric vascular pedicle is accompanied by diffuse pneumatosis intestinalis with gas in the mesenteric venous system. This indicates that significant bowel wall necrosis has already occurred.

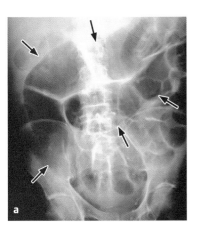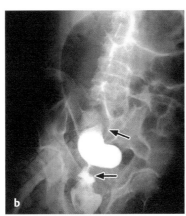

Fig. 5.21 a, b **Sigmoid volvulus.**
a Plain abdominal radiograph shows marked prestenotic dilatation of the elongated sigmoid colon.
b Contrast enema demonstrates abrupt luminal tapering due to torsion.

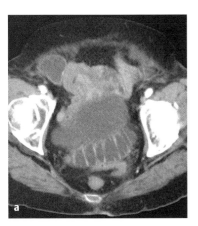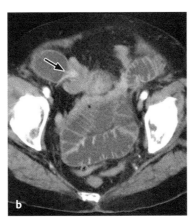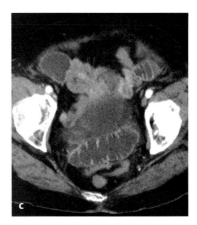

Fig. 5.22 a–c **Intussusception.**
Intussusception may be transient and asymptomatic, in which case it is noted as an incidental finding. An intussusception is considered pathologic only when associated with bowel dilatation and clinical symptoms.

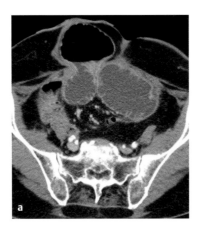
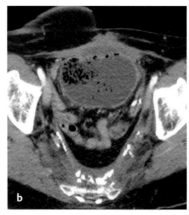

Fig. 5.23 a, b **Incarceration.**
a Small bowel has herniated through an abdominal wall defect, causing vascular strangulation (closed-loop incarceration)
b Small bowel feces sign of mechanical obstruction (see also **Fig. 5.18**, p. 166).

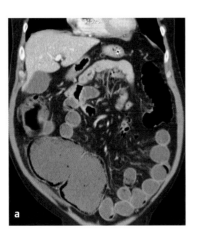
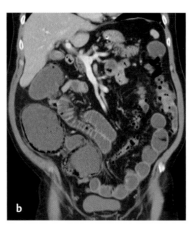

Fig. 5.24 a, b **Pneumatosis intestinalis.** The condition is characterized here by marked dilatation and pneumatosis of the ascending colon ("blowout" colon).

dominal pain, tachycardia, fever, rigidity, leukocytosis, and metabolic acidosis with an elevated LDH.

Computed Tomography

A closed-loop incarceration consists of a mechanical obstruction involving the entrapment of a bowel segment and its mesentery at two closely adjacent sites, usually due to an adhesion or herniation.

CT demonstrates signs of small bowel obstruction with fluid-filled small bowel loops arranged in a radial, C-shaped or U-shaped pattern with the mesenteric supply vessels converging toward the site of the obstruction.

When a closed-loop obstruction is associated with strangulation, causing intestinal ischemia due to vascular occlusion, the obstruction becomes an acute emergency.

A strangulated obstruction is diagnosed when two or more of the following CT signs are accompanied by signs of an obstruction (**Fig. 5.24**):
- bowel wall thickening (> 3 mm) with or without a concentric ring pattern of contrast enhancement (target or halo sign), excluding inflammatory bowel changes
- pneumatosis intestinalis

- high attenuation of the bowel wall on unenhanced CT scans (usually > 20 HU due to venous stasis)
- air in the portal vein or a mesenteric vessel
- air in the bowel wall (pneumatosis intestinalis)
- mesenteric infiltration or hemorrhage or free fluid
- decreased or heterogeneous enhancement of the bowel wall after IV contrast administration

The most specific CT signs of intestinal ischemia are gas formation in the portal vein and pneumatosis intestinalis (see **Fig. 5.20**). These signs are rarely found in a strangulated obstruction, however. At the same time, bowel wall thickening with or without a target enhancement pattern may also be seen in inflammatory bowel disease. Thus while these signs are relatively sensitive, they are not very specific.

Ischemic Bowel Obstruction

See the section Acute Intestinal Ischemia in Chapter 4, page 140.

Intestinal ischemia due to thromboembolic vascular occlusion without strangulation is among the most dreaded postoperative complications.

Complications of Specific Operations

C. Schaefer-Prokop,
S. Kreuzer, and
T. Sautner

This section deals with the detection of early complications that are typical of certain operations. As with any postoperative complication, it is important to elicit as much information as possible on the nature of the previous surgery to distinguish normal postoperative findings from pathology.

After Esophageal Surgery

Normal Postoperative Findings

After Fundoplication

One of the most common operations for gastroesophageal reflux is the *Nissen fundoplication*, which today is usually performed laparoscopically. It is important to recognize that the fundoplication creates a kind of pseudotumor close to the gastric cardia. Other "noncircumferential" fundoplication techniques (e. g., Belsey Mark IV, Hill) can mimic intrathoracic hernias.

After Tumor Resection

Various resection techniques are employed:
- With a complete esophageal resection and gastric pull-up reconstruction (Akiyama procedure), the anastomosis may be located at a cervical (extrathoracic) or intrathoracic level.
- When small bowel or colon is interposed, the cervical anastomosis is accompanied by multiple intra-abdominal anastomoses.

Complications

After Fundoplication

Perforation of the *posterior esophageal wall* is a possibility after laparoscopic procedures due to limitations of intraoperative vision (**Fig. 5.25a**). Another early complication is mediastinal or pleural *hematoma formation* (**Fig. 5.25b**). Other nonacute reasons for persistent postoperative complaints may relate to a fundoplication that is too narrow or too broad, injury to the vagus nerve, torsion of the esophagus above the fundoplication, or intrathoracic herniation of the fundoplication.

After Tumor Resection

The complication rate after esophageal surgery is higher than after other gastrointestinal surgery because it is more difficult for the esophagus to retain sutures and staples. This is due partly to the absence of a serosal layer on the esophagus and because the transposed stomach or interposed bowel segment may compromise blood flow.

Anastomotic leak. The principal complication, known as the "Achilles heel" of esophageal surgery, is anastomotic leak, which occurs in up to 20% of cases, even at experienced centers. The cervical anastomosis is more commonly affected than the mediastinal anastomosis, although a leaky thoracic anastomosis is associated with higher morbidity.

The leak itself is diagnosed by oral (intraluminal) contrast administration. CT is best for evaluating the degree of mediastinal infiltration, abscess formation, and involvement of the pleural space (empyema) (**Fig. 5.26**). While leaks accessible to external drainage can sometimes be successfully managed conservatively, large leaks with associated mediastinitis will necessitate reoperation.

> Anastomotic leak is the principal complication of esophageal surgery, occurring in up to 20% of cases, even at experienced centers.

After Gastric Surgery

It is generally best to perform a partial gastrectomy rather than a total gastrectomy if the tumor location permits it. Total gastrectomy has a significantly higher complication rate (anastomotic leak) and results in poorer postoperative quality of life (malnutrition).

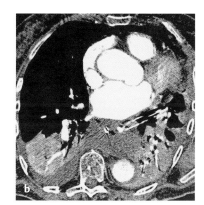

Fig. 5.25 a, b **Complications after a Nissen fundoplication.**
a Pseudotumor thickening of the cardioesophageal junction is a normal finding, but free air indicates a perforation.
b Hematoma in the posterior mediastinum, accompanied by lower lobe atelectasis and bilateral thoracostomy tubes.

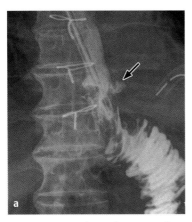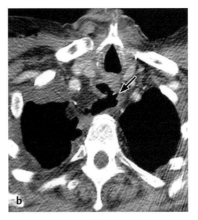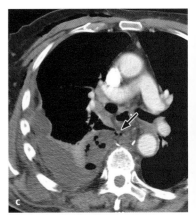

Fig. 5.26 a–c **Findings after an esophageal resection in two patients.**

a   Water-soluble oral contrast examination demonstrates a small suture-line leak.

b, c   Extensive leakage from the proximal anastomosis with pleural empyema.

Normal Postoperative Findings

The Billroth I and II operations are two types of reconstruction performed after a (partial) gastrectomy (**Fig. 5.27**).

Billroth I. This operation involves a partial gastrectomy (antrectomy) and duodenectomy followed by an end-to-end anastomosis. Variants do not utilize the entire cross-section for the anastomosis (Polya procedure), but anastomose only part of the cross-section (Hofmeister modification) and close the rest. The Billroth I anastomosis (visible on CT by metal clips or staples) is located just behind the left lobe of the liver or, if the duodenum retains its original anatomic position, in the subhepatic peripancreatic space.

Billroth II. In this operation the duodenal stump is closed and the stomach is anastomosed to the jejunum. The type of anastomosis and location of the afferent duodenal loop are variable (short retrocolic stump vs. longer antecolic stump). The adjacent jejunal limbs can be joined by a side-to-side anastomosis. Orientation is aided by restoring continuity between the residual duodenum and the jejunum. The afferent and efferent jejunal limbs may be placed anterior or just posterior to the colon.

Total gastroduodenectomy. Postoperative anatomy is similar to that of the Billroth II operation: an end-to-side or end-to-end anastomosis is created between the esophagus and jejunum (Roux-en-Y esophagojejunostomy). The orthotopic duodenal stump is closed proximally and joined to the jejunum distally by an end-to-side anastomosis (Roux-Y technique).

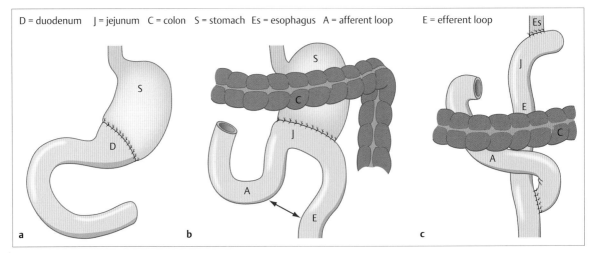

D = duodenum   J = jejunum   C = colon   S = stomach   Es = esophagus   A = afferent loop   E = efferent loop

Fig. 5.27 a–c **Types of reconstruction after gastric resections.**

a   Billroth I: gastroduodenostomy with an end-to-end anastomosis.

b   Billroth II: gastrojejunostomy.

c   Roux-en-Y esophagojejunostomy after total gastrectomy.

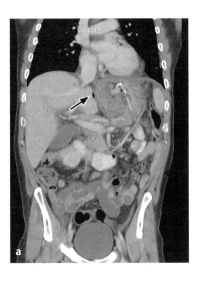 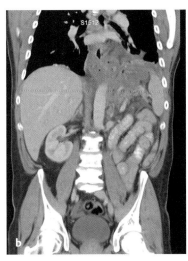

Fig. 5.28 a, b **Anastomotic leak.**
This patient underwent a Nissen fundoplication and Billroth I gastrectomy for ulcers. Subsequent total gastrectomy was performed. An anastomotic leak (**a**) is associated with free air and a large abscess that extends into the mediastinum (**b**).

Table 5.12 Complications after partial or total gastrectomy

- Intra-abdominal bleeding
- Mediastinal hematoma and hemothorax
- Wound infection
- Anastomotic leak with abscess formation (**Fig. 5.28**)
- Pancreatitis
- Afferent loop syndrome
- Mechanical obstruction (herniation, kinking, intussusception, or recurrent tumor)

Complications

Gastrectomy is associated with relatively high peri- and postoperative morbidity. Complications may result from infection or may relate to the surgical procedure (anastomotic leak, hemorrhage) (**Table 5.12**).

Leaks

Leaks may occur at any anastomosis. Dehiscence is particularly common in the efferent limbs of a Billroth II or Roux-en-Y reconstruction. The imaging modality of choice is CT after oral and IV contrast administration.

The mesentery and ligaments are mobilized during the operation, compromising their function as natural anatomical barriers. As a result, postoperative fluid collections may be found at unusual sites:

- Mobilizing the gastrocolic and gastrosplenic ligaments creates a direct communication between the lesser sac and subphrenic space.
- Mobilizing or resecting the gastrohepatic ligament creates a communication between the lesser sac, gastrohepatic space, and gastrosplenic space. This "neocompartment" between the lesser sac, liver, gastric remnant, and spleen is a frequent site of postoperative abscess formation.

- Smaller collections are usually located in the *left* subphrenic space (negative abdominal pressure during respiration).

Leakage from the duodenal stump is likely to produce complications because the escaping pancreatic and biliary fluid may incite a chemical peritonitis and infection. Fluid collections and abscesses are most commonly located in the right subhepatic space or at peripancreatic sites. Duodenal stump leaks should be surgically repaired!

After Pancreatic Surgery (Whipple Operation)

The most common surgical procedure on the pancreas, called the Kausch–Whipple operation (pancreaticoduodenectomy, PD), includes a duodenectomy, a partial or complete pancreatectomy, resection of the gastric antrum, and the resection of a short segment of jejunum in most cases (**Fig. 5.29a**). Gastrointestinal continuity is restored by:

- pancreaticojejunostomy (after partial resections)
- choledochojejunostomy
- gastrojejunostomy

When the pylorus is preserved (pylorus-preserving pancreaticoduodenectomy, PPPD), an anastomosis is created between the jejunum and the postpyloric duodenal stump (**Fig. 5.29b**).

Leaks may occur at any anastomotic site. The imaging modality of choice is contrast-enhanced CT.

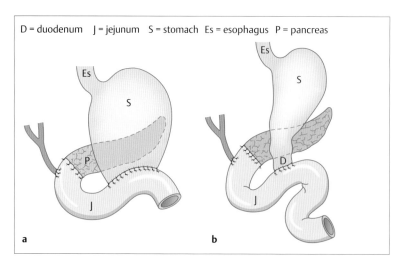

D = duodenum   J = jejunum   S = stomach   Es = esophagus   P = pancreas

Fig. 5.29 a, b **Types of reconstruction after pancreatic resections.**

a   A Whipple pancreaticoduodenectomy with resection of the pancreatic head, antrum, and duodenum is followed by the creation of three anastomoses: a gastrojejunostomy, a pancreaticojejunostomy, and a choledochojejunostomy.

b   In a pylorus-preserving pancreaticoduodenectomy (PPPD), the pylorus and a short segment of duodenum are preserved.

Normal Postoperative Findings

Owing to the frequent delay of gastric emptying that occurs after pancreatic surgery and poor retrograde opacification with contrast medium, the proximal jejunal limb (Roux limb) is poorly visualized and the bilioenteric or pancreaticoenteric anastomosis is correspondingly difficult to evaluate. The proximal jejunal limb is often located in the gallbladder bed or porta hepatis after the operation and should not be mistaken for an abscess.

— **Practical Recommendation** —————

The afferent limb may be mistaken at follow-up for an abscess or tumor unless the specifics of the operation are known. Small bowel is identified by the presence of valvulae conniventes. Oral contrast opacification of the afferent limb can be improved by the IV administration of 1 mg glucagon (see **Fig. 5.31**).

More than 80% of patients undergoing PD are found to have postoperative fluid collections in the pancreatic bed, Morison pouch, and right paracolic gutter. In most cases these collections are reabsorbed within a matter of days. Clinical suspicion of infection should be investigated by follow-up and by fine-needle aspiration if necessary.

Up to 80% of patients undergoing PD have postoperative fluid collections in the pancreatic bed, Morison pouch, and right paracolic gutter.

Complications

Anastomotic Leaks

The *pancreaticoenteric anastomosis* has a particularly high complication rate (ca. 15%) in nonfibrotic pancreatic parenchyma (tumor surgery). A leak is evidenced by a change in the composition of the drainage material (lipase and amylase detection). Adequate drainage of the anastomotic site should significantly improve or relieve systemic symptoms. The placement of additional drains

may be indicated. Reoperation and revision of the anastomosis are associated with a high risk of further leakage.

Leakage from a biliary-enteric anastomosis is confirmed by the presence of bile in the drainage material (**Fig. 5.30**).

Abscesses can be positively identified only by detecting small air bubbles within the lesion. Basically any fluid collection may become superinfected (suspicious clinical signs, needle aspiration). Abscesses may form at various sites: subphrenic, intrahepatic, in the cul-de-sac, in the gallbladder bed (the gallbladder is usually removed!), or in the lesser sac. It is common to find multiple abscesses that do not communicate with one another and thus require separate drainage.

— **Practical Recommendation** —————

Helpful criteria for distinguishing a fluid-filled loop of jejunum from an abscess are oral contrast opacification (**Fig. 5.31**, not always successful), air–fluid levels, IV contrast administration to detect bowel wall enhancement, and the identification of

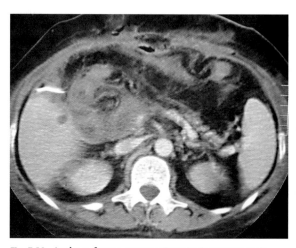

Fig. 5.30 **Leakage from a pancreaticoenteric anastomosis** after partial pancreatectomy and drain insertion.

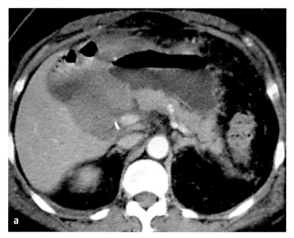

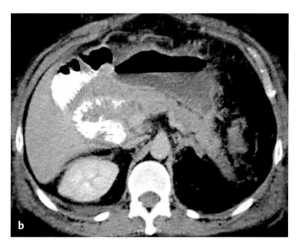

Fig. 5.31 a, b   CT findings after a Whipple operation.

a   Axial scan demonstrates a large abscess with a fluid level in the lesser sac. Parahepatic evaluation is difficult without opacification of the bowel loops.

b   Oral contrast opacification of the afferent bowel loop shows no parahepatic abnormalities. The abscess is confined to the lesser sac.

intestinal folds. Follow-up images are helpful in doubtful cases, as the jejunal loop will change its shape whereas an abscess will not.

After Biliary Tract Surgery

Complications

The bile ducts are very sensitive to ischemic complications, which may include intrahepatic or subhepatic biliomas and leakage from a biliary–enteric anastomosis (hepaticojejunostomy). Adequate transabdominal and/or transhepatic drainage is essential for the prevention of sepsis (**Fig. 5.32**).

Some surgeons fix the blind jejunal loop (into which the bile duct drains) to the abdominal wall to facilitate percutaneous access to the anastomosis.

After Cholecystectomy

Complications

Postoperative complications in cholecystectomy patients are an important issue for radiologists due to the sheer number of cholecystectomies that are performed. Today most hospitals offer laparoscopic cholecystectomy as a preferred alternative to open techniques (**Table 5.13**). ERCP (endoscopic retrograde cholangiopancreatography) is used in both the diagnosis and treatment of biliary tract diseases.

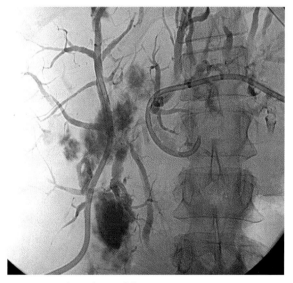

▶ Jejunum is distinguished from the abscess by noting changes in the shape of bowel loop on serial images.

Fig. 5.32   **Leakage from a biliary–enteric anastomosis** with extensive contrast extravasation and a percutaneous biliary drain.

Table 5.13   Complications of gallbladder operations

Complications after laparoscopy (trocar placement)
- Abdominal wall hematoma
- Vascular injuries (intra- and retroperitoneal)
- Gastrointestinal perforation
- Perforation of the bladder or ureter
- Infection
- Parenchymal injuries (liver, kidneys)

Complications after cholecystectomy
- Bleeding
- Biliary tract injury
- Leak, bilioma
- Infection

Impacted Stones

Stones impacted in the bile ducts are most easily detected by T-drain cholangiography in cases where a T-drain was placed during the initial biliary surgery. The bile ducts should also be visualized by MRCP (magnetic resonance cholangiopanceatography).

Bile Leaks

Bile leakage most commonly occurs from the *cystic duct stump* or from *aberrant bile ducts* (6% incidence), and therefore bile leaks can be recognized primarily as free fluid located at a typical site. Postoperative bile leak is confirmed by the presence of bile in the drainage fluid. It may result from faulty clip placement or postischemic necrosis of the biliary stump. Most bile leaks will close spontaneously in response to decompression (drainage).

A small bile leak is reabsorbed or evacuated through the subhepatic drain. Fluid collections in the gallbladder bed after cholecystectomy are found in 20% of patients without drainage of the gallbladder bed and in less than 5% of patients with drainage (normal finding in the first 5 postoperative days).

Superinfection (e. g., with *Escherichia coli*) is a potentially serious complication. Even a small amount of bile leaking into the abdominal cavity can lead to *abscess formation*, which may occur even at distant sites.

The more acute the gallbladder surgery (cholecystitis, perforation), the greater the risk of a leak (poor ligation of the cystic duct stump, injury due to atypical biliary anatomy). CT can detect drain dislodgement or the spread of a bile leak past the subhepatic space to other compart-

ments (**Fig. 5.33a**). Bile peritonitis is a life-threatening complication with a mortality rate of up to 50%.

Leakage from a biliary–enteric anastomosis (e. g., after resection of gallbladder cancer or Klatskin tumor) is confirmed by the presence of bile in the drain output.

— Practical Recommendation ———

A *massive primary bile leak* requires immediate revision. For example, the anastomosis for a high resection at the hepatic bifurcation may have missed a segmental bile duct, which will requires reexposure and definitive drainage via the anastomosis.

Biliomas

Biliomas at a subhepatic location can be distinguished from hematomas by their density (10–20 HU) and their configuration, as they are rarely loculated (**Fig. 5.33b**).

Hematomas

Hematomas may form after open and laparoscopic cholecystectomy and may become superinfected (**Figs. 5.33c, 5.34**). They are usually accessible to percutaneous drainage.

After Colorectal Surgery

Proctectomes are associated with a higher complication rate than colon resections. Two main types of proctectomy are performed:

- *Anterior resection* with an end-to-end coloanal anastomosis (usually with staples) or the creation of a

> **▶** Leaks are more likely after acute gallbladder surgery for cholecystitis or perforation than after elective operations.

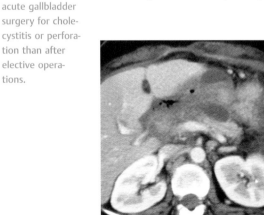 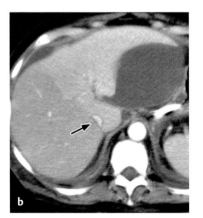 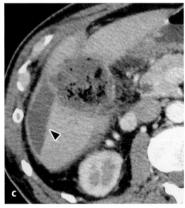

Fig. 5.33 a–c **Complication after cholecystectomy.**

a Infected bile leak with contralateral spread and reactive infiltration of the left perirenal space.

b Uninfected subcapsular bilioma. Note the swelling of the liver with compression of the inferior vena cava and hypoperfusion of the right hepatic lobe due to compression of the right portal vein branch.

c Infected sub(extra)hepatic hematoma accompanied by an uninfected subcapsular hematoma (arrowhead).

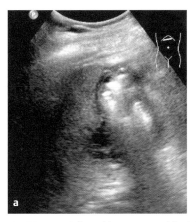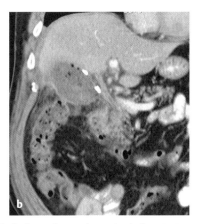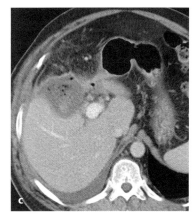

Fig. 5.34 a–c **Infected hematoma with air inclusions after endoscopic cholecystectomy.**

colon pouch (Kock pouch, TS pouch, J or W pouch constructed from the distal colon), which yields a better functional result, or the creation of a temporary stoma.

- *Abdominoperineal resection* (T4 tumors), which involves an en-bloc resection of the rectum (total mesorectal excision) and the creation of a colostomy.

Complications

Possible complications after colon surgery are abscess formation, obstructive strictures, bleeding, anastomotic dehiscence, and urinary retention due to ureteral stenosis.

Anastomotic Leak

Reoperation is indicated in patients with an intra-abdominal anastomotic leak and signs of peritonitis.

Approximately 10% of anterior resections develop an anastomotic leak due to tension created by inadequate mobilization of the left colic flexure or as a result of diminished blood flow (**Figs. 5.35, 5.36**).

— Practical Recommendation —————

A small leak not associated with systemic inflammatory signs can be treated conservatively (percutaneous drainage). Persistent leakage and persistent abscesses (**Fig. 5.36**) require the construction of a protective stoma. This is particularly indicated in patients with an underlying inflammatory bowel disease (diverticulitis, ulcerative colitis, or Crohn disease).

Bleeding

Colorectal surgery is associated with an increased risk of *intra- and perioperative bleeding* (e.g., due to mobilization of the left flexure, splenic injury, or bleeding from the sacral venous plexus in a mesorectal excision). The risk of bleeding after a proctectomy increases with involvement of the presacral venous plexus.

Anastomotic bleeding is somewhat rare in colon surgery. An exception is subtotal colectomy for ulcerative

Up to 10% of anterior resections develop an anastomotic leak. A protective stoma should be created if the leak persists during drainage.

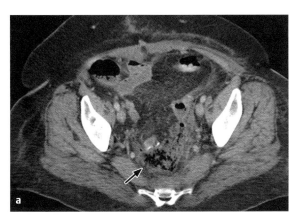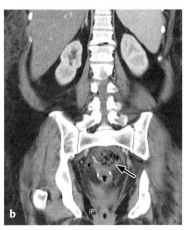

Fig. 5.35 a, b **Anastomotic leak with local abscess formation after a sigmoid colon resection for diverticulitis.**

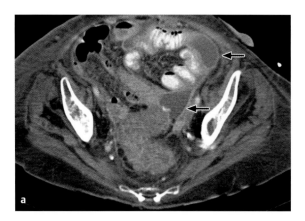
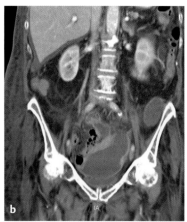

Fig. 5.36 a, b **Anastomotic leak with diffuse peritonitis and multiple loop abscesses following a sigmoid colon resection for perforated diverticulitis.**

colitis, where serious bleeding may occur from the remaining portion of the rectum. Bleeding after an appendectomy most commonly occurs from the divided mesoappendix (especially after a mass ligation).

After (Partial) Nephrectomy

Complications

Postoperative complications after renal surgery or interventions include subcapsular, perirenal and pararenal hematomas (with or without parenchymal injury), injuries to the renal collecting system, and the faulty placement of ureteral stents and nephrostomy tubes.

Imaging

Extracorporeal shock-wave lithotripsy (ESWL) is often followed by a latent period that precedes hematoma formation. Imaging is done to evaluate the extent of the hematoma and the distribution of blood. Small subcapsular hematomas may be missed on ultrasound scans. Fresh hematomas are echo-free and show increasing echogenicity over time. They are initially hyperdense on CT (60–80 HU) and show a steady decline of attenuation values during subsequent days and weeks. Large hematomas are often inhomogeneous. Injuries to the collecting system are extremely rare (< 1%).

Postoperative imaging modalities after *pyeloplasty* (e. g., for ureteropelvic or subpelvic stenosis), *ureteroneocystostomy*, or *ureteral reconstruction* (e. g., for distal ureteral stenosis) include ultrasonography and contrast visualization of the collecting system via a pyelostomy. An intravenous pyelogram (IVP) to evaluate outflow should be delayed until the drains have been removed on postoperative day 10–12. Dilatation is normally present and

should not be interpreted as evidence of a new obstruction. A relative constriction due to edema is often present at the level of the anastomosis. Hematomas and leaks are detectable by ultrasonography or CT, depending on their extent.

The initial imaging studies after total or partial nephrectomy or nephroureterectomy are ultrasonography (hematoma, urinoma) and IVP (outflow, leakage), which are performed at ca. 10 days. Equivocal cases require further evaluation by contrast-enhanced CT (delayed scans). Vascular complications that present with persistent bleeding or hematuria (e. g., aneurysm, AV fistula) are usually managed by endovascular therapy. It is normal to find perirenal or pararenal air inclusions for up to 10 days postoperatively. Imaging findings must be interpreted within the context of clinical and laboratory findings to distinguish simple fluid collections from infected collections during this period. If contrast use is contraindicated, imaging should rely on MRI (T1-weighted imaging with and without fat saturation to differentiate fluid infiltration from fat).

Postoperative mechanical small bowel obstruction develops in ca. 5% of patients following the construction of an ileal conduit.

After Renal Transplantation

Acute Complications

Early surgical and nephrologic complications after renal transplantation may compromise the function of the renal allograft.

Surgical complications include perirenal fluid collections (hematoma, abscess, lymphocele, urinoma), vascular problems (anastomotic stricture, renal vein thrombo-

■ Ultrasonography and IVP are the imaging studies of choice for evaluating outflow after renal surgery, generally on postoperative day 10–12. CT should be used in equivocal cases.

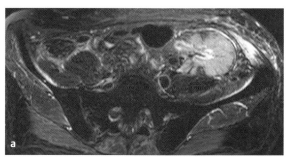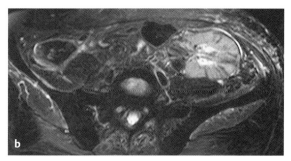

Fig. 5.37 a, b **Acute renal allograft rejection presenting as acute nephritis.**
Note the streaky, inhomogeneous signal pattern of the renal parenchyma with wedge-shaped subcapsular signal voids (with kind permission of H. Shin, Hannover Medical College).

sis), and ureteral problems (urine leakage, stenosis of the neo-ostium).

Ureteral outflow obstruction in the early postoperative period may be caused by kinking, intraluminal thrombi, edema, or inflammation. Ureteral obstruction at later stages may result from scarring, ischemia, or extraluminal compression of the ureter (lymphocele).

Nephrologic complications are acute graft rejection (**Fig. 5.37**), acute tubular necrosis, and cyclosporin A toxicity.

Diagnostic Strategy

Ultrasonography is the imaging modality of choice for defining the renal allograft, perirenal/periureteral fluid collections, or a urinary tract obstruction. Duplex scanning can detect narrowing or occlusion of the renal artery, thrombosis of the renal vein, or obstructive vasopathy in the setting of allograft rejection.

IVP, conventional angiography, CT or MR angiography, and CT or MR urography are second-line adjunctive studies in patients with suspected complications involving blood vessels or the excretory portion of the urinary tract.

Imaging

Perirenal Fluid Collections

Perirenal fluid collections are a common finding after renal transplantation. The differential diagnosis includes hematomas, seromas, urinomas, lymphoceles, and abscesses in cases of infection. Often the fluid cannot be identified by its echogenicity, but the collections can be differentiated by taking into account other morphologic criteria and postoperative time of occurrence. Ultrasound-guided fine-needle aspiration is diagnostic.

Hematoma. A hematoma is echogenic in the acute stage and becomes less echogenic over time. Internal septa-

tions are frequently present. With an extraperitoneal graft placement, the hematoma is usually loculated and may compress the organ. The hematoma associated with an intraperitoneal graft can spread freely. Postoperative enlargement of the hematoma over time is suggestive of a complication, so it is imperative to document the initial size. Hematomas have high T1- and T2-weighted signal intensity on MRI, which serves to distinguish them from other collections.

Abscess. An abscess after renal transplantation typically presents as a perirenal fluid collection in a febrile patient. CT and MRI are more sensitive than ultrasonography for detecting air inclusions in the perirenal collection and demonstrating rim enhancement.

Urinoma. Urinomas may result from an ischemic leak in the ureter or may form at the ureterovesical anastomosis. They develop in 3–10% of patients during the first five postoperative weeks and require immediate radiologic or surgical intervention. Less common than hematomas, they present with pain and urine in the drainage fluid. The diagnosis is confirmed by scintigraphy (leakage of ^{99m}Tc-DTPA into the peritoneal cavity) or by noting contrast extravasation on delayed MR images or CT scans.

Lymphocele. Lymphoceles occur in ca. 15% of transplant recipients 4–8 weeks after the operation. Because most patients are asymptomatic, lymphoceles are often an incidental finding. Treatment (aspiration, drainage, surgery) is necessary only if the lymphocele produces a mass effect causing ureteral compression and outflow obstruction. The late occurrence of a lymphocele is commonly associated with allograft rejection. A lymphocele has fluid attenuation on CT scans and does not enhance after IV contrast administration. It is devoid of signal on T1-weighted MRI and hyperintense on T2-weighted MRI.

> Ultrasonography is the imaging study of choice initially for evaluating the renal allograft.

Vascular Complications

Acute tubular necrosis. Acute tubular necrosis results from prolonged ischemia and is a cause of delayed graft function, which should resolve spontaneously within the following 2 weeks. The diagnosis is confirmed by scintigraphy.

Rejection. The stages of acute allograft rejection are diagnosed by scintigraphy or biopsy. A resistance index (RI) > 0.8 by Doppler ultrasound imaging is an indicator with a reported sensitivity and specificity ranging from 14% to 98% in the literature. A reversal of diastolic flow is another indicator of graft rejection. Depending on the stage, ultrasound imaging may show diffuse organ swelling, mild hydronephrosis, increased or decreased echogenicity of the parenchymal rim, loss of corticomedullary differentiation, and increased prominence of the medullary pyramids.

Renal artery stenosis. Renal artery stenosis (< 10%) can lead to refractory hypertension and organ dysfunction. Most stenoses are close to the anastomosis and a few are located further peripherally on the recipient side.

Renal vein thrombosis. Renal vein thrombosis is a rare complication that usually occurs during the first postoperative week. It may be caused by stenosis close to the anastomosis, hypovolemia, or extrinsic compression by extrarenal fluid collections. Absence of venous flow and a plateaulike inversion of diastolic flow in the renal artery are diagnostic.

AV fistula and pseudoaneurysm. Arteriovenous (AV) fistulas (**Fig. 5.38**) or an arterial pseudoaneurysm are complications of percutaneous biopsy. Most are small and will often resolve spontaneously. Renal ischemia may develop as an adverse sequela. A "machine sound" on Doppler ultrasound scanning combined with a focal zone of increased turbulence are pathognomonic.

Obstruction of the Renal Collecting System and Ureter

Fewer than 5% of renal transplant recipients develop a urinary tract obstruction caused by ureteral kinking, extraureteral compression (hematoma, lymphocele, etc.), an ischemic or edema-related stricture, or other causes. Affected patients are asymptomatic, and the obstruction is diagnosed by (routine) ultrasonography.

It should be noted that the ureter and collecting system of the graft are normally somewhat dilated due to the denervated, hypotonic condition of the transplanted organ. A rising creatinine level or progressive hydronephrosis are indicators of pathologic obstruction.

After Liver Transplantation

Acute Complications

While imaging has no role in the diagnosis of graft rejection, it plays a key role in the diagnosis of vascular and biliary complications (**Table 5.14**). The primary imaging modality is ultrasonography, including Doppler. Multidetector CT has established itself as a sensitive modality that is less dependent on patient constitution.

In early imaging after liver transplantation, special attention is given to the *anastomoses. Arterial complications* are the most important differential diagnosis in early postoperative complications. They may necessitate retransplantation, depending on their severity, and have a high mortality. Arterial complications are more frequent than venous complications. All complications, whether vascular or biliary, are more common in split-liver transplantations.

Since the bile ducts are supplied entirely by the hepatic artery, any biliary complication is suspicious for some type of hepatic artery pathology (**Fig. 5.39**).

The following are common postoperative findings that do not necessarily indicate a serious problem: right-sided pleural effusion, pulmonary segmental atelectasis, peri-

Vascular complications are acute tubular necrosis, acute and chronic rejection (occlusive vasculopathy), and the stenosis or thrombotic occlusion of an artery or vein.

Since the bile ducts are supplied entirely by the hepatic artery, any biliary complication is suspicious for hepatic artery pathology.

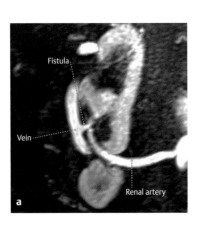
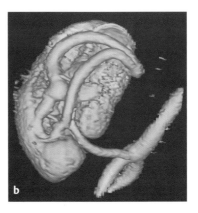

Fig. 5.38 a, b **AV fistula after renal biopsy, demonstrated by MR angiography (with kind permission of H. Shin, Hannover Medical College).**

Table 5.14 **Complications after liver transplantation**

Operating technique	Type of complication	Symptoms	Diagnosis
Hepatic artery: "fish-mouth" reconstruction, Carrell patch between celiac trunk (recipient) and hepatic artery at the origin of the gastroduodenal artery (donor) or hepatic bifurcation (donor)	Thrombosis (4–12%): typical early complication, more common in children (42%) Stenosis (5–11%) and secondary thrombosis, usually near the anastomosis	Bile duct necrosis, biliary stricture, bile leak, intrahepatic biliomas, hepatic infarction, hepatic necrosis or abscess (sepsis)	▪ Doppler: peak flow velocity > 2 m/s, turbulent flow with flattened and broadened waveform, RI decreased to < 0.55, SAT increased to > 0.08 s ▪ MDCTA
Portal vein: end-to-end anastomosis (often difficult to locate)	Thrombosis/stenosis in 1–3% due to mismatch of vascular diameters	Portal hypertension, ascites, edema, hemorrhage, organ failure	▪ MDCTA ▪ Transhepatic venography
Inferior vena cava: (1) resection of the recipient retrohepatic vena cava with a double end-to-end anastomosis, or (2) end-to-side or end-to-end anastomosis of the donor hepatic veins directly to the recipient vena cava (piggy-back technique)	Thrombosis/stenosis in < 1% due to coagulopathy or faulty anastomosis	Acute Budd–Chiari syndrome: hepatomegaly, ascites, limb edema	
	Arterioportal fistula after biopsy, usually closes spontaneously within weeks		MDCTA: early opacification of portal branches before the mesenteric veins, wedge-shaped area of increased blood flow
Anastomosis between common bile duct (recipient) and hepatic duct (donor) after cholecystectomy via T-drain; if the recipient duct is abnormal, the donor duct is implanted directly into the bowel via a stent after creating a Roux limb	Biliary complications: ▪ Strictures (6–34%, most in the first 3 months) ▪ Leak (4%) at the anastomosis or due to ischemia after occlusion/stenosis of the hepatic artery	Cholestasis is often absent! This does *not* exclude stenosis. Strictures close to the anastomosis caused by a cast or intraductal debris should raise suspicion of an hepatic artery stenosis. Strictures at sites farther from the anastomosis (10%), such as the hepatic bifurcation, may be caused by: ▪ arterial ischemia ▪ infection ▪ primary sclerosing cholangitis	▪ MRCP (Teslascan) ▪ T-drain cholangiography ▪ Scintigraphy (99 mTc-IDA)
	Ischemia of hepatic parenchyma ▪ Subcapsular focal areas due to surgery or transport are innocent and should regress in weeks ▪ Peripheral wedge-shaped areas or more central areas are suspicious for arterial ischemia		
	Ascites, bilioma, hematoma		

SAT: systolic acceleration time = time between end diastole and systolic peak.
RI: resistance index = peak systolic velocity – peak diastolic velocity/peak systolic velocity.
MRCP: magnetic resonance cholangiopancreaticography.
MDCTA: multidetector computed tomographic angiography.

hepatic fluid (ascites, seroma, small hematoma), right-sided adrenal hematoma (surgically induced), and periportal edema due to impaired lymphatic drainage.

After Surgery or Stenting of an Aortic Aneurysm

Complications

CT angiography is the method of choice for detecting complications following stent-graft implantation or a vascular intervention (**Table 5.15**). Both precontrast and de-layed scans are necessary for the documentation of slow and delayed contrast extravasation from an endoleak.

As a general rule, a significant amount of periaortic *fluid* should not be present after the stenting of an aortic aneurysm. A significant fluid collection indicates a complication.

Postoperative CT scans immediately after stent grafting may demonstrate *air bubbles* in the thrombus. The bypassed lumen should become fully thrombosed and may shrink over time but should at least maintain a constant diameter.

Any size increase over time (relative to prior images) is suspicious for the presence of an *endoleak*, defined as reperfusion of the aneurysm despite stent grafting. Five

▣ Periaortic fluid after stent grafting indicates a complication.

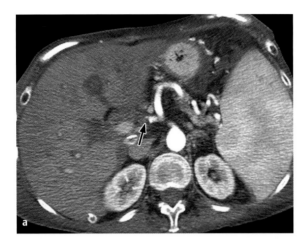

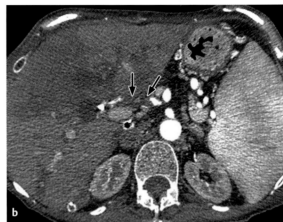

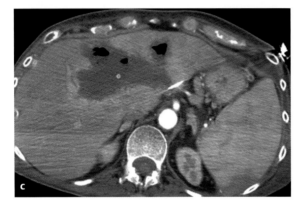

Fig. 5.39 a–c **Thrombosis of the hepatic artery following liver transplantation.**
- **a** Thrombotic occlusion of the hepatic artery with bile leakage and periportal edema.
- **b** Scan 2 days later shows increasing demarcation of a bilioma with a drain in place. Partial arterial occlusion is still present.
- **c** Air inclusions following drainage of the bilioma. (With kind permission of H. Shin, Hannover Medical College.)

Table 5.15   Complications after a vascular graft or bypass

Acute anastomotic leak
- Pseudoaneurysm
- Perigraft perfusion
- Confined perforation
- Suture-line leak with hemorrhage

Chronic anastomotic leak
- Pseudoaneurysm

Hemorrhagic complications
- Local hematoma
- Retroperitoneal or mediastinal hematoma
- Cardiac tamponade
- Hemorrhagic pleural effusion
- Hemoperitoneum

Infection
- Prosthetic infection
- Abscess
- Mycotic aneurysm
- Aortotracheal or aortoenteric fistula

Malperfusion
- Dissection (iatrogenic)
- Vascular occlusion (thrombosis)
- Stenosis (anastomosis)
- Organ infarction (especially of the cerebrum, bowel, or kidney)

types are distinguished according to the cause and location of the leak (**Table 5.16**).

The following points should be noted:

- *Type I and type III leaks* may require immediate intervention, even in acute cases, depending on clinical symptoms or documented enlargement of the aneurysm sac. Other types of leak are treated electively.

- *Anastomotic complications* may present as a confined perforation, a pseudoaneurysm, perigraft perfusion, or a free perforation. A pseudoaneurysm appears on CT as a circumscribed dilatation with thin walls.

- *Perigraft infection* is characterized by periprosthetic fluid, air inclusions, contrast enhancement of the fluid layer, and perifocal infiltration. A gap of more than 5 mm between the prosthesis and surrounding wall (usually the original vessel wall) after the first postoperative week is considered suspicious for an infection. Since hemostatic agents (e.g., Tabotamp) are packed into the opened sac at the conclusion of aneurysm surgery, the vascular surgeon should be consulted to avoid mistaking that material for a postoperative infection.

- Vascular prostheses always have smooth margins, and any contour irregularities are considered a suspicious sign. Autologous graft materials (veins) do not always have smooth margins, and contour irregularities in

Table 5.16 Endoleak after stent grafting

Type		Description, cause	Treatment
I		Leak at the proximal or distal end of the graft through a gap between the aortic wall and stent graft	Always
	A	Leak at the proximal end (stent migration, stent graft too short, progression of aneurysm)	
	B	Leak at the distal end	
	C	Incomplete occlusion of the iliac artery by the occluder of a monoiliac stent graft	
II		Retrograde perfusion due to an aortic side branch (e. g., from lumbar arteries, inferior mesenteric artery, or accessory renal arteries)	Often
	A	Inflow and outflow through the same artery	
	B	Inflow and outflow through different arteries	
III		Leak or disconnect between stent graft components or tears in the synthetic material	Always
IV		Leak through initially porous material (should stop by 4–6 weeks)	Rarely
Endotension		Increase in the outer diameter of the aneurysm and rising pressure in the aneurysm due to an occult leak (not detectable by imaging)	Always

this case are considered most suspicious when located at the anastomotic site. *Occlusion* of the prosthesis or an occluded Y-limb of an abdominal prosthesis is easily identified by the lack of enhancement after contrast administration. CT angiography cannot supply functional information, however (outflow, collaterals).

Summary

Abdominal drains consist of overflow drains, suction drains, and special drains such as percutaneous biliary drains and catheters for chronic abdominal peritoneal dialysis. Feeding tubes consist of stomach tubes, duodenal tubes, PEG (percutaneous endoscopic gastronomy) tubes, and jejunostomy catheters. The position of PEG tubes and jejunostomy catheters is evaluated by the instillation of water-soluble, nonionic, iodinated contrast medium. The correct placement of urinary tract drains can be confirmed by contrast instillation under fluoroscopic guidance.

Normal postoperative findings include postoperative intra-abdominal fluid collections, which occur in ca. 20% of patients without an abscess or hemorrhage. Peristalsis generally resumes spontaneously on the third postoperative day. Small amounts of free intraperitoneal air do not signify an anastomotic leak or perforation when detected before the 18th postoperative day. Only large or increasing amounts of free air are considered suspicious.

The principal **complications after abdominal surgery** are bleeding, sepsis, peritonitis, abscesses, and bowel obstruction. "Four P's" should be considered in the differential diagnosis of sepsis in ICU patients: pneumonia, peritonitis, phlebitis, and pyelitis.

■ The leading cause of postoperative peritonitis is anastomotic leakage. CT in acute peritonitis shows ascites with dilatation of the mesenteric vessels and diffusely increased density of the mesenteric fat.

■ Intraperitoneal abscesses most commonly form at subphrenic, subhepatic and paracolic sites, in the lesser pelvis, in the Morison pouch, between bowel loops, or at intraparenchymal sites. An abscess may be drained if it is reasonable to expect spontaneous resolution of its cause.

■ The plain abdominal radiograph in mechanical bowel obstruction generally shows dilatation of the small bowel. The stomach and colon are additionally dilated in paralytic ileus. An abrupt caliber change at the transition zone is the main CT-criterion for distinguishing a mechanical obstruction from paralysis.

To detect **complications associated with specific operations**, the radiologist should be cognizant of the type of surgery that was performed.

■ Anastomotic leaks may occur after any gastric reconstructive procedure. The imaging modality of choice is contrast-enhanced CT.

■ The afferent limb following a pancreaticoduodenectomy should not be mistaken for an abscess or tumor.

■ Biliary leaks may occur after biliary surgery and cholecystectomy. The more acute the gallbladder operation (cholecystitis, perforation), the greater the risk.

- Approximately 10% of low anterior resections develop an anastomotic leak. A protective stoma should be created if the leak persists during drainage.
- Ultrasonography is the imaging study of choice for evaluating a renal allograft. Vascular complications are the most serious complications that follow renal transplantation.

- B-mode and Doppler ultrasound imaging and multi-detector CT are used after liver transplantations to diagnose vascular and biliary complications.
- CT angiography is the method of choice for detecting complications after stent grafting or vascular interventions. The presence of periaortic fluid after stent grafting indicates a complication.

Thoracic Imaging of the Pediatric Intensive Care Patient

6

Normal Thoracic Findings in Newborns 183
Catheter Position: Normal Findings and Malposition . 185
Transient Tachypnea of the Newborn (Wet Lung) . . . 187
Infantile Respiratory Distress Syndrome 188
Meconium Aspiration Syndrome 190
Neonatal Pneumonia 190
Complications during or after Mechanical Ventilation 191

Congenital Lung Diseases with Respiratory
Failure at Birth 194
Acute Obstruction of the Upper Airways 197
Asthma 200
(Viral) Bronchiolitis 201
Pneumonia 203

Acute respiratory failure in children may be due to a variety of causes, depending on the age of the patient. Accordingly, an accurate knowledge of patient age is a key factor in the interpretation of radiologic findings.

This chapter deals solely with acquired acute diseases and congenital thoracic diseases that may necessitate treatment in an intensive care unit. Issues relating to congenital heart disease may be found in the specialized literature.

The imaging modality of choice is the chest radiograph, usually limited to the anteroposterior (AP) projection, and it may be supplemented by ultrasonography. Computed tomography (CT) (with age-adapted protocols) is reserved for cases with complications and equivocal radiographic findings.

A. Smets and
C. Schaefer-Prokop

Normal Thoracic Findings in Newborns

The correct interpretation of thoracic findings in newborns requires an accurate knowledge of the patient's *age* at the time of the imaging study. It is also essential to know the timeline of normal radiologic findings. This applies particularly to the interpretation of chest radiographs during the first days of life. Moreover, there are several pitfalls that may cause difficulties for the less experienced examiner (**Table 6.1**).

Fetal lung fluid. Normally, the first new postnatal breaths leads to good aeration of both lungs, and it may take several hours for the fetal lung fluid to be completely absorbed from the alveoli. This absorption takes place through the pulmonary interstitium and lymphatic vessels. It is marked by an increasing radiographic lucency which starts at the center of the lungs and spreads to the upper lobes and then to the lower lobes. Fetal lung fluid appears radiographically as a diffuse haziness in both lungs or an increase in perihilar markings.

In ca. 50% of cases the small right interlobar fissure is visible on the first day, but as fluid absorption progresses

Table 6.1 Pitfalls in the interpretation of chest radiographs in newborns, infants, and small children

Findings	Possible misinterpretations
Skin folds	Pneumothorax
Air in the suprasternal notch	Esophageal atresia
Funnel chest	Pneumomediastinum or cardiomegaly
Oblique projection that omits the pectoral muscle	Unilateral hyperlucent lung
Apparent opacity in the right paracardiac area	Infiltration
Nipple-areola	Nodular mass
Sternal ossification shifted from the midline due to an oblique projection	Nodular mass
Expiratory radiograph (e. g., due to crying, evidenced by elevation of the diaphragm and tracheal bowing to the right)	Diffuse infiltration based on increased lung density, heart failure (**Fig. 6.1**)

An accurate knowledge of patient age and the timeline of normal findings are necessary for the correct interpretation of thoracic findings in newborns.

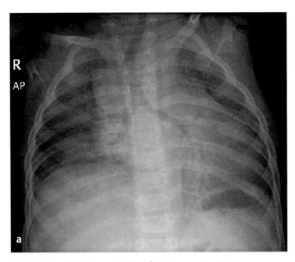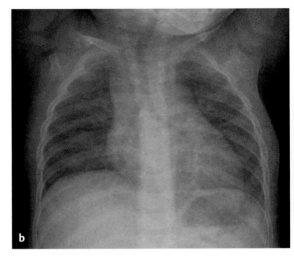

Fig. 6.1 a, b **Misinterpretation due to poor inspiration.**
A poor inspiratory view (a) cannot exclude bilateral pulmonary opacities and cardiomegaly. The findings disappear at full inspiration (b).

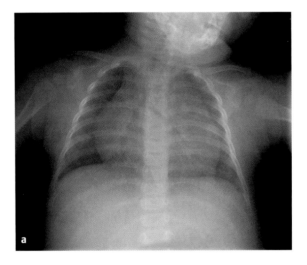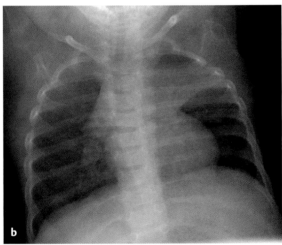

Fig. 6.2 a–c **The neonatal thymus.**
The thymus has the same density as the heart. It should not be misinterpreted as cardiomegaly (a), and its typical "sail" configuration should not be mistaken for atelectasis (b). On ultrasound scan, the thymus shows moderate homogeneous echogenicity with small white spots.

it becomes less pronounced or may disappear completely. In a normal inspiratory view the diaphragm leaflets are projected over the posterior portions of the eighth and ninth ribs and the anterior portion of the sixth rib.

Thymus. The thymus appears as a hoodlike structure overlapping the cardiac silhouette and should not be mistaken for cardiomegaly (**Fig. 6.2**). Typically the thymus has the same radiographic density as the heart. The pulmonary vessels are visible within the thymic shadow much as they are in the retrocardiac space. On the ultrasound scan the thymus presents a characteristic homogeneous echo pattern with multiple interspersed "white dots" that resemble snowflakes.

The thymus is relatively large through 4 years of age (with considerable anatomic variation) and undergoes a steady involution after 9 years. Even if the thymus appears large on radiographs and covers the cardiac border and hila, normally it will *never* compress or displace mediastinal structures. This serves to distinguish a normal thymus from pathologic thymic dysplasia or a mediastinal tumor, which may become symptomatic if they compress or displace vessels or respiratory passages.

Cardiac size. Measurements for estimating cardiac size, like those performed in adults, are much less useful in children due to variables introduced by the thymus and variations in inspiratory position (a cardiothoracic ratio <0.65 can serve as a guideline).

During Mechanical Ventilation

The tip of the endotracheal tube should be above the carina at the level of the T2 vertebral body. The chin and head position should be noted during imaging: When the head is flexed, the tip of the tube is about 1 cm above the carina. Extending the head or tilting it to one side raises the tip to approximately the level of T1 or the head of the clavicle.

In infants with normal lung expansion during mechanical ventilation (e. g., high-frequency oscillatory ventilation), the right hemidiaphragm is projected between the posterior portions of the eighth and ninth ribs.

▮▮ The normal thymus is relatively large through age 4 years but *never* compresses or displaces mediastinal structures.

▮▮ The tip of the endotracheal tube is ca. 1 cm above the carina when the head is flexed, rising to the level of T1 or the head of the clavicle when the head is extended or tilted to one side.

Catheter Position: Normal Findings and Malposition

The anatomy of the fetal circulation is shown schematically in **Fig. 6.3**. The *umbilical artery catheter* (UAC) initially descends into the lesser pelvis. It enters the systemic circulation through the internal iliac artery or common iliac artery and runs toward the aorta. Its tip may be positioned above the aortic bifurcation, distal to the origin of the renal arteries ("*low* position" at the L3/L4 level), or at the level of the midthoracic aorta above the origins of the visceral arteries ("*high* position" at the T7/T8 level). The catheter tip should not be located between

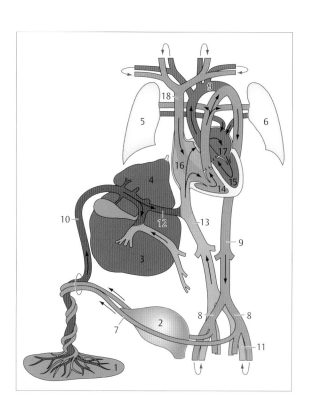

Fig. 6.3 **Anatomy of the fetal circulation.**
The umbilical vein arises from the placenta and opens into the inferior vena cava via the ductus venosus. The umbilical artery arises from the internal iliac artery and runs back along the bladder to the placenta. Because of this arrangement, an umbilical arterial catheter (UAC) first descends into the lesser pelvis whereas an umbilical venous catheter (UVC) runs cephalad to the liver.

1 Placenta	10 Umbilical vein
2 Bladder	11 Iliac vein
3 Right lobe of liver	12 Ductus venosus
4 Left lobe of liver	13 Inferior vena cava
5 Right lung	14 Right ventricle
6 Left lung	15 Left ventricle
7 Umbilical artery	16 Right atrium
8 Iliac artery	17 Left atrium
9 Aorta	18 Superior vena cava

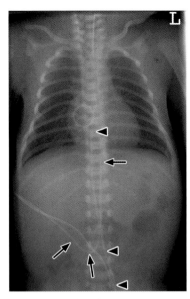

Fig. 6.4 **Normal catheter position in a newborn.**
The umbilical artery catheter (UAC, arrowheads) first dips into the lesser pelvis. Its tip is placed at the level of the T8 vertebra (high position). The umbilical vein catheter (UVC, arrows) runs directly cephalad with its tip just below the diaphragm.

the origins of the visceral or renal arteries ("*no* position" between T 10 and L 3 levels) (**Fig. 6.4**).

The *umbilical vein catheter* (UVC) runs directly upward through the ductus venosus and left portal venous system into the inferior vena cava. The tip should be just below the diaphragm, occupying a level that is cranial to the level of the liver veins and caudal to the right atrium (**Fig. 6.4**). The catheter tip should not be intrahepatic, as it might cause liver injury (**Fig. 6.5**).

Irrespective of whether the *central venous catheter* has been introduced through the inferior or superior vena cava, the tip should be just outside the right atrium. The same applies to the very thin peripheral venous catheters (silastic catheters), which are difficult to locate radiographically because of their small diameter. Their tip should also be outside the right atrium.

The tip of the *gastric tube* should be below the diaphragm!

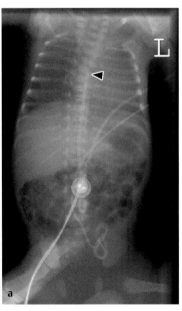
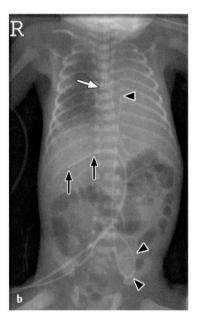
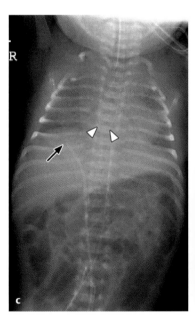

Fig. 6.5 a–c **Malpositioned catheters.**
a The UAC is positioned too high (T5 level).
b The UVC is in the portal vein. The endotracheal tube is in the right main bronchus, causing atelectasis of the left lung. The gastric tube and UAC are correctly positioned.
c The UVC is in the portal vein, and the UAC is correctly positioned. The gastric tube is looped in the stomach, and the endotracheal tube is correctly positioned.

Transient Tachypnea of the Newborn (Wet Lung)

This condition (TTN or wet lung) is characterized by its transient nature with a typical correlation between the history, clinical manifestations, and radiographic findings. It most commonly occurs in preterm infants or children delivered swiftly or by cesarean section, which results in little or no opportunity for natural mechanical expulsion of the fetal fluid from the lung during delivery. Venous and lymphatic reabsorption of the fetal lung fluid is delayed, impairing the distensibility of the lungs. Transient left-sided heart failure may also play a role.

The diagnosis is suggested by the transient nature of the condition, continuous clinical and radiographic improvement within hours to a maximum of 2–3 days, and the relatively good clinical condition of the affected newborn.

Clinical Aspects

Children with TTN develop a (usually) mild respiratory dysfunction with tachypnea (90–140 breaths/min) during the first 6 hours of postnatal life (the normal range is up to 90 breaths/min). Oxygen may be administered by nasal cannula for a brief time, but generally the children are not intubated (in contrast to infantile respiratory distress syndrome [IRDS]).

Imaging

Radiographs taken during the first 2–6 hours of postnatal life usually show a symmetrical, hazy pattern of interstitial fluid accumulation in the lungs, small pleural effusions, and thickened septa outlined by fluid (**Fig. 6.6**). The heart is of normal size or may show transient slight enlargement. The lung volume is normal or slightly increased.

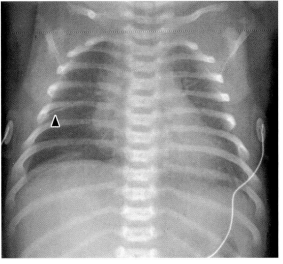

Fig. 6.6 **Child with wet lung 6 hours after cesarean delivery.** Chest radiograph shows hazy lung opacity and a fluid-outlined septum on the right side. The lung volume is normal (the child is not intubated).

TTN is a transient condition marked by rapid clinical and radiographic improvement and relatively mild respiratory dysfunction.

Reabsorption of the opacities begins peripherally and spreads centrally. As a result, radiographs taken ca. 10–12 hours after birth show increased symmetrical, linear markings in the perihilar region. All radiographic signs normally resolve within a maximum of 72 hours without additional therapeutic efforts.

Differential Diagnosis

Rapid improvement and the relatively mild degree of respiratory dysfunction are the main criteria that distinguish wet lung from neonatal pneumonia and hyaline membrane disease (see **Table 6.2**).

Table 6.2 Differential diagnostic criteria for evaluating the neonatal thorax

	Wet lung (TTN) *	IRDS/HMD *	Neonatal pneumonia	Meconium aspiration
Lung volume	Normal or increased	Decreased	Normal	Increased
Pulmonary opacities	Inhomogeneous	Uniform	Inhomogeneous	Irregular patchy opacities
Pleural effusion	+	–	++	+
Heart	Slight transient enlargement	Enlarged	Normal	Slight transient enlargement
History	Cesarean section or prematurity		Prematurity (increased risk), may also affect mature newborns	Postdate infants (10 days average), previous intrauterine stress
Clinical presentation	Mild respiratory dysfunction	Severe respiratory dysfunction		Severe respiratory dysfunction

* For explanation of abbreviations, see text.

Infantile Respiratory Distress Syndrome

Synonyms for IRDS are surfactant deficiency disease (SDD) and hyaline membrane disease (HMD).

There is some confusion of terminology in that several terms are applied to the same condition. One states the cause (SDD), one the result (HMD), and another the resulting functional deficit (IRDS).

Respiratory distress syndrome is a common disease of preterm infants (< 37 weeks gestation, < 2500 g) caused by immaturity of the lungs and is the leading cause of death in this group. Surfactant deficiency prevents adequate expansion of the acini, leading to alveolar collapse and diffuse microatelectasis with impairment of gas exchange.

IRDS, in which surfactant deficiency prevents adequate expansion of the acini, is the leading cause of death in preterm infants (< 37 weeks, < 2500 g).

Imaging

Staging. Radiographs show general hypovolemia (!) of both lungs and a diffusely granular lung structure with an air bronchogram extending far into the periphery. Atelectasis is classified into four stages of severity (**Table 6.3**), although the findings are usually masked by

Table 6.3 Radiographic stages of infantile respiratory distress syndrome (IRDS)

Stage	Characteristics
Stage I	Reticulogranular opacities, hypovolemia
Stage II	Like stage I, plus an air bronchogram (the large bronchi do not collapse)
Stage III	Like stage II, plus blurring of the cardiac border (increasing alveolar opacities)
Stage IV	Homogeneous opacity of both lungs (white lung)

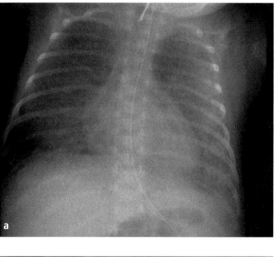
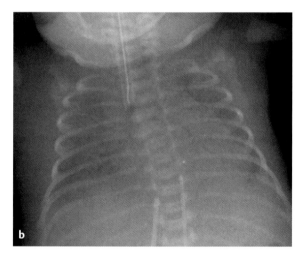
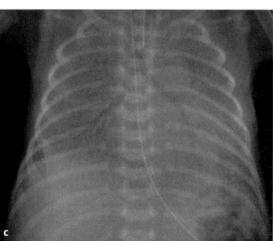
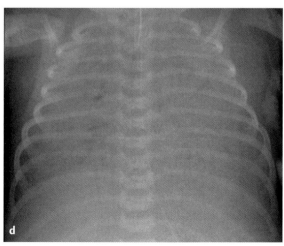

Fig. 6.7 a–d **Different children with IRDS.**
All of these infants are intubated and show pulmonary hypovolemia.
a   Stage I–II: fine granular opacities with an air bronchogram (1 day after birth).
b   Stage II: like stage I, but with a more conspicuous air bronchogram (1 day after birth).
c   Stage III: like stage II, but with increasing unsharpness of the cardiac border (1 day after birth, same child as in a).
d   Stage IV: white lung and air bronchogram.

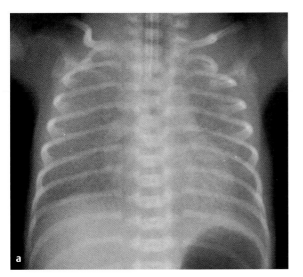

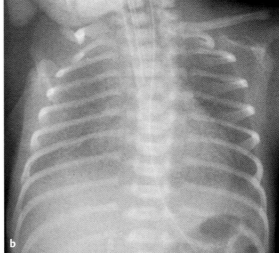

Fig. 6.8 a–c   **Preterm infant with IRDS on ventilation.**
a   After birth.
b   Ten hours after surfactant therapy.
c   Two days after surfactant therapy. Note that improvement is more pronounced in the left lung. This asymmetry results from uneven intrapulmonary distribution of the surfactant.

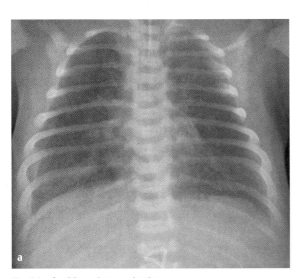

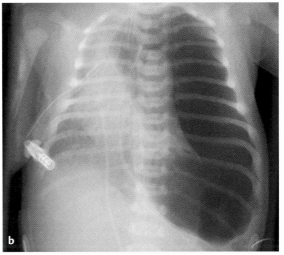

Fig. 6.9 a, b   **Meconium aspiration.**
a   Radiograph after meconium aspiration shows diffuse pulmonary hyperinflation (flattened diaphragm leaflets) with patchy opacities (1 day after birth).

b   Massive tension pneumothorax after meconium aspiration in a different child (1 day after birth).

immediate intubation and surfactant therapy (see below). Morphologic changes are often more pronounced in the lower lobes than in the upper lobes (**Fig. 6.7**).

Course. Affected infants who are not intubated immediately after birth develop full-blown IRDS within ca. 12–24 hours. Today, however, it is rare to encounter fully developed IRDS or witness its staged progression because affected infants are intubated immediately after birth and surfactant is administered through the endotracheal tube, often without prior imaging. Surfactant therapy in responders leads to increased lung volumes and clearing of granular opacities (**Fig. 6.8**), at which point the findings may resemble pulmonary interstitial emphysema. With an uneven intrapulmonary distribution of surfac-

tant (e. g., right > left), radiographic findings may be very asymmetrical and mimic the appearance of neonatal pneumonia or meconium aspiration (see **Fig. 6.9**). These cases require close cooperation with the pediatrician to ensure that the images are interpreted correctly.

Differential Diagnosis

Pleural effusion is not a feature of IRDS and would be more consistent with neonatal pneumonia. Resolution of radiographic findings within a few hours would also be inconsistent with IRDS. Reappearance of pulmonary haziness after an interval of improvement is a sign of pulmonary edema (see also **Table 6.2**).

Meconium Aspiration Syndrome

The intrauterine or intrapartum aspiration of meconium-stained amniotic fluid occurs mainly in children who are delivered several days postterm, or in patients where intrauterine or perinatal stress has caused vagal stimulation leading to increased intestinal peristalsis and premature passage of meconium into the amniotic sac.

Meconium aspiration syndrome (MAS) is a very serious condition. Many infants with MAS have pulmonary dysfunction that is severe enough to require extracorporeal membrane oxygenation (ECMO).

> The aspiration of meconium-stained amniotic fluid leads to pulmonary dysfunction, which may be severe enough to require ECMO.

Imaging

The radiographic changes caused by the aspiration of meconium or amniotic fluid with a high cellular content are highly variable. The following signs may be found, depending on the site of the bronchial obstruction and quantity of aspirated fluid:

- An asymmetric hyperinflation of one or both lungs or lung areas with associated depression of the hemidiaphragm (**Fig. 6.9a**)
- Perihilar linear opacities with a radial distribution

- Coarse, sometimes nodular opacities surrounded by cystlike lung areas correspond to focal zones of atelectasis surrounded by areas of compensatory hyperinflation

Up to 40% of patients have a (small) effusion and an associated pneumothorax, the latter as a complication from the combination of airway obstruction and hyperinflation, plus the need for relatively aggressive suctioning (**Fig. 6.9b**). Hypoxemia and hypercapnia lead to pulmonary vasoconstriction with secondary pulmonary hypertension.

Rarely, children show no pulmonary opacities at all after meconium aspiration but develop solely a pneumothorax: they usually have such poor respiratory function that mechanical ventilation is required.

Course. A chemical pneumonitis may develop within 48 hours, especially when large amounts of meconium have been aspirated. Secondary infections are common; the main causative organisms are gram-negative bacteria. Secondary surfactant deficiency may lead to a secondary respiratory distress syndrome that is difficult to distinguish radiographically from neonatal pneumonia.

Neonatal Pneumonia

> The neonatal lung responds initially to bacterial infection with an increased density of interstitial structures.

Preterm infants are at particularly high risk for developing neonatal pneumonia. The infection may be acquired in utero (e. g., transplacental listeriosis or CMV infection) or during delivery, due to aspiration of infected amniotic fluid. The causative agents are more often bacterial than viral. Even mature newborns may develop neonatal pneumonia.

Imaging

Because the interstitium predominates over aerated parenchyma in newborns, the initial response of the neonatal lung to various pathogens is an increased density of interstitial structures (**Fig. 6.10**). The most frequent type

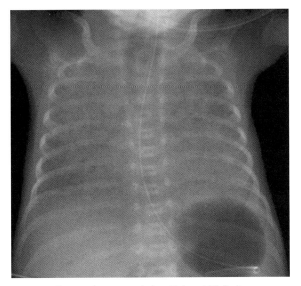

Fig. 6.10 **Neonatal pneumonia in a 5-day-old infant.** Note the diffuse alveolar opacity. (Differentiating features from IRDS: child is not intubated, IRDS occurs in the immediate postnatal period.)

of infection is streptococcal pneumonia, but other causative agents such as staphylococci, fungi, and viruses also occur.

Course. Subsequent radiographs show patchy, usually bilateral and sometimes confluent foci in addition to diffuse alveolar opacities. The opacities may show an asymmetrical arrangement..

Usually significant hyperinflation of the lungs is present. Mild cardiomegaly is another common finding.

Differential Diagnosis

The findings are difficult to distinguish from IRDS. The most important criterion is the presence of pleural effusion that is more frequently seen in infants with neonatal pneumonia. Note that IRDS and neonatal pneumonia may also coexist.

Complications during or after Mechanical Ventilation

Pulmonary Interstitial Emphysema

Pulmonary interstitial emphysema (PIE) is a result of mechanical ventilation using a high transpulmonary pressure (barotrauma). The high pressure causes overexpansion of the terminal bronchioles and alveolar ducts.

The diagnosis of PIE has special implications for ventilation therapy (high-frequency ventilation) (**Table 6.4**) and is considered a precursor of other, more serious complications such as pneumothorax and pneumomediastinum. Frequent radiographic follow-ups are needed.

Table 6.4 Various ventilation methods used in newborns

Ventilation method	Features
CPAP (continuous positive airway pressure)	Administered during spontaneous respiration
HFV (high-frequency ventilation)	Small volumes and high frequency (e. g., in pulmonary interstitial emphysema)
CMV (conventional mechanical ventilation)	Infants that cannot tolerate HFV (e. g., after asphyxia)

Imaging

Radiographs show uniformly small (millimeter-size), rounded lucencies diffusely distributed throughout both lungs. They should not be misinterpreted as increased transparency and thus indication of improvement.

If these bullae are emptied on expiration, this means that the air is still intra-alveolar. Following rupture of the alveoli, the air becomes distributed in the perivascular space toward the hila and periphery of the lungs. This stage is marked by the presence of small, cystlike lucencies ca. 2 mm in diameter along with meandering or vermiform lucencies that persist on expiration (**Fig. 6.11**). The involved lung becomes increasingly static, showing no volume change during inspiration and expiration, even when unaffected lung areas continue to show respiratory volume change.

Pneumomediastinum

Pneumomediastinum is usually preceded by interstitial pulmonary emphysema.

Since PIE is a precursor of pneumothorax and pneumomediastinum, it requires frequent radiographic follow-ups.

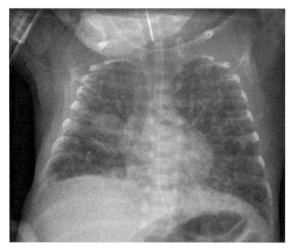

Fig. 6.11 **Pulmonary interstitial emphysema.**
Same child as in **Fig. 6.10**, now on mechanical ventilation (19 days after birth) with pulmonary interstitial emphysema (PIE) due to barotrauma. Note the cystlike lucencies caused by (confluent) interstitial air.

Imaging

Pneumomediastinum in the neonate is characterized by a sail-shaped elevation of the thymus (spinnaker sail sign, angel's wing) in the frontal (AP) chest radiograph (**Fig. 6.12**).

Pneumothorax

Pneumothorax in newborns generally results from positive-pressure ventilation in IRDS with an air leak. Less often it is secondary to bronchial obstruction or hyperinflation following meconium aspiration.

Pneumothorax in a supine newborn tends to collect anteromedially in the angle between the heart and lung. The thymus is *not* elevated, unlike a pneumomediastinum.

Pneumothorax at an atypical location is sometimes easier to detect by repositioning and refilming the patient. A lateral view, expiratory view, or lateral decubitus view may be helpful in questionable cases.

Imaging

Because the newborn is supine, the air tends to collect anteromedially in the angle between the heart and lung. This should not be misinterpreted as pneumomediastinum (elevated thymus in lateral decubitus view, see **Fig. 6.12b**). A line of air separates the basal cardiac border from the diaphragm (normally a separating line is not seen). The main pitfall is skin folds, which typically extend past the lung borders, are projected over the abdomen, or run in a mediolateral rather than craniocaudal direction.

- An *anterior pneumothorax* is characterized by a unilateral hyperlucent lung, accentuated sharpness of the cardiac border, and anteromedial herniation of the affected lung toward the healthy side (**Fig. 6.13**).
- A *medial pneumothorax* appears as a unilateral or bilateral, bandlike paramediastinal zone of increased lucency. The thymus is *not* sharply demarcated or elevated, which is in contrast to a pneumomediastinum.
- A subpulmonary basal pneumothorax appears as a crescent-shaped subpulmonary air collection (**Fig. 6.14**).

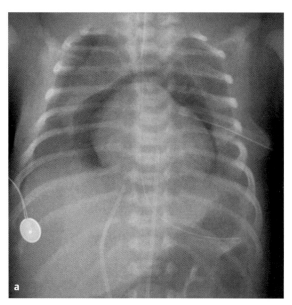

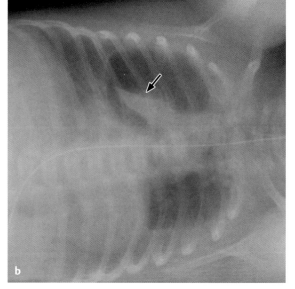

Fig. 6.12 a, b **Pneumomediastinum as a complication of barotrauma.**
Lateral decubitus view shows elevation of the thymus (**b**).

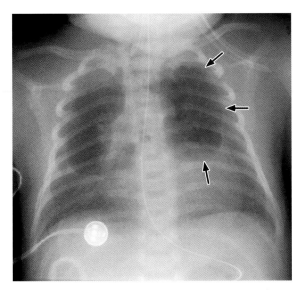

Fig. 6.13 **Left-sided pneumothorax appears as a rounded anterior lucency.**

Postextubation Atelectasis

Postextubation atelectasis is a common condition following long-term ventilation in newborns. The most common site of occurrence is the right upper lobe (note: this lobe is also most commonly affected by postaspiration atelectasis).

Hemorrhage

Diffuse intrapulmonary hemorrhage may occur in ventilated neonates (e.g., may cause a new lung opacity in infants with IRDS). The radiographic opacity correlates with the extent of the hemorrhage. The pattern ranges from that of pulmonary edema to a complete white lung with nondelineation of the diaphragm and lung. Clinically, a bloody discharge is noted from the endotracheal tube.

Bronchopulmonary Dysplasia

Bronchopulmonary dysplasia (BPD), also known as chronic lung disease of *preterm* infants, is considered a sequel to neonatal respiratory dysfunction necessitating prolonged ventilation at high pressures and/or a high oxygen concentration (*ventilator lung*).

The distal alveoli normally develop between weeks 24 and 26 of gestation. Preterm delivery and ventilation preempt normal development of the alveoli and capillaries. This incites an inflammatory process leading to capillary dysmorphia, increased interstitial fibrosis, and emphysematous changes in the distal alveoli.

IRDS or oxygen-rich ventilation does not necessarily precede the development of bronchopulmonary dysplasia. The prognosis has improved significantly in recent years.

Imaging

Radiographic abnormalities appear by 3–4 weeks after birth. Besides hyperinflated lung areas, radiographs show variable degrees of atelectasis and focal fibrosis (**Fig. 6.15**).

The dominant finding in cases with superinfection—usually by respiratory syncytial virus (RSV)—is hyperin-

Bronchopulmonary dysplasia may develop even in the absence of prior IRDS or oxygen-rich ventilation.

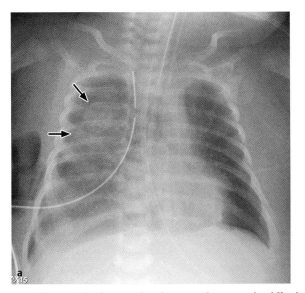

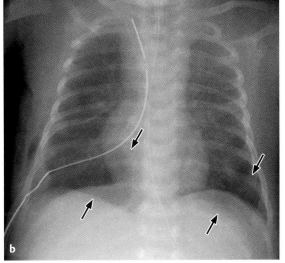

Fig. 6.14 a, b **Subpulmonary basal pneumothorax can be difficult to detect.**
a Subtle pneumothorax adjacent to an apical drain.　　**b** Bilateral pneumothorax.

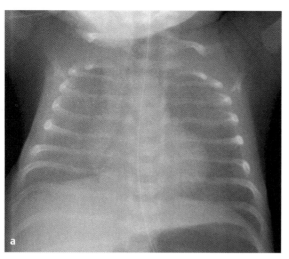 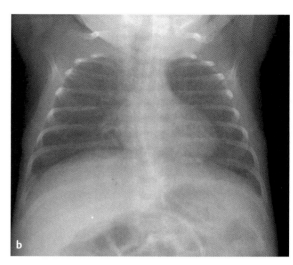

Fig. 6.15 a, b **Bronchopulmonary dysplasia (BPD).**

a Early stage of BPD in a 3-week-old infant, marked by fine granular opacities distributed diffusely in both lungs.

b Late stage of BPD in a 7-week-old infant, marked by cystlike lucencies and streaky opacities (sponge pattern).

flation. The mixed pattern of cystic hyperinflation and fibrotic atelectasis is always difficult to interpret unless the radiologist knows the details of mechanical ventilation during the neonatal period.

Staging. Affected infants typically have an increased oxygen requirement. The chest radiograph underestimates the extent of pulmonary changes. Four radiographic stages are defined based on the original description by Northway. Stage II is also called the regenerative stage, while stages III and IV are known, respectively, as the transitional and the chronic stages (**Table 6.5**). In practice, however, these stages can no longer be clearly identified

Table 6.5 Radiographic stages of bronchopulmonary dysplasia

Stage	Characteristics
Stage I	Diffuse granular lung pattern with an air bronchogram (interstitial opacities)
Stage II (days 4–10)	Complete opacification of both lungs with effaced cardiac borders
Stage III (days 10–20)	Diffuse distributed coarse vesicular and cystlike lucencies (sponge pattern)
Stage IV (> 30 days)	Enlargement of coarse vesicular lucencies and coarse striate densities

today due to superimposed therapeutic effects and infections.

Congenital Lung Diseases with Respiratory Failure at Birth

This section is limited to congenital lung changes that may cause respiratory failure at birth or during the first months of life. Congenital heart defects will not be addressed.

Tracheoesophageal Fistulas

Tracheoesophageal fistulas, with or without esophageal atresia, result from faulty separation of the esophagus from the primitive trachea during early embryonic development. By far the most common type of this anomaly (type IIIb, 90%) consists of a proximal esophageal blind pouch and a fistulous communication between the distal

esophagus and trachea. The second most common type is esophageal atresia without a fistula (type II, 5%).

Imaging

The frontal radiograph shows the *proximal esophageal blind pouch* as an air-filled, pear-shaped structure located at the cervicothoracic junction and displacing the trachea slightly toward the right side. The lateral radiograph shows that the trachea is displaced anteriorly and compressed by the esophageal blind pouch. Because of the *fistula* between the trachea and distal esophagus, the gastrointestinal tract is distended by air. A frequent complication of esophageal atresia is aspiration pneumonia.

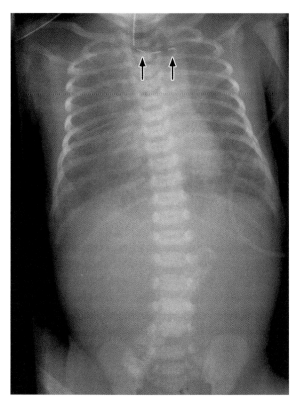

Fig. 6.16 **Esophageal stricture in a 1-day-old infant.**
The gastric tube cannot be advanced past the stricture. The abdomen is airless, indicating absence of a tracheoesophageal fistula. Wet lung is also present.

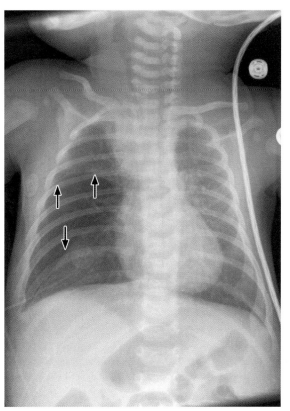

Fig. 6.17 **Congenital lobar emphysema.**
A 2-month-old infant with congenital emphysema of the middle lobe and increased lung volume (note displacement of the interlobar fissure on the right side).

The abdomen is airless in *esophageal atresia without a fistula* (type II), distinguishing this condition from the type described above (**Fig. 6.16**).

Congenital Lobar Emphysema

Congenital emphysema most commonly occurs in the upper lobes. It is caused by air-trapping and hyperinflation of a lung area due to a focal bronchial obstruction based on bronchial atresia, bronchial stenosis, a cartilage defect in the bronchial wall, or extrinsic compression by a mediastinal tumor or bronchogenic cyst. The most common sites of involvement are the left upper lobe (43%) followed by the middle lobe (32%) and right upper lobe (20%). Congenital emphysema rarely affects the lower lobes. The hyperinflated lung area may be initially filled with fluid but becomes increasingly lucent over time as the fluid is reabsorbed.

A common association exists between lobar emphysema and congenital heart disease (ventricular septal defect or patent ductus arteriosus).

Children with congenital lobar emphysema present with dyspnea or cyanosis during the first months of life.

Imaging

Radiographs typically show complete opacification of the affected lung (due to persistence of fetal fluid), which becomes increasingly aerated over time and expands. The volume increase may be sufficient to cause life-threatening compression of the rest of the lung (**Fig. 6.17**). The vessels in the affected lobe appear attenuated and spread apart, while the vessels in the remaining (healthy) lung may be compressed. Although this condition is called lobar emphysema, it may actually involve only part of the lobe. In other cases lobar emphysema may have a multilobar or multifocal distribution.

Differential Diagnosis

The differential diagnosis in a newborn should include the following:

- Pneumothorax (does not contain vessels)
- Congenital diaphragmatic hernia (usually on the left side, partial absence of the diaphragm, herniated air-filled bowel loops)
- Congenital cystic adenomatoid malformation (air-filled cysts of varying size)

With a proximal esophageal blind pouch and a fistula between the trachea and distal esophagus, the abdomen is filled with air. In esophageal atresia without a fistula, the abdomen is airless.

Lobar emphysema generally shows complete opacification of one lobe, but it may affect only part of a lobe or may have a multilobar distribution.

Congenital Cystic Adenomatoid Malformation

This condition (CCAM) is a congenital, multicystic hamartomatous lung malformation that is confined to one lobe. It involves all or part of one lobe, and bilateral changes are very rare.

Affected infants present immediately after birth with respiratory distress and recurrent infections.

Imaging

The cysts are of variable size and, with few exceptions, are confined to one lobe. Because the cysts already communicate with the bronchi at birth, the bronchi are at least partially air-filled at birth or become so within a few hours (**Fig. 6.18**). The cysts may still be fluid-filled at birth (solid appearance) and show increasing aeration during the postnatal period.

The following types are distinguished:
- Type 1: one or more large cysts 2–10 cm in diameter (most common type)
- Type 2: multiple uniformly small cysts
- Type 3: appear grossly and radiographically solid but consist of microscopic cysts (very rare)
- Type 4: one large, solitary cyst

Differential Diagnosis

Differentiation is required from sequestration, cavitating pneumonia, and congenital diaphragmatic hernia. The latter is suggested by a peridiaphragmatic location of the cysts.

Congenital Diaphragmatic Hernia (Bochdalek Hernia)

In congenital diaphragmatic hernia (CDH) abdominal organs herniate into the chest through a posterior defect in the diaphragm. Left-sided occurrence predominates by a 5 : 1 ratio. The herniation may involve the stomach, small intestine, colon, kidney, or liver. Children with extensive herniations and pronounced pulmonary hypoplasia present with severe respiratory failure at birth. Herniation of the stomach indicates the presence of a large diaphragmatic defect and is a poor prognostic sign.

Imaging

The chest radiograph shows intrathoracic air-filled bowel loops, a mediastinal shift, and compression of the lung (**Fig. 6.19**). Initially the bowel loops may be completely filled with fluid. Typically there is a reduction of intra-abdominal bowel gas. An atypical course of the umbilical vein catheter or gastric tube may also suggest the correct diagnosis.

Ultrasonography can clearly demonstrates the anatomical features of CDH.

Differential Diagnosis

The main differential diagnosis is CCAM (air bubbles). If the bowel is still completely fluid-filled, the herniated intrathoracic organs will appear solid, making this condition difficult to distinguish from a pleural effusion or solid intrapulmonary lesion. Over time, however, multiple air–fluid levels will usually appear within the herniated bowel loops.

CDH mainly requires differentiation from CCAM (air bubbles) and from pleural effusion in cases where herniated bowel loops are still fluid-filled.

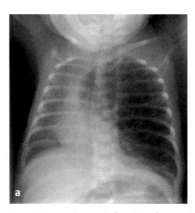
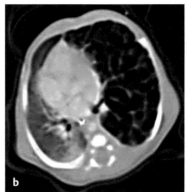
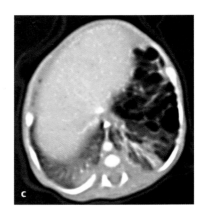

Fig. 6.18 a–c **Congenital cystic adenomatoid malformation (CCAM).** The chest radiograph (a) and axial CT scans (b, c) from a 3-week-old infant with CCAM show cystic malformation of the entire left upper lobe and atelectasis of the lower lobe due to the mass effect of the increased upper lobe volume.

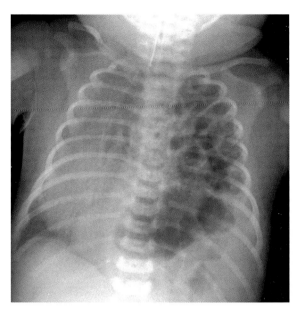

Fig. 6.19 **Congenital diaphragmatic hernia (CDH).**
Air-filled bowel loops have herniated into the left side of the chest causing a contralateral mediastinal shift in a newborn with CDH.

Congenital Lymphangiectasia and Chylothorax

Pleural effusions are very rare in newborns. When present, they may be an expression of:

- infection (pneumonia),
- malabsorption (impaired lymphatic drainage due to a thoracic duct anomaly, described as congenital lymphangiectasia), or may be associated with
- generalized edema (fetal hydrops).

Pleural effusions that are present over long periods of intrauterine development usually cause lung anomalies. They have a high association with congenital heart disease.

Chylothorax is the most frequent cause of an isolated unilateral or bilateral pleural effusion not associated with an anomaly. Most cases resolve spontaneously with multiple aspirations. A delay in the maturation and function of the thoracic duct has been postulated as a cause.

Acute Obstruction of the Upper Airways

All acute airway obstructions present with stridor. It is essential to diagnose the cause swiftly and institute appropriate management. In most cases the diagnosis is made clinically without imaging evaluation.

The *causes* include the following (**Table 6.6**):

- Acute retropharyngeal abscess
- Acute epiglottitis
- Laryngotracheobronchitis (croup)
- Exudative tracheitis
- Tonsillitis
- Foreign-body aspiration

Acute epiglottitis and exudative tracheitis are life-threatening emergencies that require immediate action and leave no time for diagnostic imaging! Imaging studies are appropriate only in patients with a retropharyngeal abscess (ultrasonography or CT) or foreign-body aspiration.

Table 6.6 Differential diagnosis of acute upper airway obstruction

- Pseudothickening of the retropharyngeal space
- Lymphangioma
- Foreign-body aspiration
- Croup
- Exudative tracheitis
- Epiglottitis

Acute Retropharyngeal Abscess

Acute retropharyngeal abscess is more common in infants and small children than in adults and may lead to acute airway obstruction. The peak age incidence is 6–12 months. It is caused by bacterial infection.

Clinical Aspects

Children with an acute retropharyngeal abscess present with diffuse swelling of the neck accompanied by symptoms of pharyngitis, otitis media, or an upper respiratory infection.

Imaging

The initial imaging study of choice is *ultrasound scan*, which shows diffusely increased echogenicity (cellulitis) or a focal fluid collection (abscess).

When the inflammation is located in the deep cervical soft tissues, even pediatric patients are currently evaluated by *CT*. The *lateral soft-tissue radiograph* (with the neck extended, as flexion mimics enlargement of the retropharyngeal space) shows swelling of the prevertebral soft tissues with anterior displacement of the trachea, but this view is rarely obtained today due to lack of patient compliance and poor specificity.

Acute epiglottitis and exudative tracheitis are life-threatening emergencies in which there is no time for imaging studies.

197

Serious potential complications are the spread of inflammation to the mediastinum and jugular vein thrombosis.

Foreign Body Aspiration

Foreign body aspiration is the *leading household emergency* with a potentially fatal outcome in children. It may occur at any age, but children between 6 months and 3 years of age are most commonly affected.

Only 5% of aspirated foreign bodies become lodged at the subglottic or laryngeal level. In up to 15% of cases the foreign body is within the trachea, and the majority (up to 80%) are in the main bronchi (about 55% in the right main bronchus, 33% in the left main bronchus, 10% bilateral).

In cases with a typical history, flexible bronchoscopy should be used for definitive diagnosis and treatment. Imaging is important in children with an *equivocal* history and—especially when the diagnosis is *delayed*—in children with nonspecific respiratory symptoms that may result from a foreign body aspirated some time before presentation.

> Foreign body aspiration is the leading household emergency in children and is most common between 6 months and 3 years of age.

Pathogenic Mechanism

Several mechanisms may occur depending on the size of the object relative to the diameter of the airways and on the degree of airway obstruction:

- *Partial airway obstruction* by a small foreign body that does not impede inspiration or expiration (two-way check-valve mechanism). No imaging abnormalities are found (< 1% of cases).
- *Complete airway obstruction* during inspiration and expiration (no-way check-valve mechanism) by a large foreign body. Postobstructive atelectasis occurs (in ca. 20% of cases).
- *Partial airway obstruction* by a medium-sized foreign body that allows full or partial inspiration but obstructs expiration (one-way check-valve mechanism). This leads to overinflation of the lung area distal to the affected airway (in > 80% of cases) (**Fig. 6.20a**).

Clinical Aspects

The classic clinical presentation, seen in up to 90% of cases, consists of stridor and a sudden cough. Cyanosis and severe respiratory failure may also be present, depending on the degree of airway obstruction. If the foreign body is subglottic or within the larynx, the situation may deteriorate dramatically as a result of laryngospasm.

Even an object lodged in the esophagus may cause secondary tracheal obstruction and clinical symptoms such as stridor as a result of inflammatory esophageal swelling.

Diagnostic Strategy

Chest radiographs are diagnostic in more than 60% of cases (**Fig. 6.20b**). Sensitivity is increased by obtaining inspiratory *and* expiratory views. Because expiratory views are not obtained routinely, the radiologist should be aware of the patient history and the indication.

A *lateral radiograph* is taken to differentiate between foreign body aspiration into the trachea, which requires bronchoscopy, and a foreign body lodged in the esophagus, which is removed by endoscopy (**Fig. 6.20c**).

— **Practical Recommendation** —

Bilateral *decubitus radiographs* can be taken in uncooperative children as an alternative to inspiratory and expiratory views. Normally the basal lung has a smaller volume and the vessels appear compressed. Hyperinflation of the basal lung is a sign of airway obstruction.

Oblique radiographs can track the central airways into the mediastinal shadow and confirm truncation or nonvisualization of the affected bronchus. Fluoroscopy can increase confidence by showing asymmetrical or diminished motion of the diaphragm.

Imaging

Because less than 10% of foreign bodies are radiopaque, it is essential to look for secondary signs.

The most common finding is unilateral hyperinflation on the affected side, possibly accompanied by decreased volume of the unaffected contralateral lung (**Fig. 6.20a**). While the inspiratory view is often normal or nearly normal, the expiratory view can more sensitively detect air trapping on the affected side. Ipsilateral vascularity is decreased (obstructive emphysema), the diaphragm is flattened, the costophrenic angle is blunted, and the mediastinum is shifted toward the opposite side. The normal lung, on the other hand, shows a (relative) increase in vascularity.

Hyperinflation of the basal lung on *decubitus radiographs* signifies an obstruction. *Oblique radiographs* may show absence or truncation of the affected bronchus.

A complete obstruction leads to segmental, lobar, or occasional complete atelectasis. The unaffected lung areas show compensatory overinflation and may be hyperlucent while showing normal or increased vascular markings (differentiating feature from obstructive emphysema).

Note that mediastinal shift is not a criterion in patients with bilateral foreign bodies.

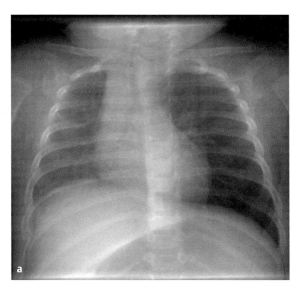
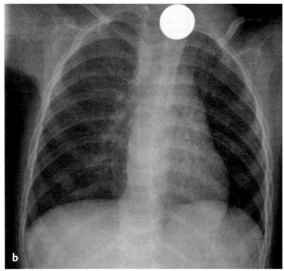
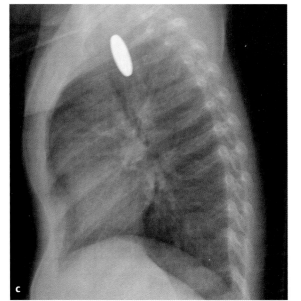

Fig. 6.20 a–d **Foreign bodies.**

a   Aspirated radiolucent foreign body in the left (!) main bronchus of a 6-month-old child. The check-valve mechanism has caused hyperinflation of the affected lung.

b–d This 1-year-old child swallowed a coin (**b, c**), which caused tracheal narrowing due to edematous swelling of the esophageal wall and surrounding edema (**d**).

Complications

It is rare for foreign body aspirations to cause immediate *asphyxia*.

Complete atelectasis of the right lung may lead to *upper venous inflow obstruction* resulting from massive displacement and kinking of the superior vena cava.

Pneumonia develops in ca. 30% of cases where more than 3 days pass before the aspirated foreign body is removed. It predominantly involves the lower lobes and is most often caused by unusual organisms that respond poorly to antibiotics. Foreign body aspiration should be considered in every child under 4 years of age who presents with pneumonia..

The sudden rise of alveolar pressure produces an air leak that leads to *interstitial emphysema*, pneumomediastinum, or pneumothorax. Foreign-body aspiration should be considered in children under 2 years of age who have mediastinal emphysema and no apparent history of trauma.

The removal of an airway obstruction may be followed by the development of *reactive pulmonary edema*.

The *ingestion of hydrocarbon liquids* (e.g., furniture polish, gasoline, kerosene) may also cause aspiration due to the low viscosity of the liquid. This incites the

The possibility of foreign-body aspiration should be considered in every child under 4 years of age with pneumonia.

development of a chemical pneumonitis within 6–12 hours, marked radiographically by faint, patchy opacities with ill-defined margins that are usually located in the basal lung zones. These findings may persist for weeks or months.

Differential Diagnosis

A foreign body lodged in the *esophagus* may also cause laryngospasm and symptoms of airway obstruction. A coin in the esophagus usually appears as a round object in the lateral projection and as an edge-on line in the PA projection. This is why a lateral radiograph is recommended before proceeding with further tests (**Fig. 6.20c**).

The *complete atelectasis* of a lung may also be caused by mucus plugging in pediatric patients. Foreign-body aspiration should always be excluded in children showing no signs of infection.

Complete consolidation is a rare cause of an opaque hemithorax in children. The differential diagnosis should include lobar emphysema, pulmonary lymphangiectasia, and a type III cystic adenomatoid malformation.

Imaging is not instrumental in the diagnosis of croup, acute epiglottitis, exudative tracheitis, or tonsillitis.

Acute Epiglottitis, Croup, Exudative Tracheitis, and Tonsillitis

All of these conditions are diagnosed clinically and do not require radiologic evaluation.

Croup. Also called laryngotracheobronchitis, this is the most frequent cause of upper airway obstruction in small children. It is generally caused by a viral infection (parainfluenza type A). The peak age incidence is between 6 months and 3 years and shows seasonal variations. Most cases run a mild course.

Acute epiglottitis. This occurs mainly from 3 to 4 years of age (older than the typical "croup child") and is caused by a type B haemophilus infection. Immediate treatment is indicated, and many patients require intubation.

Exudative tracheitis. This disease is characterized by a purulent infection of the trachea with exudative plaque formation that may cause upper airway obstruction. Since the advent of haemophilus vaccinations, exudative tracheitis has replaced the downward-trending epiglottitis as a life-threatening complication. It is caused by a staphylococcal or polymicrobial infection. The diagnosis is not based on imaging but is made by examining suspected cases endoscopically to confirm the diagnosis and remove potentially obstructive membranes.

Tonsillitis. Occasionally the tonsils may be so greatly enlarged due to inflammation that they obstruct the upper airway. Affected children often present with obstructive sleep apnea, recurrent otitis media, and recurrent upper respiratory infections. A diameter of 12 mm is considered the upper limit of normal. The diagnosis is made clinically.

Asthma

Asthma is the leading cause of hospitalization in the pediatric age group. It may be the result of an allergic reaction to various agents. Asthma requires differentiation from viral bronchiolitis. Asthma is rare before 2 years of age, whereas bronchiolitis is fairly common before 1 year of age.

Asthma is rare before 2 years of age, whereas bronchiolitis is common before 1 year of age.

Diagnostic Strategy

Asthma is diagnosed clinically. A chest radiograph should be obtained only in cases refractory to treatment or with presumed local pathology (e.g., pneumothorax). Routine chest films are *not* necessary. The main purpose of chest radiographs in asthmatic children is to identify complications such as pneumonia or dystelectasis in obstructive emphysema, and to detect pneumothorax or pneumomediastinum.

Imaging

The radiographic hallmark of both asthma and bronchiolitis is *hyperinflation* (**Fig. 6.21**).

Radiographs show bilateral hyperinflation, peribronchial opacities due to mucosal edema, and atelectasis secondary to bronchial plugging. Atelectasis or collapse should not be misinterpreted as consolidation due to infection.

Mild hyperinflation is detectable only by comparison with prior radiographs. More severe hyperinflation leads to flattening of the diaphragm and enlargement of the retrosternal space. Peribronchial densities may persist in children who have chronic recurrent attacks. Lymph node enlargement is generally absent, but the hila are enlarged due to prominent pulmonary vessels or central atelectasis.

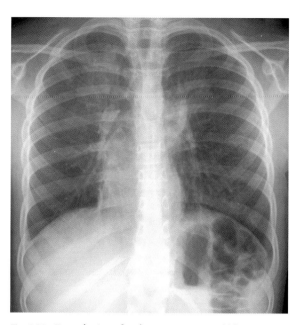

Fig. 6.21 **Exacerbation of asthma in a 10-year-old boy.**
Chest radiograph shows compression atelectasis of the upper lobes by the hyperinflated lower lobes and accentuation of bronchial wall structures.

Table 6.7 Causes of spontaneous pneumomediastinum in children

Respiratory maneuvers, Valsalva maneuver
- Coughing, crying, screaming
- Vomiting
- Hyperventilation (in ketoacidosis)
- Defecation
- Lifting heavy objects
- Inflating a balloon
- Sports
- Drug inhalation (e. g., marijuana, cocaine)
- Smoke exposure

Associated diseases
- Asthma
- Cystic fibrosis
- Bronchiolitis
- Retropharyngeal abscess
- Laryngitis
- Seizure

Esophagus
- Foreign-body ingestion
- Esophageal rupture

Iatrogenic
- Tooth extraction
- Heimlich maneuver
- Respiratory function studies

Barotrauma
- Flying
- Diving

Complications

Pneumomediastinum. An asthma attack may be complicated by a pneumomediastinum due to ruptured alveoli. The chest radiograph shows bilateral demarcation of the thymus (spinnaker sail sign). Pneumomediastinum in older children is marked by vertical lucent air streaks distributed along the aorta or cardiac border and is often more apparent in the lateral projection (retrosternal, precardial, peritracheal, and periaortic). The air spreads outside the pleura (between the pleura and diaphragm) and dissects into the soft tissues of the neck and chest wall. The diaphragm is visualized across the central mediastinal shadow, producing a "continuous diaphragm sign."

Table 6.7 lists other potential causes of a spontaneous pneumomediastinum (not associated with trauma or an endotracheal or endoesophageal procedure) in children. It should be noted that the children present with a variety of nonspecific complaints that may include respiratory distress; neck, back, or chest pain; dyspnea and dysphagia.

An asthma attack may be complicated by pneumomediastinum due to ruptured alveoli.

(Viral) Bronchiolitis

Bronchiolitis is a seasonal disease that occurs mainly during the winter months and is usually caused by a viral infection (e. g., > 50% RSV, 20% parainfluenza, 5% influenza, 15% adenovirus, < 10% mycoplasma or chlamydia after conjunctivitis). Any age group may be affected, but more than 90% of cases with a viral etiology occur in children under 5 years of age. Mycoplasma and bacterial infections are more common in school-age children.

The imaging modality of choice is the *chest radiograph* for detection or exclusion of an infiltrate that may require antibiotic therapy (differentiation of viral from bacterial infection, but note: viral infections may also cause confluent infiltrates).

Most children with bronchiolitis recover completely. Only a few develop *chronic lung disease* with recurrent bouts of pneumonia, atelectasis, bronchiolitis obliterans, or Swyer–James syndrome. Asthmoid hyperreactivity of the small airways may persist, especially after an RSV infection.

Clinical Aspects

Children present clinically with cough, respiratory distress, and fever. Only extreme cases develop hypoxia, requiring ventilation.

Pathogenesis

Inflammatory edema and mucus hypersecretion lead to narrowing of the peripheral airways. A check-valve mechanism may cause hyperinflation due to air trapping, or there may be a complete obstruction leading to atelectasis. Because collateral air drift (via Lambert channels and Kohn pores) is not yet fully developed in children, it cannot compensate for increased intra-alveolar pressure, and the air cannot be exhaled through unaffected bronchioles.

Imaging

Radiographs show a hyperlucent lung with flattening or even inversion of the diaphragm (below the posterior 10th rib). The mediastinal and cardiac shadows are narrowed, and the sagittal thoracic diameter is increased. Peribronchial thickening—most prominent in the perihilar region—and segmental atelectasis give rise to linear opacities radiating from the hilum (**Fig. 6.22**). Areas of central atelectasis sometimes mimic hilar lymphadenopathy (although lymph node enlargement may actually be present). The central lung zones have a "dirty" appearance, although this is largely a subjective assessment.

Hyperinflation (flattened diaphragms, increased AP diameter) may be the only sign of a viral infection (especially with RSV) and is an expression of acute bronchiolitis.

Subsegmental atelectases tend to migrate and should not be mistaken for bacterial infiltrates (one of the most common errors in pediatric radiology). Bacterial infiltrates are not accompanied by peribronchial densities but are frequently associated with pleural effusion. Atelectases may be widespread, resulting in acute respiratory failure.

Bacterial contamination leads to focal opacities and (subsegmental) consolidation. A bacterial superinfection following a viral infection should be considered in cases where clinical improvement is delayed.

Hyperinflation may be the only sign of acute bronchiolitis. Migrating subsegmental atelectases should not be mistaken for bacterial infiltrates.

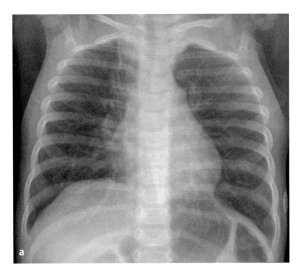

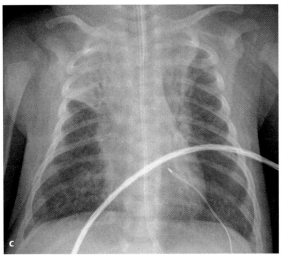

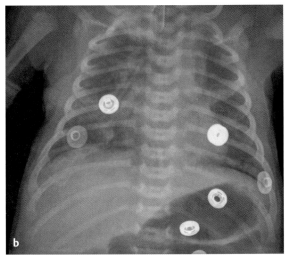

Fig. 6.22 a–c **Children with viral bronchiolitis.**
a Diffuse hyperinflation with increased perihilar peribronchial opacities.
b Hyperinflation coexisting with segmental atelectases.
c Complete bilateral upper lobe atelectasis with patchy peribronchial infiltrates in the rest of the lung, which is hyperinflated.

Pneumonia

Infections of the respiratory tract are very common in children. Most lung inflammations in children under 5 years of age have a viral etiology, and less than 5% are caused by bacteria. The most frequent causative viruses of pneumonia in children are RSV, rhinovirus, parainfluenza virus, and adenovirus. The incidence of bacterial and nonviral atypical infections (mycoplasma, chlamydia) rises with increasing age. By school age, ca. 30% of lung infections are caused by mycoplasma.

Imaging

Due to the absence of collateral air drift, children under 8 years of age rarely develop lobar consolidation, even with a bacterial infection. The absence of collateral ventilation predisposes to the development of *round pneumonia*, which occurs chiefly in the posterior lower lobe (**Fig. 6.23a**). While an air bronchogram is often absent on radiographs, it can be clearly demonstrated by ultrasound scan (important differentiating feature from solid pulmonary nodules in children over 8 years of age) (**Fig. 6.23b, c**). Typically, pneumonia changes its morphology quickly and shows immediate response to antibiotic therapy. Significant clinical improvement is noted within 48 hours.

It should be emphasized that the *spectrum of causative organisms* cannot be determined based on radiographic morphology alone (interstitial vs. acinar–alveolar pattern, **Fig. 6.24**). Even viruses may produce acinar shadows. Conversely, bacteria may cause an interstitial pattern (see also Pneumonia in Chapter 2). *Mycoplasma pneumoniae* may develop focal opacities (confined to one lobe) as well as bilateral reticulonodular opacities.

Recurrent infections, infections of unusual extent, and infections by unusual organisms in children should raise suspicion of a primary or secondary *immunodeficiency*. The history may suggest the cause of a secondary immune deficiency (**Table 6.8**).

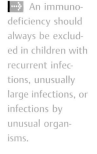 An immunodeficiency should always be excluded in children with recurrent infections, unusually large infections, or infections by unusual organisms.

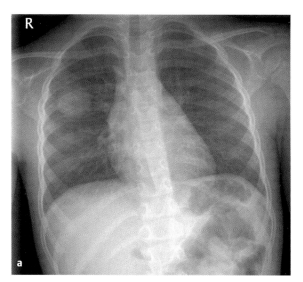

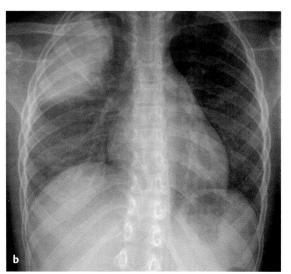

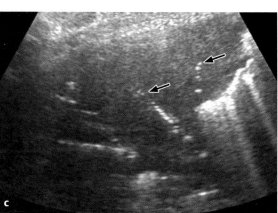

Fig. 6.23 a–c **Children with pneumonia.**
a   Rounded area of consolidation in a 3-year-old girl (so-called "round pneumonia").
b, c   Extensive upper lobe consolidation without an air bronchogram in an 8-year-old girl (differential diagnosis: pleural vs. pulmonary). Ultrasound scan shows aerated bronchi and identifies the consolidation as pneumonia.

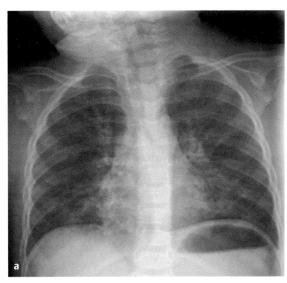
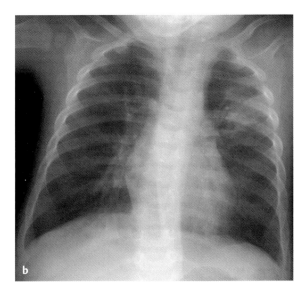

Fig. 6.24 a, b **Patterns of opacity.**
Alveolar (**a**) and interstitial (**b**) patterns of radiographic opacity are not useful in children for determining the spectrum of causative organisms.

Table 6.8 Infections associated with immunodeficiency in children (modified from Markowitz and Kramer 2000)

	T cell defect*	B cell defect*	Granulocyte defect	Complement defect
Pathology	▪ DiGeorge syndrome (thymic hypoplasia) ▪ HIV	▪ Bruton agammaglo-bulinemia ▪ Hyper-IgE syndrome ▪ General agammaglo-bulinemia ▪ Sickle cell anemia	▪ Chediak–Higashi syndrome ▪ Leukemia, lymphoma on chemotherapy	
Bacteria	Sepsis	Streptococci Staphylococci *Haemophilus*	Staphylococci *Pseudomonas*	*Neisseria* Pyogenic bacteria
Viruses	CMV EBV VZV Rhinoviruses	*Enterovirus*		
Fungi, parasites	*Candida* *Pneumocystis*	*Candida* *Nocardia* *Aspergillus*		

* Combined T and B cell deficits: in SCID (severe combined immunodeficiency) syndromes, Wiskott–Aldrich syndrome, ataxia-telangiectasia, and ciliary hypokinesia.
CMV, cytomegalovirus; EBV, Epstein-Barr virus; HIV, human immunodeficiency virus; VZV, varicella-zoster virus.

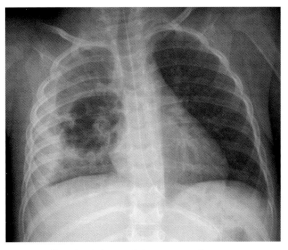

Fig. 6.25 **Complicated necrotizing pneumonia.**
A large pleural effusion (differential diagnosis: emphysema) in a 2-year-old child.

Complications

Possible complications of pneumonia include parapneumonic pleural effusion, empyema formation, abscess formation, and cavitation (cavitary necrosis, **Fig. 6.25**).

Pleural Effusion

The most frequent cause of pleural effusion is bacterial infection (pneumococci in newborns, staphylococci in small children). Pleural effusions in newborns are rarely large enough to compromise pulmonary function. The absence of air bronchograms (ultrasound scan!) is a useful criterion for distinguishing a layered-out pleural effusion from pneumonia. Interlobar fluid collections are less common in children than in adults but may appear radiographically as an elliptical intrapulmonary focus which is similar to that seen in adults.

Empyema

The most frequent cause of complete hemithoracic opacity is an empyema occurring as a complication of underlying pneumonia. A diagnosis of pleural empyema should be considered in every child who responds poorly to treatment. Not infrequently, the cause is a previously unrecognized foreign body aspiration. Septations and increased echogenicity on ultrasound scanning suggest the correct diagnosis.

Pneumatocele (Cavitary Necrosis)

Pneumatoceles are cavitary lesions that result from alveolar destruction in an area of pneumonic consolidation. The inflammation leads to the thrombosis of small arterioles with consequent ischemia and necrosis. Most patients have a streptococcal infection, which leads to pneumatocele formation in up to 60% of cases. The condition is rarely caused by *Klebsiella*, staphylococci, or *Haemophilus*.

This complication should mainly be considered in children who respond poorly to antibiotics. Ischemia and necrosis may elude radiographic detection and are an indication for contrast-enhanced CT.

Imaging. Pneumatocele is characterized by a loss of normal bronchial structures and by necrosis, which shows lack of contrast enhancement. An air-filled cyst will form only after the necrotic area has established a communication with aerated lung tissue (alveoli or bronchi).

Unlike the thick walls of a pulmonary abscess, the *cyst walls* are thin and do not enhance after IV contrast administration. Generally an air–fluid level is absent. With treatment, the lesion should resolve completely within 40 days leaving a residual scar. Generally there is *no* need for CT follow-up.

A pneumatocele is different from "pseudocavitation," which refers normally aerated lung within a consolidated area. Differentiation is required from sequestration, a (potentially superinfected) CCAM, and a lung abscess.

Abscess

An abscess is a complication of suppurative pneumonia, generally following an infection with aerobic bacteria such as *Staphylococcus aureus*. Rarely, abscess formation is caused by foreign body aspiration and superinfection or by an endobronchial tumor.

Most abscesses respond to appropriate antibiotic treatment. Surgical resection is rarely necessary.

Imaging. Unlike a pneumatocele (cavitary necrosis), an abscess consists of a circumscribed fluid collection with a thick, enhancing wall. An abscess communicating with a bronchial passage may also contain air.

— Practical Recommendation ————

Ultrasonography can help to confirm the intrapulmonary location of an abscess by demonstrating movement with respiratory excursions, distinguishing it from a pleural lesion. Additionally, pleural effusion is often present.

Cyst walls are thin and nonenhancing after contrast administration, whereas an abscess has thick walls that do enhance.

Summary

An accurate knowledge of patient age is essential for the correct interpretation of **thoracic images in newborns**. The **normal thymus** is relatively large through 4 years of age but will not compress or displace mediastinal structures unless abnormal thymic hyperplasia or a mediastinal tumor is present.

Transient tachypnea of the newborn, caused by the delayed reabsorption of fetal lung fluid, is a transient condition marked by rapid clinical and radiologic improvement and a relatively mild degree of respiratory dysfunction.

Infantile respiratory distress syndrome is a typical disease of preterm infants that is caused by immaturity of the lungs. It presents with general hypovolemia of both lungs and a diffuse granular pulmonary structure with an air bronchogram extending far into the periphery of the lung.

Meconium aspiration syndrome is a serious condition characterized by poor oxygenation and variable radiographic signs.

Pulmonary interstitial emphysema results from mechanical ventilation at a high transpulmonary pressure (barotrauma) and is characterized by uniformly small, rounded lucencies distributed diffusely in both lungs. Frequent complications are **pneumomediastinum** and **pneumothorax**.

The most important **congenital lung diseases with respiratory failure at birth** are tracheoesophageal fistulas, congenital lobar emphysema, congenital cystic adenomatoid malformation, congenital diaphragmatic hernia, and congenital lymphangiectasia.

Acute obstruction of the upper airways due to acute epiglottitis or exudative tracheitis is a life-threatening emergency that leaves no time for diagnostic imaging. Foreign-body aspiration is the leading household emergency in children and is most prevalent between 6 months and 3 years of age. Pneumonia may develop in cases where several days pass before a partially obstructive foreign body is removed.

Chest radiographs are not routinely indicated in children with **asthma**. They are obtained if there are suspected complications such as pneumonia or dystelectasis due to obstructive emphysema, pneumothorax, or pneumomediastinum.

Hyperinflation may be the only sign of **acute (viral) bronchiolitis**. Migrating subsegmental atelectases are common and should not be mistaken for bacterial infiltrates.

Pneumonia in children tends to present as round pneumonia, typically occurring in the posterior lower lobe, due to the absence of collateral air drift. Possible complications are pleural effusion, empyema, pneumatocele, and abscess formation.

7

Acute Abdomen in the Pediatric Intensive Care Patient

Meconium Ileus 208
Necrotizing Enterocolitis 209
Malrotation and Volvulus 211
Gastrointestinal Atresia and Stenosis 213

Congenital Megacolon (Hirschsprung Disease) 214
Hypertrophic Pyloric Stenosis 215
Intussusception 215

The differential diagnosis of diseases that present with an "acute abdomen" in children is very broad and varies with the age of the patient (**Table 7.1**). Acute abdominal pain is one of the most frequent indications for radiographic examinations in children. Diseases of the gastrointestinal tract are the leading cause, but extra-abdominal diseases such as basal pneumonia may also underlie an acute abdomen. Moreover, it is sometimes difficult in children to distinguish somatic pain from pain due to a psychosocial conflict. The limited ability of these young patients to cooperate and communicate makes it difficult to take an accurate history and conduct a radiologic evaluation.

This chapter deals with the differential diagnosis and imaging of an acute abdomen that may occur in pediatric intensive care patients, may prompt admission to an intensive care unit, or may require evaluation by a radiologist in an acute emergency.

Abdominal emergencies in school-age children show a broad overlap with diseases and findings in adults, and so the discussions in this chapter will be limited to diseases in neonates and small children.

M. Hoermann

Examination Technique

Ultrasonography

Ultrasonography is the primary imaging modality for evaluating an acute abdomen in children, even after trauma. Ultrasound scans have replaced plain abdominal radiographs and contrast examinations in many cases. A basic rule is the smaller the patient, the higher the operating frequency of the ultrasound transducer (**Table 7.2**).

Plain Abdominal Radiograph

Upright abdominal radiographs are poorly tolerated by most small children and tend to be of poorer quality than comparable supine radiographs. On the whole, however, plain films of an acute abdomen are nonspecific and may contribute little to making a diagnosis. Given these limi-

Table 7.1 Overview of the most common causative diseases of acute abdomen in different age groups

Neonates	Infants and small children	School-age children
▪ Atresia and stenosis	▪ Pyloric hypertrophy	▪ Appendicitis
▪ Meconium ileus	▪ Intussusception	▪ Diseases of adnexa
▪ Malrotation and volvulus	▪ Duplications	▪ Urologic diseases
▪ Necrotizing enterocolitis	▪ Foreign-body ingestion	▪ Blunt abdominal trauma
▪ Hirschsprung disease	▪ Gastroenteritis	▪ Cholecystitis
▪ Biliary diseases	▪ Mesenteric lymphadenitis	▪ Pancreatitis (in the setting of biliary tract anomalies)
▪ Gastroenteritis	▪ Febrile urinary tract infection	▪ Gastroenteritis
▪ Tumors	▪ Meckel diverticulum	

Table 7.2 Transducer frequencies recommended for different groups of pediatric patients

Age	GI tract	Parenchymal organs
Newborn	12–15 MHz	10–12 MHz
Small child	12–15 MHz	7 MHz
School-age child	10–12 MHz	5–7 MHz

Table 7.3 Exposure parameters for plain abdominal radiographs

Age	kV	mA	Grid
Newborn	55	2.0	None
Infant	58	2.2	None
School-age child, 7–9 years	64	2.5	None

tations, strict criteria should be applied in selecting children for plain abdominal radiographs (**Table 7.3**).

Coverage should always include the basal lung zones and inguinal region so that basal pneumonia or an incarcerated hernia can be recognized. If free air is suspected, a chest radiograph should be obtained in the upright or cross-table supine position (see **Figs. 7.5b** and **7.6b**).

> Gastrografin should not be used in children, owing to the risk of dehydration and its toxicity to gastrointestinal mucosa in newborns.

Meconium Ileus

Meconium ileus is the initial manifestation of cystic fibrosis in ca. 15% of affected newborns. The inspissation of bowel contents due to abnormal intestinal secretions prevents the normal passage of meconium.

Imaging

The *plain abdominal radiograph* shows signs of a low obstruction as in atresia or stenosis but without significant prestenotic dilatation. Air–fluid levels are very rarely seen owing to the inspissated condition of the meconium. The viscous meconium sometimes contains small air bub-

Oral Contrast Examinations

Contrast examinations of the gastrointestinal tract are rarely necessary. The contrast medium may consist of barium or a nonionic water-soluble material.

Gastrografin should *not* be used in children, as its hyperosmolarity may lead to life-threatening dehydration and cause toxic injury to the gastrointestinal mucosa in neonates.

bles. This may suggest the correct diagnosis but is *nonspecific*, as it may also result from a distal obstruction due to other causes.

The *contrast enema* is both therapeutic and diagnostic and demonstrates a poorly distensible microcolon ("unused colon," **Fig. 7.1**). When contrast medium enters the terminal ileum, the radiograph shows irregular filling defects caused by inspissated meconium.

Therapeutic contrast enema with a hypertonic medium is successful in up to 60% of cases. Attention must be given to avoiding perforations (up to 5% of cases) and to the maintenance of fluid balance.

Complications

Calcifications in the abdominal radiograph suggest an intrauterine perforation, possibly associated with pseudocyst formation, as a possible complication of meconium ileus. Other potential complications are volvulus and atresia.

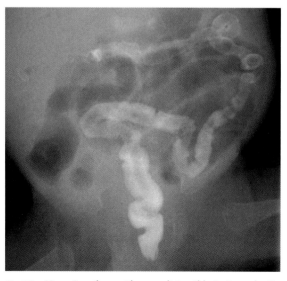

Fig. 7.1 **Meconium ileus with a nondistensible "microcolon" and dilatation of the small bowel.**

Necrotizing Enterocolitis

Necrotizing enterocolitis (NEC) occurs in immature newborns (>90% of NEC patients are delivered before 35 weeks' gestation) several days after the start of enteral feeding; symptoms never appear before feeding is initiated. Very rarely, NEC may also occur in mature newborns. The etiology is uncertain, but NEC has a multifactorial pathogenesis based on damage to the mucosal barrier.

Sites of predilection for NEC are the terminal ileum and ascending colon, although radiographic changes are often first noted in the sigmoid colon.

Diagnostic Strategy

NEC is a clinical diagnosis. The primary imaging modality is *plain abdominal radiography.*

Ultrasonography is being used increasingly in the diagnosis of NEC. It can detect air in the portal veins (pneumoportogram) earlier than radiography. Ultrasound scanning can also detect a (small) pneumoperitoneum more easily and with greater sensitivity (indication for surgery!).

Imaging

The imaging findings of NEC lag well behind its clinical manifestations. Almost invariably, the child has already been placed on antibiotics by the time of radiologic evaluation and the appearance of initial x-ray signs.

Radiography

The *plain abdominal radiograph* shows separated and distended bowel loops (bowel wall edema). All morphologic imaging findings are nonspecific, however, and there are no specific radiographic criteria for NEC.

Pneumatosis. Pneumatosis of the bowel wall is strongly suggestive of NEC but is not specific and may be found in other inflammatory bowel diseases. For example, it may occur in the setting of a rotavirus infection, which is the most frequent cause of enteritis in infants.

— Practical Recommendation —————————

Intestinal pneumatosis can be confirmed by obtaining a cross-table view or a short-interval follow-up that confirms pneumatosis by showing a constant location of the air collections.

Subsequent air migration through the mesenteric veins leads to a pneumoportogram (in about 10% of cases), which does not correlate with the severity of the disease (**Fig. 7.2**).

Perforation. NEC is responsible for more than 50% of pediatric abdominal perforations. Pneumoperitoneum is an indication for surgical treatment (**Fig. 7.3**).

The *supine abdominal radiograph* will show the following signs of "free air" in cases where perforation has occurred (**Table 7.4**):

- Air bordering the falciform ligament on both sides
- Continuity of the diaphragm shadow across the midline (unlike pneumothorax, which is confined to one side) (**Fig. 7.4**)
- Intramural and extramural air marking both sides of the bowel wall (Rigler sign, **Fig. 7.5b**)
- Triangular air collections between the bowel loops (triangle sign, **Fig. 7.5**)
- Rounded midabdominal lucency (football sign) on the supine radiograph caused by anterior migration of large amounts of free air (**Fig. 7.6**)

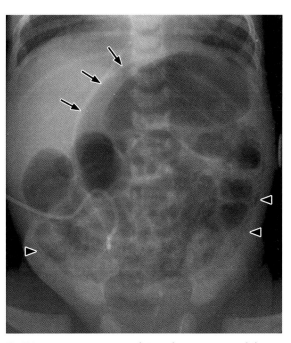

🔲 Pneumatosis of the bowel wall is suggestive of NEC, but the disease does not have specific radiographic signs.

Fig. 7.2 **Necrotizing enterocolitis with pneumatosis of the colon wall (arrowheads) and a rounded collection of free air (football sign) due to a perforation (arrows).**
Note the displacement of the arterial umbilical catheter.

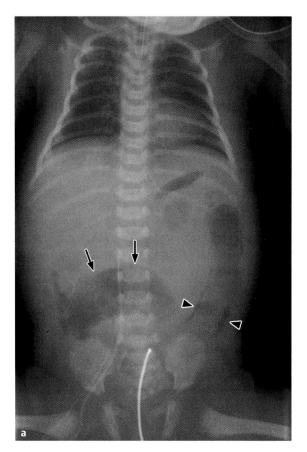

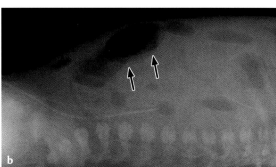

Fig. 7.3 a, b **Necrotizing enterocolitis.**
a Pneumatosis of the colon wall (arrowheads) and free air following a perforation (football sign, arrows).
b Cross-table view confirms the free-air collection along the anterior abdominal wall.

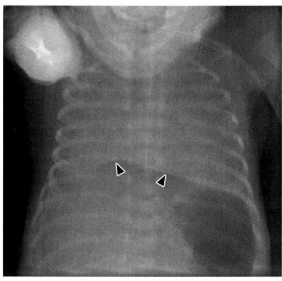

Fig. 7.4 **Continuous diaphragm sign caused by intraperitoneal free air.**

Table 7.4 Signs of free air on supine abdominal radiographs

- Lucencies over the upper abdomen
- Air outlining the falciform ligament
- Subhepatic or subphrenic air
- Rounded central lucency (football sign)
- Air outlining both sides of the bowel wall (Rigler sign)
- Delineation of the umbilical vessels and ligament
- Air in the scrotum
- Triangular air collections between bowel loops

Ultrasonography

Thickening of the bowel wall, intramural air, and free fluid are demonstrated equally well by ultrasound scanning. *Doppler sonography* of the superior mesenteric artery is an important study that will show an increased resistance index in NEC. This examination should be done in the fasted state, however, to avoid a physiologic postprandial rise in the resistance index.

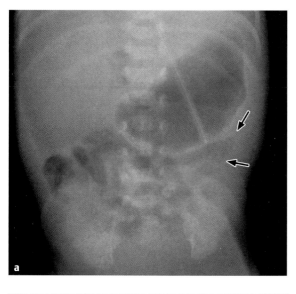

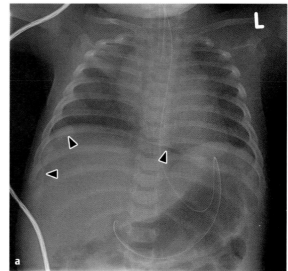

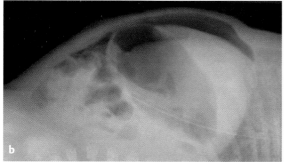

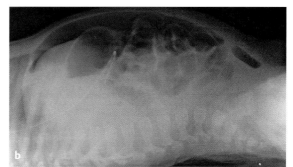

Fig. 7.5 a, b **Triangle sign.**
Triangular free-air collection between the bowel loops (a) with intramural and extramural air bordering both sides of the bowel wall (**b**, cross-table view).

Fig. 7.6 a, b **Football sign.**
a   With a very large collection of free air, it is possibly to miss the diffuse increase in lucency.
b   Lateral projection demonstrates free air along the anterior abdominal wall.

Malrotation and Volvulus

In normal intrauterine development, the gut undergoes three 90° counterclockwise rotations before reaching its definitive position. If these rotations are absent or incomplete, the result is nonrotation or malrotation of the intestines. Malrotation is a major developmental anomaly in children because it may lead to duodenal atresia and stenosis, volvulus, and perforation.

In newborns with a normally rotated bowel, the mesenteric root extends from the duodenojejunal loop to the distal ileum and thus provides for a long, stable fixation of the bowel. With malrotation, however, the mesenteric root is significantly shortened and offers less resistance to volvulus, which leads to vascular and intestinal stenosis. Fibrous peritoneal thickenings called Ladd bands stretch from the cecum to the liver or to the posterior abdominal wall, additionally causing duodenal stenosis (**Fig. 7.7**).

Clinical Aspects

More than 70% of affected children present with bilious vomiting and abdominal pain, possibly accompanied by muscular guarding. Less dramatic symptoms are anorexia, nausea, and vomiting. All children who present with bilious vomiting should undergo a small bowel contrast study to exclude volvulus.

Imaging

Radiography

Malrotation. Malrotation is difficult to recognize in the abdomen plain film of small children. The colon does not yet show the normal haustrations of adults, making it difficult to distinguish between large and small bowel. In most cases the cecum cannot be accurately localized.

> Every child with bilious vomiting should undergo a small bowel contrast study to exclude volvulus.

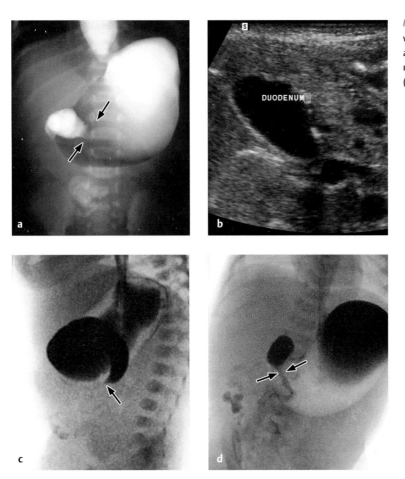

Fig. 7.7 a–d **Malrotation** with massive dilatation of the stomach and distal esophagus secondary to duodenal stenosis caused by a Ladd band (arrows).

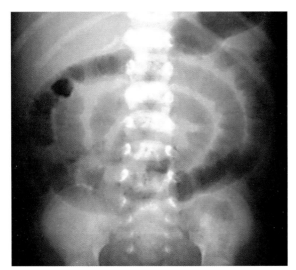

Fig. 7.8 **Volvulus.**
Plain radiograph shows gas-distended whorled bowel loops in the midabdomen (whirlpool sign). Decreased blood flow causes signs of wall thickening with separation of bowel loops (thumbprinting).

Diagnosis is aided by *contrast examination*. This may consist of a contrast enema, which will confirm that the cecum is outside the right lower quadrant of the abdomen. Another option is to administer contrast medium by gastric tube to define the location of the Treitz ligament: With a normally rotated bowel, the Treitz ligament occupies a left paravertebral location at the level of the duodenal bulb. With malrotation, the Treitz ligament has a variable location but usually occupies an inferior position on the right side.

Volvulus. The most serious complication of malrotation besides perforation is volvulus, which must be diagnosed quickly because vascular compromise may cause extensive, life-threatening intestinal necrosis.

The *plain abdominal radiograph* is nonspecific in the great majority of cases. Ideally the film will show a "whirlpool sign," or a whorled arrangement of gas-distended bowel loops in the midabdomen (**Fig. 7.8**). A gas-less abdomen on plain radiography signifies an incomplete vascular obstruction in which gas is still absorbed, while the picture of a distal obstruction (dilated air-/fluid-filled bowel loops) associated with malrotation indicate severe intestinal ischemia.

The diagnosis is established by contrast administration via gastric tube, which demonstrates the corkscrew-like configuration of the small bowel and cutoff of the contrast column. Note that complete obstruction of the duodenum by peritoneal bands does not produce this classic configuration, but it should still be assumed that malrotation is present.

With malrotation, the cecum is located in the right upper quadrant. This is also true in ca. 20% of normal cases, however, and so the diagnosis of malrotation requires *additional* signs such as abrupt "bird-beak" tapering of the contrast column in the twisted small bowel.

Ultrasonography

In most cases ultrasound scanning can verify the diagnosis by showing the inverted arrangement of the mesenteric vessels (the mesenteric vein is to the left of the mesenteric artery). Sonograms can also demonstrate the twisted mesenteric root. Additional sonographic signs are a dilated duodenum with hyperperistalsis, a thickened bowel wall in the right flank, and free fluid.

Although the detection of positive sonographic criteria is diagnostic, volvulus *is not excluded* by negative ultrasonographic findings.

> Volvulus can be diagnosed by ultrasound scanning but is not excluded by negative sonographic findings.

Gastrointestinal Atresia and Stenosis

Atresias of the gastrointestinal tract are much more common in the small bowel than in the colon (1 : 750 births in the small bowel, ileum > jejunum, 1 : 3500 in the duodenum, 1 : 40 000 in the colon). The anomalies are believed to result from a disturbance of intrauterine blood flow.

Gastrointestinal *stenoses* may have an extraintestinal cause such as malrotation, Ladd bands, a thickened Treitz ligament, or an annular pancreas. Stenoses are less common than atresias and are generally less impressive in their symptoms and imaging findings, depending on the degree of obstruction.

Clinical Aspects

The onset and course of clinical manifestations depend on the site of the obstruction. Duodenal atresia presents very early with bile-stained vomiting, whereas ileal atresia does not become symptomatic until several days after birth. Anal atresia is usually diagnosed in utero and rarely leads to an acute abdomen.

Diagnostic Strategy

Contrast examination is *not* indicated for the evaluation of high atresias and stenoses due to the risk of aspiration. In these cases the diagnosis is established by plain abdominal radiographs and ultrasonography, unless the condition has already been identified by prenatal tests.

An incomplete stenosis may present with (misleading) air distension of the bowel distal to the stenosis, in which case (oral) contrast examination can confirm the diagnosis.

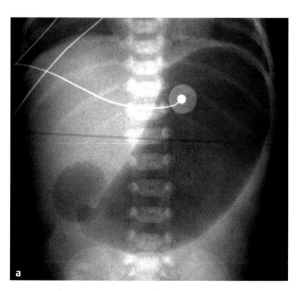
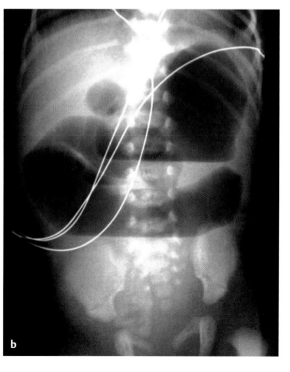

Fig. 7.9 a, b **Congenital causes of an acute abdomen.**
Duodenal stenosis (double bubble sign, **a**) and jejunal atresia (**b**) are each associated with massive distension of the proximal gastrointestinal tract and absence of air distal to the stenosis.

Contrast studies are indicated for distal stenoses and atresias to localize the obstruction and differentiate the cause (e.g., malrotation vs. atresia vs. stenosis).

Imaging

The plain abdominal radiograph in *duodenal atresia* shows a double-bubble sign caused by the air-filled stomach and duodenum with an absence of air distally (**Fig. 7.9a**).

— Practical Recommendation ——————————

Careful air insufflation through the gastric tube can support a diagnosis of duodenal atresia or stenosis. A positive test shows distension of the stomach and duodenum with an absence of bowel gas distal to the atresia.

The more aboral the site of the atresia, the less pronounced the distension. In *jejunal atresia* the stomach and duodenum are greatly dilated (**Fig. 7.9b**) while the colon is of normal size, because the ileum is producing sufficient fluid so that the colon remains "used."

Atresia of the ileum is characterized by multiple dilated small bowel loops (distal obstruction). Only the adjacent proximal bowel segment may have a "bulbous" appearance.

In *colonic atresia* the cecum and ascending colon are greatly distended, especially with a competent ileocecal valve. Contrast enema demonstrates a normal-sized colon with meconium in the presence of a distal stenosis, and an empty, unused microcolon in the presence of a proximal stenosis.

Complicated ileal atresia. In complicated ileal atresia or "apple-peel syndrome," large portions of the ileum and the distal superior mesenteric artery are absent. The small bowel mesentery is hypoplastic, and the bowel remnant distal to the atresia is wrapped around the vessels of the right colon. The abdominal radiograph shows a high obstruction with dilatation of the stomach, duodenum, and jejunum. Contrast enema demonstrates a microcolon with a coiled ileal attachment that mimics volvulus. The cecum may occupy a high subhepatic location in these cases, and malrotation may also be present. The survival rate of complicated ileal atresia is less than 50%.

Congenital Megacolon (Hirschsprung Disease)

Congenital disturbances of the autonomic nervous system (myenteric plexus) may occur anywhere in the lower gastrointestinal tract (small and large bowel). One of the most common forms is Hirschsprung disease, which is characterized by an aganglionic segment in the rectum (> 75%). The diagnosis is confirmed by anorectal biopsy and manometry.

Clinical Aspects

The cardinal symptom of Hirschsprung disease is constipation. The disease may also present in newborns as neonatal ileus or bowel obstruction after weaning, resulting in an acute abdomen.

Imaging

The abdominal radiograph shows marked distension of the colon (**Fig. 7.10**). Contrast medium should be administered carefully, as an overvigorous contrast enema could mask the easily distended aganglionic segment. Contrast enema can demonstrate the aganglionic segment and especially the transition zone from the aganglionic to dilated segment.

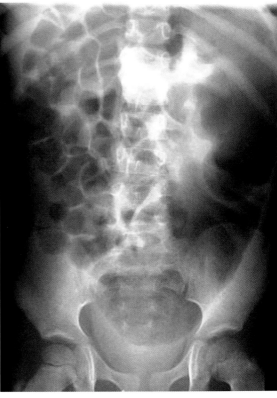

Fig. 7.10 **Congenital megacolon (Hirschsprung disease).** Note the massive dilatation of the descending colon and complete absence of air (!) in the distal rectum.

Hypertrophic Pyloric Stenosis

Hypertrophic pyloric stenosis (HPS) is caused by local thickening of the pylorus muscle. The etiology is unknown. It predominantly affects males (4 : 1), and is diagnosed between 4 and 6 weeks of age. HPS has a familial disposition with an incidence of 1 in 3000 live births.

Clinical Aspects

The clinical presentation of HPS ranges from nonbilious projectile vomiting to life-threatening dehydration in severe cases.

Diagnostic Strategy

Although the diagnosis of HPS once relied on abdominal radiographs and oral contrast examination, *ultrasonography* has now become the primary imaging study. The gallbladder is imaged in longitudinal section, and the transducer is then angled medially to define the pylorus.

— **Practical Recommendation** ————————

If the air-filled stomach obstructs vision, the child can be given tea to drink or the examiner can scan through the liver from the right side to define the pylorus in coronal section. The pylorus can also be scanned from the posterior side, again using the liver as an acoustic window. The anterior approach is the most practical as it permits the use of a high-frequency probe.

The sensitivity, specificity, and positive predictive value of ultrasound scanning is in the high 90's (96%, 99%, and 99%, respectively). Nondefinitive cases should be reexamined in 24–48 hours. The indication for surgical treatment is based mainly on clinical findings, with ultrasonography serving as an adjunct.

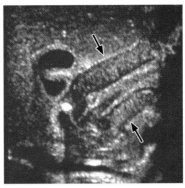

Fig. 7.11 **Pyloric stenosis.**
Ultrasonographic appearance of hypertrophic pyloric stenosis. The pyloric channel is longer than 16 mm with a wall thickness greater than 3 mm.

Imaging

The *ultrasound scan* typically shows a target sign. The pyloric channel is more than 16 mm long and its wall is thickened to more than 3 mm (**Fig. 7.11**). Additional findings are absence of pyloric relaxation, hyperperistalsis of the stomach, and absent or greatly delayed passage of liquid through the pylorus (drink test).

Radiographs after *oral contrast administration* demonstrate the filiform stenosis and the curved and elongated pylorus with markedly delayed passage of contrast medium.

Differential Diagnosis

Differentiation is required from pylorospasm, in which follow-up images will again show a normal wall thickness of the pylorus. If the stomach is empty, the collapsed antrum may mimic a thickened pylorus (drink test to distend the antrum).

▶ Hypertrophic pyloric stenosis is diagnosed by ultrasound scanning, which shows a pyloric canal longer than 16 mm with a wall thickness greater than 3 mm.

Intussusception

Intussusception occurs when one bowel segment invaginates into the lumen of the adjacent distal segment. Ileocolic intussusception, in which the terminal ileum invaginates into the cecum, is by far the most common form (85%). Colocolic and ileoileal intussusceptions are less common and may be secondary to the ileocolic form.

An obstructing lesion creating a lead point for the intussusception (duplication cyst, enlarged lymph nodes, polyps, etc.) should be excluded. An increased seasonal incidence in the spring and fall suggests an infectious etiology relating to lymph node enlargement in the cecal region. Intussusceptions are more common in children with Peutz–Jeghers syndrome and Henoch–Schönlein purpura.

Intussusception may occur in children of *any* age. It is most common between 3 months and 1 year and shows a 2 : 1 predilection for males. In children more than 6 years old, a tumor (lymphoma) should definitely be excluded as a possible lead point for the intussusception.

Clinical Aspects

Typical symptoms are colicky abdominal pain (80%), bile-stained vomiting (75%), and bilious stool (60%). Children diagnosed *very* late may present with clinical signs of meningism while abdominal complaints are less prominent.

Diagnostic Strategy

The diagnosis and treatment of intussusception formerly relied on contrast enema under fluoroscopic guidance, but today both functions can be accomplished using ultrasound scanning (5–7.5 MHz). Plain abdominal radiographs are obtained to exclude free air (indication for surgery).

Table 7.5 Absolute and relative contraindications to the hydrostatic reduction of intussusception

Absolute contraindications
- Severe dehydration
- Severe muscular guarding (peritonism)
- Clinical signs of peritonitis
- Signs of free air on the plain abdominal radiograph

Relative contraindications
- History longer than 48 hours
- Patient younger than 3 months or older than 2 years (underlying cause), signs of small bowel obstruction on the abdominal radiograph
- Wall thickness greater than 10 mm by ultrasound scan

■■■ The absence of Doppler flow signals indicates vascular obstruction and is an immediate indication for surgery.

A nonsurgical hydrostatic reduction requires cooperation among the radiologist, pediatrician, and (pediatric) surgeon. Absolute and relative contraindications to this procedure should be noted (**Table 7.5**). Signs of small bowel obstruction are not a contraindication.

Imaging

Ultrasonography

The longitudinal ultrasound scan shows a "pseudo-kidney" with a hypoechoic rim (edematous bowel wall) and an echogenic center (mucosa of the intussusceptum). High-resolution probes will show multiple ringlike structures representing the different wall layers. A transverse scan displays the "crescent-in-doughnut" sign, in which the intussuscepted bowel and indrawn mesentery appear in cross-section as a swirled echogenic structure (**Figs. 7.12**, **7.13**).

The absence of detectable *Doppler flow signals* indicates vascular obstruction and is an indication for immediate surgery. A small amount of free fluid has no effect on management. The detection of fluid in the intussuscepted bowel segment often correlates with an unsuccessful nonsurgical reduction attempt. Even so, a radiological reduction should always be attempted first. Ultrasonography can also identify the cause of the intussusception (Meckel diverticulum, lymph node, duplication cyst).

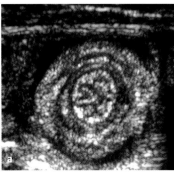
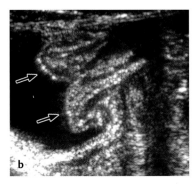

Fig. 7.12 a, b **Intussusception.** Transverse and longitudinal ultrasonographic findings. Arrows indicate the intussuscepted bowel.

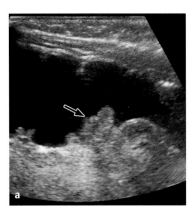
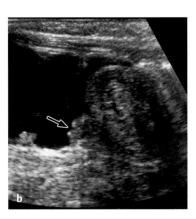

Fig. 7.13 a, b **Intussusception.** Appearance of an ileocecal intussusception as per ultrasound scan (arrow indicates the ileocecal valve).

Radiography

Plain radiographic findings are typical in about 50% of cases, nonspecific in 25%, and normal in 25%. "Typical" radiographic signs are a soft-tissue structure with small lucencies (fat) or a peripheral ring of air accompanied by signs of intestinal obstruction.

Reduction Methods

Fluid instillation. Hydrostatic reduction is performed under ultrasound guidance. A highly diluted, warmed solution of contrast medium in water (1 : 20 to ca. 500 mL of water-soluble contrast medium) is administered through an enema tube to reduce the intussuscepted segment by mechanical pressure. The use of a water/contrast mixture makes it possible to switch later from a sonographically to a fluoroscopically guided technique.

The fluid is suspended at a height of 100–130 cm above the table top (equivalent to about 70–100 mmHg) to generate the necessary pressure. Occasionally the reservoir can be raised to 160 cm to produce a maximum pressure of about 120 mmHg (a 30-cm water column cor-

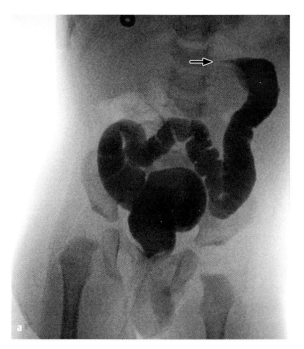

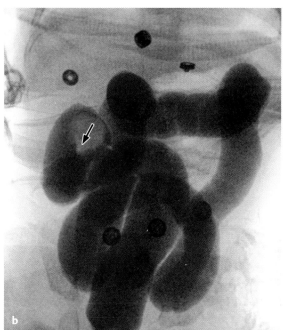

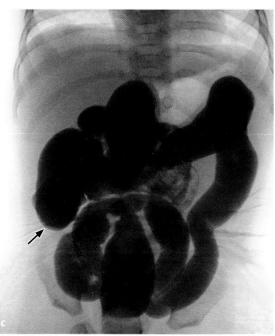

Fig. 7.14 a–c **Reduction of intussusception.**
Documentation of a successful reduction from the splenic flexure toward the ileocecal valve.

responds to ca. 22 mmHg). A total fluid volume of 500 mL to a maximum of 1000 mL is instilled under ultrasound guidance.

Sedation. Hydrostatic reduction requires the presence of a pediatric surgeon who can administer the sedation and be ready to intervene if complications arise. Sedation is controversial in the literature. On the one hand, the reduction is very painful for the child, but the Valsalva maneuver in nonsedated patients is believed to protect against perforation. Glucagon is not administered.

Reduction. A fluoroscopically guided reduction is supported by manual pressure while an sonographically guided reduction is aided by probe pressure. The criterion for a successful reduction is the passage of fluid into the terminal ileum.

The therapeutic result is documented by a sonogram or a plain radiograph. Both must demonstrate free fluid passage into the proximal bowel segment (e.g., from the cecum as far into the ileum as possible) (**Fig. 7.14**).

Pneumatic reduction. An alternative to hydrostatic reduction (sonographically or fluoroscopically guided) is pneumatic reduction, in which air is insufflated under fluoroscopic guidance to reduce the invaginated bowel. Both methods are well tested and effective; the preferred method is the one that is more familiar to the radiologist.

Complications

The recurrence rate after a successful nonsurgical reduction is 5–10%, with most recurrences developing within the first 72 hours. An intussusception may recur several times, but multiple nonsurgical reductions (up to five) may be performed. The perforation rate with hydrostatic reduction is less than 0.5%.

▄ Summary

The differential diagnosis of acute abdominal pain in children is very broad and varies with the age of the patient. Extra-abdominal diseases may also underlie an **acute abdomen**. Ultrasonography is the primary imaging modality for evaluating an acute abdomen in children.

Meconium ileus is often the initial manifestation of cystic fibrosis. Therapeutic contrast enema is successful in up to 60% of cases.

Pneumatosis of the bowel wall is strongly suggestive of **necrotizing enterocolitis** (NEC) but is also seen in other inflammatory bowel diseases. There are no specific radiographic signs for NEC.

In every child who presents with bilious vomiting, **volvulus** should be excluded by contrast administration via gastric tube or confirmed by detecting a corkscrew-like configuration of the small bowel and cutoff of the contrast column. Volvulus can also be detected by ultrasound scanning but is not excluded by negative sonographic findings.

The more aboral the site of an **atresia**, the less the distension of more proximal gastrointestinal structures. Contrast examination is appropriate for locating a distal stenosis or atresia and determining its cause.

The main symptom of **Hirschsprung disease** is constipation. The disease may cause intestinal obstruction in newborns. Contrast enema should be performed carefully, as it can easily distend the aganglionic segment.

Today, **hypertrophic pyloric stenosis** is diagnosed sonographically. The pyloric channel is more than 16 mm long and its wall is thickened to more than 3 mm. Pylorospasm can be excluded by follow-up scans.

Intussusception can also be diagnosed by ultrasound scanning. The longitudinal scan demonstrates a "pseudo-kidney" while the transverse scan shows a "crescent-in-doughnut" sign. Treatment consists of hydrostatic or pneumatic reduction. The absence of Doppler flow signals indicates vascular obstruction, however, and is an indication for immediate surgery.

Further Reading

Basic Principles: Radiologic Techniques and Radiation Safety

Radiologic Techniques in the Intensive Care Unit

Book Chapters / Review Articles
MacMahon H, Giger M. Portable chest radiography: techniques and teleradiology. Radiol Clin North Am 1996;34(1):1–20

Digital Radiography
Eisenhuber E, Stadler A, Prokop M, Fuchsjager M, Weber M, Schaefer-Prokop C. Detection of monitoring materials on bedside chest radiographs with the most recent generation of storage phosphor plates: dose increase does not improve detection performance. Radiology 2003;227(1):216–221

Prokop M, Neitzel U, Schaefer-Prokop C. Principles of image processing in digital chest radiography. J Thorac Imaging 2003;18(3):148–164

Schaefer-Prokop C, Uffmann M, Eisenhuber E, Prokop M. Digital radiography of the chest: detector techniques and performance parameters. J Thorac Imaging 2003;18(3):124–137

Schaefer-Prokop C, Uffmann M, Sailer J, Kabalan N, Herold C, Prokop M. Digital thorax radiography: flat-panel detector or storage phosphor plates. [Article in German] Radiologe 2003;43(5):351–361

Radiation Exposure to Patients and Staff
Ciraulo DL, Marini CP, Lloyd GT, Fisher J. Do surgical residents, emergency medicine physicians, and nurses experience significant radiation exposure during the resuscitation of trauma patients? J Trauma 1994;36(5):703–705

Cupitt JM, Vinayagam S, McConachie I. Radiation exposure of nurses on an intensive care unit. Anaesthesia 2001;56(2):183

Duetting T, Foerste B, Knoch T, Darge K, Troeger J. Radiation exposure during chest X-ray examinations in a premature intensive care unit: phantom studies. Pediatr Radiol 1999;29(3):158–162

Grazer RE, Meislin HW, Westerman BR, Criss EA. Exposure to ionizing radiation in the emergency department from commonly performed portable radiographs. Ann Emerg Med 1987;16(4):417–420

Grazer RE, Meislin HW, Westerman BR, Criss EA. A nine-year evaluation of emergency department personnel exposure to ionizing radiation. Ann Emerg Med 1987;16(3):340–342

Leppek R, Bertrams SS, Holtermann W, et al. Radiation exposure during thoracic radiography at the intensive care unit. Dose accumulation and risk of radiation-induced cancer in long-term therapy. [Article in German] Radiologe 1998;38:730–736

Mostafa G, Sing RF, McKeown R, Huynh TT, Heniford BT. The hazard of scattered radiation in a trauma intensive care unit. Crit Care Med 2002;30(3):574–576

Radiation Exposure during Pregnancy
Ames Castro M, Shipp TD, Castro EE, Ouzounian J, Rao P. The use of helical computed tomography in pregnancy for the diagnosis of acute appendicitis. Am J Obstet Gynecol 2001;184(5):954–957 PubMed

Damilakis J, Perisinakis K, Voloudaki A, Gourtsoyiannis N. Estimation of fetal radiation dose from computed tomography scanning in late pregnancy: depth-dose data from routine examinations. Invest Radiol 2000;35(9):527–533

Kennedy A. Assessment of acute abdominal pain in the pregnant patient. Semin Ultrasound CT MR 2000;21(1):64–77

Lowdermilk C, Gavant ML, Qaisi W, West OC, Goldman SM. Screening helical CT for evaluation of blunt traumatic injury in the pregnant patient. Radiographics 1999;19(Spec No):S 243–S 255, discussion S 256–S 258

Macklon NS. Diagnosis of deep venous thrombosis and pulmonary embolism in pregnancy. Curr Opin Pulm Med 1999;5(4):233–237

Radiation Exposure in Children
American Academy of Pediatrics. Committee on Environmental Health. Risk of ionizing radiation exposure to children: a subject review. Pediatrics 1998;101(4 Pt 1):717–719

Berdon WE, Slovis TL. Where we are since ALARA and the series of articles on CT dose in children and risk of long-term cancers: what has changed? Pediatr Radiol 2002;32(10):699

Frush DP. Pediatric CT: practical approach to diminish the radiation dose. Pediatr Radiol 2002;32(10):714–717, discussion 751–754

Frush DP, Slack CC, Hollingsworth CL, et al. Computer-simulated radiation dose reduction for abdominal multidetector CT of pediatric patients. AJR Am J Roentgenol 2002;179(5):1107–1113

Hall EJ. Lessons we have learned from our children: cancer risks from diagnostic radiology. Pediatr Radiol 2002;32(10):700–706

Hollingsworth C, Frush DP, Cross M, Lucaya J. Helical CT of the body: a survey of techniques used for pediatric patients. AJR Am J Roentgenol 2003;180(2):401–406

McParland BJ, Gorka W, Lee R, Lewall DB, Omojola MF. Radiology in the neonatal intensive care unit: dose reduction and image quality. Br J Radiol 1996;69(826):929–937

Slovis TL. The ALARA concept in pediatric CT: myth or reality? Radiology 2002;223(1):5–6

Suess C, Chen X. Dose optimization in pediatric CT: current technology and future innovations. Pediatr Radiol 2002;32(10):729–734, discussion 751–754

Dose Reduction in Computed Tomography
Prokop M. Optimizing dosage in thoracic computerized tomography. [Article in German] Radiologe 2001;41(3):269–278

Prokop M. Radiation dose and image quality in computed tomography. [Article in German] Rofo 2002;174(5):631–636

Prokop M. Radiation dose and Image Quality. In: Prokop M, Galanski M, ed. Spiral and Multidetektor Computed Tomography of the body. Stuttgart: Thieme; 2003

Dose Reduction in Digital Radiography
Eisenhuber E, Stadler A, Prokop M, Fuchsjager M, Weber M, Schaefer-Prokop C. Detection of monitoring materials on bedside chest radiographs with the most recent generation of storage phosphor plates: dose increase does not improve detection performance. Radiology 2003;227(1):216–221

Communication, Reporting of Findings, and Teleradiology
Redfern RO, Kundel HL, Polansky M, Langlotz CP, Horii SC, Lanken PN. A picture archival and communication system shortens delays in obtaining radiographic information in a medical intensive care unit. Crit Care Med 2000;28(4):1006–1013

Steckel RJ, Batra P, Johnson S, et al. Chest teleradiology in a teaching hospital emergency practice. AJR Am J Roentgenol 1997;168(6):1409–1413

Thoracic Imaging of the Intensive Care Patient

Review Articles / Book Chapters
Bankier A, Fleischmann D, Aram L, Heimberger K, Schindler E, Herold CJ. Imaging in intensive care. Methods, indications, diagnostic signs. I. [Article in German] Radiologe 1998;38(11):972–986

Bankier A, Fleischmann D, Aram L, Heimberger K, Schindler E, Herold CJ. Imaging in intensive medicine. Techniques. Indications, diagnostic signs. II. [Article in German] Radiologe 1998;38(12):1089–1099

Goodman LR. Acute pulmonary disease. In: Goodman LR, Putman CE, eds. Critical Care Imaging. Philadelphia: Saunders; 1992

Henschke CI, Yankelevitz DF, Wand A, Davis SD, Shiau M. Accuracy and efficacy of chest radiography in the intensive care unit. Radiol Clin North Am 1996;34(1):21–31

Maffessanti M, Berlot G, Bortolotto P. Chest roentgenology in the intensive care unit: an overview. Eur Radiol 1998;8(1):69–78

Miller WT Sr. The chest radiograph in the intensive care unit. Semin Roentgenol 1997;32(2):89–101

Wandtke JC. Bedside chest radiography. Radiology 1994;190(1):1–10

Portable Chest Radiography—Efficiency

Brainsky A, Fletcher RH, Glick HA, Lanken PN, Williams SV, Kundel HL. Routine portable chest radiographs in the medical intensive care unit: effects and costs. Crit Care Med 1997;25(5):801–805

Fong Y, Whalen GF, Hariri RJ, Barie PS. Utility of routine chest radiographs in the surgical intensive care unit. A prospective study. Arch Surg 1995;130(7):764–768

Greenbaum DM, Marschall KE. The value of routine daily chest x-rays in intubated patients in the medical intensive care unit. Crit Care Med 1982;10(1):29–30

Hall JB, White SR, Karrison T. Efficacy of daily routine chest radiographs in intubated, mechanically ventilated patients. Crit Care Med 1991;19(5):689–693

Silverstein DS, Livingston DH, Elcavage J, Kovar L, Kelly KM. The utility of routine daily chest radiography in the surgical intensive care unit. J Trauma 1993;35(4):643–646

Adult Respiratory Distress Syndrome (ARDS)

Bernard GR, Artigas A, Brigham KL, et al. The American-European Consensus Conference on ARDS. Definitions, mechanisms, relevant outcomes, and clinical trial coordination. Am J Respir Crit Care Med 1994;149(3 Pt 1):818–824

Krafft P, Fridrich P, Pernerstorfer T, et al. The acute respiratory distress syndrome: definitions, severity and clinical outcome. An analysis of 101 clinical investigations. Intensive Care Med 1996;22(6):519–529

Montgomery AB, Stager MA, Carrico CJ, Hudson LD. Causes of mortality in patients with the adult respiratory distress syndrome. Am Rev Respir Dis 1985;132(3):485–489

Navarrete-Navarro P, Rodriguez A, Reynolds N, et al. Acute respiratory distress syndrome among trauma patients: trends in ICU mortality, risk factors, complications and resource utilization. Intensive Care Med 2001;27(7):1133–1140

Pathophysiology, Imaging

Bankier A, Fleischmann D, Aram L, Heimberger K, Schindler E, Herold CJ. Imaging in intensive care. Methods, indications, diagnostic signs. I. [Article in German] Radiologe 1998;38(11):972–986

Bankier A, Fleischmann D, Aram L, Heimberger K, Schindler E, Herold CJ. Imaging in intensive medicine. Techniques. Indications, diagnostic signs. II. [Article in German] Radiologe 1998;38(12):1089–1099

Bink A, Marksteller K, Birkenkamp K, et al. Multi-rotation CT and acute respiratory distress syndrome. Animal experiment studies. [Article in German] Radiologe 2001;41:195–200

Bombino M, Gattinoni L, Pesenti A, Pistolesi M, Miniati M. The value of portable chest roentgenography in adult respiratory distress syndrome. Comparison with computed tomography. Chest 1991;100(3):762–769

Desai SR. Acute respiratory distress syndrome: imaging of the injured lung. Clin Radiol 2002;57(1):8–17

Desai SR, Hansell DM. Lung imaging in the adult respiratory distress syndrome: current practice and new insights. Intensive Care Med 1997;23(1):7–15

Desai SR, Wells AU, Rubens MB, Evans TW, Hansell DM. Acute respiratory distress syndrome: CT abnormalities at long-term follow-up. Radiology 1999;210(1):29–35

Gattinoni L, Bombino M, Pelosi P, et al. Lung structure and function in different stages of severe adult respiratory distress syndrome. JAMA 1994;271(22):1772–1779

Gattinoni L, Pelosi P, Suter PM, Pedoto A, Vercesi P, Lissoni A. Acute respiratory distress syndrome caused by pulmonary and extrapulmonary disease. Different syndromes? Am J Respir Crit Care Med 1998;158(1):3–11

Goodman LR, Fumagalli R, Tagliabue P, et al. Adult respiratory distress syndrome due to pulmonary and extrapulmonary causes: CT, clinical, and functional correlations. Radiology 1999;213(2):545–552

Goodman PC. Radiographic findings in patients with acute respiratory distress syndrome. Clin Chest Med 2000;21(3):419–433, vii

Greene R. Adult respiratory distress syndrome: acute alveolar damage. Radiology 1987;163(1):57–66

Halperin BD, Feeley TW, Mihm FG, Chiles C, Guthaner DF, Blank NE. Evaluation of the portable chest roentgenogram for quantitating extravascular lung water in critically ill adults. Chest 1985;88(5):649–652

Henschke CI, Yankelevitz DF, Wand A, Davis SD, Shiau M. Accuracy and efficacy of chest radiography in the intensive care unit. Radiol Clin North Am 1996;34(1):21–31

Howling SJ, Evans TW, Hansell DM. The significance of bronchial dilatation on CT in patients with adult respiratory distress syndrome. Clin Radiol 1998;53(2):105–109

Meade MO, Cook RJ, Guyatt GH, et al. Interobserver variation in interpreting chest radiographs for the diagnosis of acute respiratory distress syndrome. Am J Respir Crit Care Med 2000;161(1):85–90

Nöbauer-Huhmann IM, Eibenberger K, Schaefer-Prokop C, et al. Changes in lung parenchyma after acute respiratory distress syndrome (ARDS): assessment with high-resolution computed tomography. Eur Radiol 2001;11(12):2436–2443

Owens CM, Evans TW, Keogh BF, Hansell DM. Computed tomography in established adult respiratory distress syndrome. Correlation with lung injury score. Chest 1994;106(6):1815–1821

Pelosi P, Crotti S, Brazzi L, Gattinoni L. Computed tomography in adult respiratory distress syndrome: what has it taught us? Eur Respir J 1996;9(5):1055–1062

Pelosi P, D'Andrea L, Vitale G, Pesenti A, Gattinoni L. Vertical gradient of regional lung inflation in adult respiratory distress syndrome. Am J Respir Crit Care Med 1994;149(1):8–13

Pesenti A, Tagliabue P, Patroniti N, Fumagalli R. Computerised tomography scan imaging in acute respiratory distress syndrome. Intensive Care Med 2001;27(4):631–639

Puybasset L, Cluzel P, Gusman P, Grenier P, Preteux F, Rouby JJ; CT Scan ARDS Study Group. Regional distribution of gas and tissue in acute respiratory distress syndrome. I. Consequences for lung morphology. Intensive Care Med 2000;26(7):857–869

Rubenfeld GD, Caldwell E, Granton J, Hudson LD, Matthay MA. Interobserver variability in applying a radiographic definition for ARDS. Chest 1999;116(5):1347–1353

Tagliabue M, Casella TC, Zincone GE, Fumagalli R, Salvini E. CT and chest radiography in the evaluation of adult respiratory distress syndrome. Acta Radiol 1994;35(3):230–234

Therapeutic Measures

Amato MBP, Barbas CSV, Medeiros DM, et al. Effect of a protective-ventilation strategy on mortality in the acute respiratory distress syndrome. N Engl J Med 1998;338(6):347–354

Blanch L, Mancebo J, Perez M, et al. Short-term effects of prone position in critically ill patients with acute respiratory distress syndrome. Intensive Care Med 1997;23(10):1033–1039

Brower RG, Fessler HE. Mechanical ventilation in acute lung injury and acute respiratory distress syndrome. Clin Chest Med 2000;21 (3):491 – 510, viii

Brower RG, Ware LB, Berthiaume Y, Matthay MA. Treatment of ARDS. Chest 2001;120(4):1347 – 1367

Dambrosio M, Roupie E, Mollet JJ, et al. Effects of positive end-expiratory pressure and different tidal volumes on alveolar recruitment and hyperinflation. Anesthesiology 1997;87(3):495 – 503

Dellinger RP, Zimmerman JL, Taylor RW, et al; Inhaled Nitric Oxide in ARDS Study Group. Effects of inhaled nitric oxide in patients with acute respiratory distress syndrome: results of a randomized phase II trial. Crit Care Med 1998;26(1):15 – 23

Domenighetti G, Stricker H, Waldispuehl B. Nebulized prostacyclin (PGI2) in acute respiratory distress syndrome: impact of primary (pulmonary injury) and secondary (extrapulmonary injury) disease on gas exchange response. Crit Care Med 2001;29(1):57 – 62

Fridrich P, Krafft P, Hochleuthner H, Mauritz W. The effects of long-term prone positioning in patients with trauma-induced adult respiratory distress syndrome. Anesth Analg 1996;83(6):1206 – 1211

Gattinoni L, D'Andrea L, Pelosi P, Vitale G, Pesenti A, Fumagalli R. Regional effects and mechanism of positive end-expiratory pressure in early adult respiratory distress syndrome. JAMA 1993;269(16):2122 – 2127

Gattinoni L, Mascheroni D, Torresin A, et al. Morphological response to positive end expiratory pressure in acute respiratory failure. Computerized tomography study. Intensive Care Med 1986;12 (3):137 – 142

Gattinoni L, Pelosi P, Crotti S, Valenza F. Effects of positive end-expiratory pressure on regional distribution of tidal volume and recruitment in adult respiratory distress syndrome. Am J Respir Crit Care Med 1995;151(6):1807 – 1814

Gattinoni L, Pesenti A, Avalli L, Rossi F, Bombino M. Pressure–volume curve of total respiratory system in acute respiratory failure. Computed tomographic scan study. Am Rev Respir Dis 1987;136 (3):730 – 736

Johnson MM, Ely EW, Chiles C, et al. Radiographic assessment of hyperinflation: correlation with objective chest radiographic measurements and mechanical ventilator parameters. Chest 1998;113(6):1698 – 1704

Ketai LH, Godwin JD. A new view of pulmonary edema and acute respiratory distress syndrome. J Thorac Imaging 1998;13 (3):147 – 171

Parker JC, Hernandez LA, Peevy KJ. Mechanisms of ventilator-induced lung injury. Crit Care Med 1993;21(1):131 – 143

Vincent JL, Brase R, Santman F, et al. A multi-centre, double-blind, placebo-controlled study of liposomal prostaglandin E1 (TLC C-53) in patients with acute respiratory distress syndrome. Intensive Care Med 2001;27(10):1578 – 1583

Walmrath D, Schneider T, Pilch J, Grimminger F, Seeger W. Aerosolised prostacyclin in adult respiratory distress syndrome. Lancet 1993;342(8877):961 – 962

Walmrath D, Schneider T, Schermuly R, Olschewski H, Grimminger F, Seeger W. Direct comparison of inhaled nitric oxide and aerosolized prostacyclin in acute respiratory distress syndrome. Am J Respir Crit Care Med 1996;153(3):991 – 996

Zwissler B, Kemming G, Habler O, et al. Inhaled prostacyclin (PGI2) versus inhaled nitric oxide in adult respiratory distress syndrome. Am J Respir Crit Care Med 1996;154(6 Pt 1):1671 – 1677

Differential Diagnosis

Goodman LR. Congestive heart failure and adult respiratory distress syndrome. New insights using computed tomography. Radiol Clin North Am 1996;34(1):33 – 46

Ketai LH, Godwin JD. A new view of pulmonary edema and acute respiratory distress syndrome. J Thorac Imaging 1998;13 (3):147 – 171

Milne EN, Pistolesi M, Miniati M, Giuntini C. The radiologic distinction of cardiogenic and noncardiogenic edema. AJR Am J Roentgenol 1985;144(5):879 – 894

Pistolesi M, Miniati M, Milne ENC, Giuntini C. The chest roentgenogram in pulmonary edema. Clin Chest Med 1985;6(3):315 – 344

Tomiyama N, Müller NL, Johkoh T, et al. Acute respiratory distress syndrome and acute interstitial pneumonia: comparison of thin-section CT findings. J Comput Assist Tomogr 2001;25(1):28 – 33

Complications

Pingleton SK. Complications of acute respiratory failure. Am Rev Respir Dis 1988;137(6):1463 – 1493

Seidenfeld JJ, Pohl DF, Bell RC, Harris GD, Johanson WG Jr. Incidence, site, and outcome of infections in patients with the adult respiratory distress syndrome. Am Rev Respir Dis 1986;134(1):12 – 16

Tocino I, Westcott JL. Barotrauma. Radiol Clin North Am 1996;34 (1):59 – 81

Tocino IM, Miller MH, Fairfax WR. Distribution of pneumothorax in the supine and semirecumbent critically ill adult. AJR Am J Roentgenol 1985;144(5):901 – 905

Vieira SR, Puybasset L, Richecoeur J, et al. A lung computed tomographic assessment of positive end-expiratory pressure-induced lung overdistension. Am J Respir Crit Care Med 1998;158(5 Pt 1):1571 – 1577

Winer-Muram HT, Rubin SA, Ellis JV, et al. Pneumonia and ARDS in patients receiving mechanical ventilation: diagnostic accuracy of chest radiography. Radiology 1993;188(2):479 – 485

Winer-Muram HT, Steiner RM, Gurney JW, et al. Ventilator-associated pneumonia in patients with adult respiratory distress syndrome: CT evaluation. Radiology 1998;208(1):193 – 199

Pneumonia

Nosocomial Pneumonia

Celis R, Torres A, Gatell JM, Almela M, Rodríguez-Roisin R, Agustí-Vidal A. Nosocomial pneumonia. A multivariate analysis of risk and prognosis. Chest 1988;93(2):318 – 324

Lefcoe MS, Fox GA, Leasa DJ, Sparrow RK, McCormack DG. Accuracy of portable chest radiography in the critical care setting. Diagnosis of pneumonia based on quantitative cultures obtained from protected brush catheter. Chest 1994;105(3):885 – 887

Lipchik RJ, Kuzo RS. Nosocomial pneumonia. Radiol Clin North Am 1996;34(1):47 – 58

Lode HM, Schaberg T, Raffenberg M, Mauch H. Nosocomial pneumonia in the critical care unit. Crit Care Clin 1998;14(1):119 – 133

Santos E, Talusan A, Brandstetter RD. Roentgenographic mimics of pneumonia in the critical care unit. Crit Care Clin 1998;14(1):91 – 104

Aspiration Pneumonia

Landay MJ, Christensen EE, Bynum LJ. Pulmonary manifestations of acute aspiration of gastric contents. AJR Am J Roentgenol 1978;131(4):587 – 592

Mendelsohn CL. The aspiration of stomach contents into the lungs during obstetric anesthesia. Am J Obstet Gynecol 1946;52:191 – 205

Schwartz DJ, Wynne JW, Gibbs CP, Hood CI, Kuck EJ. The pulmonary consequences of aspiration of gastric contents at pH values greater than 2.5. Am Rev Respir Dis 1980;121(1):119 – 126

Pneumonia during Mechanical Ventilation

Butler KL, Sinclair KE, Henderson VJ, et al. The chest radiograph in critically ill surgical patients is inaccurate in predicting ventilator-associated pneumonia. Am Surg 1999;65(9):805 – 809, discussion 809 – 810

Chastre J, Fagon JY. Ventilator-associated pneumonia. Am J Respir Crit Care Med 2002;165(7):867 – 903

Craven DE, Kunches LM, Kilinsky V, Lichtenberg DA, Make BJ, McCabe WR. Risk factors for pneumonia and fatality in patients receiving continuous mechanical ventilation. Am Rev Respir Dis 1986;133 (5):792 – 796

Fagon JY, Chastre J, Hance AJ, et al. Detection of nosocomial lung infection in ventilated patients. Use of a protected specimen brush and quantitative culture techniques in 147 patients. Am Rev Respir Dis 1988;138(1):110 – 116

Fagon JY, Chastre J, Hance AJ, Domart Y, Trouillet JL, Gibert C. Evaluation of clinical judgment in the identification and treatment of nosocomial pneumonia in ventilated patients. Chest 1993;103 (2):547 – 553

Hahn U, Pereira P, Heininger A, Laniado M, Claussen CD. Value of CT in diagnosis of respirator-associated pneumonia. [Article in German] Rofo 1999;170(2):150 – 155

Jiménez P, Torres A, Rodríguez-Roisin R, et al. Incidence and etiology of pneumonia acquired during mechanical ventilation. Crit Care Med 1989;17(9):882 – 885

Johnson MM, Ely EW, Chiles C, et al. Radiographic assessment of hyperinflation: correlation with objective chest radiographic measurements and mechanical ventilator parameters. Chest 1998;113(6):1698 – 1704

Meduri GU, Mauldin GL, Wunderink RG, et al. Causes of fever and pulmonary densities in patients with clinical manifestations of ventilator-associated pneumonia. Chest 1994;106(1):221 – 235

Pugin J, Auckenthaler R, Mili N, Janssens JP, Lew PD, Suter PM. Diagnosis of ventilator-associated pneumonia by bacteriologic analysis of bronchoscopic and nonbronchoscopic "blind" bronchoalveolar lavage fluid. Am Rev Respir Dis 1991;143(5 Pt 1):1121 – 1129

Winer-Muram HT, Jennings SG, Wunderink RG, Jones CB, Leeper KV Jr. Ventilator-associated Pseudomonas aeruginosa pneumonia: radiographic findings. Radiology 1995;195(1):247 – 252

Winer-Muram HT, Steiner RM, Gurney JW, et al. Ventilator-associated pneumonia in patients with adult respiratory distress syndrome: CT evaluation. Radiology 1998;208(1):193 – 199

Wunderink RG, Woldenberg LS, Zeiss J, Day CM, Ciemins J, Lacher DA. The radiologic diagnosis of autopsy-proven ventilator-associated pneumonia. Chest 1992;101(2):458 – 463

Wunderink RG. Radiologic diagnosis of ventilator-associated pneumonia. Chest 2000;

Zimmerman JE, Goodman LR, Shahvari MB. Effect of mechanical ventilation and positive end-expiratory pressure (PEEP) on chest radiograph. AJR Am J Roentgenol 1979;133(5):811 – 815

ARDS and Pneumonia

Chastre J, Trouillet JL, Vuagnat A, et al. Nosocomial pneumonia in patients with acute respiratory distress syndrome. Am J Respir Crit Care Med 1998;157(4 Pt 1):1165 – 1172

Sutherland KR, Steinberg KP, Maunder RJ, Milberg JA, Allen DL, Hudson LD. Pulmonary infection during the acute respiratory distress syndrome. Am J Respir Crit Care Med 1995;152(2):550 – 556

Winer-Muram HT, Rubin SA, Ellis JV, et al. Pneumonia and ARDS in patients receiving mechanical ventilation: diagnostic accuracy of chest radiography. Radiology 1993;188(2):479 – 485

Winer-Muram HT, Steiner RM, Gurney JW, et al. Ventilator-associated pneumonia in patients with adult respiratory distress syndrome: CT evaluation. Radiology 1998;208(1):193 – 199

Atelectasis

Ashizawa K, Hayashi K, Aso N, Minami K. Lobar atelectasis: diagnostic pitfalls on chest radiography. Br J Radiol 2001;74(877):89 – 97

Marini JJ, Pierson DJ, Hudson LD. Acute lobar atelectasis: a prospective comparison of fiberoptic bronchoscopy and respiratory therapy. Am Rev Respir Dis 1979;119(6):971 – 978

Shevland JE, Hirleman MT, Hoang KA, Kealey GP. Lobar collapse in the surgical intensive care unit. Br J Radiol 1983;56(668):531 – 534

Pneumothorax

Beres RA, Goodman LR. Pneumothorax: detection with upright versus decubitus radiography. Radiology 1993;186(1):19 – 22

Chiles C, Ravin CE. Radiographic recognition of pneumothorax in the intensive care unit. Crit Care Med 1986;14(8):677 – 680

Galanski M, Hartenauer U, Krumme B. X-Ray diagnosis of pneumothorax in intensive care units (author's transl). [Article in German] Radiologe 1981;21:459 – 462

Gordon R. The deep sulcus sign. Radiology 1980;136(1):25 – 27

Kurlander GJ, Helmen CH. Subpulmonary pneumothorax. Am J Roentgenol Radium Ther Nucl Med 1966;96(4):1019 – 1021

Rowan KR, Kirkpatrick AW, Liu D, Forkheim KE, Mayo JR, Nicolaou S. Traumatic pneumothorax detection with thoracic US: correlation with chest radiography and CT—initial experience. Radiology 2002;225(1):210 – 214

Sivak SL. Late appearance of pneumothorax after subclavian venipuncture. Am J Med 1986;80(2):323 – 324

Tocino IM, Miller MH, Fairfax WR. Distribution of pneumothorax in the supine and semirecumbent critically ill adult. AJR Am J Roentgenol 1985;144(5):901 – 905

Tocino IM, Miller MH, Frederick PR, Bahr AL, Thomas F. CT detection of occult pneumothorax in head trauma. AJR Am J Roentgenol 1984;143(5):987 – 990

Ziter FMH Jr, Westcott JL. Supine subpulmonary pneumothorax. AJR Am J Roentgenol 1981;137(4):699 – 701

Pleural Effusion

Patel MC, Flower CDR. Radiology in the management of pleural disease. Eur Radiol 1997;7(9):1454 – 1462

Ruskin JA, Gurney JW, Thorsen MK, Goodman LR. Detection of pleural effusions on supine chest radiographs. AJR Am J Roentgenol 1987;148(4):681 – 683

Schmidt O, Simon S, Schmitt R, et al. Volumetry of pleural effusion in multi-morbidity, postoperative patients of a surgical intensive care unit. Comparison of ultrasound diagnosis and thoracic bedside image. [Article in German] Zentralbl Chir 2000;125:375 – 379

Acute Pulmonary Embolism

ACCP Consensus Committee on Pulmonary Embolism. American College of Chest Physicians. Opinions regarding the diagnosis and management of venous thromboembolic disease. Chest 1998;113(2):499 – 504

Armstrong P, Wilson AG, Dee P, Hansell DM. Imaging of Diseases of the Chest. 3rd ed. London: Mosby; 2000: 405 – 430

Bankier AA, Janata K, Fleischmann D, et al. Severity assessment of acute pulmonary embolism with spiral CT: evaluation of two modified angiographic scores and comparison with clinical data. J Thorac Imaging 1997;12(2):150 – 158

Beigelman C, Chartrand-Lefebvre C, Howarth N, Grenier P. Pitfalls in diagnosis of pulmonary embolism with helical CT angiography. AJR Am J Roentgenol 1998;171(3):579 – 585

Braunwald E, Isselbacher KJ, Petersdorfr RG, Wilson JD, Martin JB, Fauci AS. Harrison's Principles of Internal Medicine. 12th ed. New York: Mc Graw Hill; 1998

Chunilal SD, Eikelboom JW, Attia J, et al. Does this patient have pulmonary embolism? JAMA 2003;290(21):2849 – 2858

Coche E, Verschuren F, Hainaut P, Goncette L. Pulmonary embolism findings on chest radiographs and multislice spiral CT. Eur Radiol 2004;14(7):1241 – 1248

Fleischmann D, Kontrus M, Bankier AA, Wiesmayr MN, Janata-Schwatczek K, Herold CJ. Spiral CT in acute pulmonary embolism. [Article in German] Radiologe 1996;36(6):489 – 495

Fraser RS, Colman N, Müller N, Paré PD. Fraser and Pare's Diagnosis of Diseases of the Chest. Vol. III, 4th ed. Philadelphia: Saunders; 1999: 775 – 1835

Frost SD, Brotman DJ, Michota FA. Rational use of D-dimer measurement to exclude acute venous thromboembolic disease. Mayo Clin Proc 2003;78(11):1385 – 1391

Garg K, Sieler H, Welsh CH, Johnston RJ, Russ PD. Clinical validity of helical CT being interpreted as negative for pulmonary embolism: implications for patient treatment. AJR Am J Roentgenol 1999;172(6):1627 – 1631

Ghaye B, Remy J, Remy-Jardin M. Non-traumatic thoracic emergencies: CT diagnosis of acute pulmonary embolism: the first 10 years. Eur Radiol 2002;12(8):1886 – 1905

Hoffmann U, Schima W, Herold C. Pulmonary magnetic resonance angiography. Eur Radiol 1999;9(9):1745 – 1754

Kavanagh EC, O'Hare A, Hargaden G, Murray JG. Risk of pulmonary embolism after negative MDCT pulmonary angiography findings. AJR Am J Roentgenol 2004;182(2):499 – 504

Kuiper JW, Geleijns J, Matheijssen NAA, Teeuwisse W, Pattynama PM. Radiation exposure of multi-row detector spiral computed tomography of the pulmonary arteries: comparison with digital subtraction pulmonary angiography. Eur Radiol 2003;13(7):1496 – 1500

Loud PA, Grossman ZD, Klippenstein DL, Ray CE. Combined CT venography and pulmonary angiography: a new diagnostic technique for suspected thromboembolic disease. AJR Am J Roentgenol 1998;170(4):951 – 954

Miniati M, Monti S, Bauleo C, et al. A diagnostic strategy for pulmonary embolism based on standardised pretest probability and perfusion lung scanning: a management study. Eur J Nucl Med Mol Imaging 2003;30(11):1450 – 1456

Miniati M, Monti S, Pratali L, et al. Value of transthoracic echocardiography in the diagnosis of pulmonary embolism: results of a prospective study in unselected patients. Am J Med 2001;110 (7):528 – 535

Miniati M, Prediletto R, Formichi B, et al. Accuracy of clinical assessment in the diagnosis of pulmonary embolism. Am J Respir Crit Care Med 1999;159(3):864 – 871

Naidich DP, Müller NL, Zerhouni EA, Mc Guinness G. Computed Tomography and Magnetic Resonance of the Thorax. 3rd ed. Philadelphia: Lippincott-Raven; 1999: 622 – 642

Oudkerk M, van Beek EJ, Wielopolski P, et al. Comparison of contrast-enhanced magnetic resonance angiography and conventional pulmonary angiography for the diagnosis of pulmonary embolism: a prospective study. Lancet 2002;359(9318):1643 – 1647

Perrier A, Roy PM, Aujesky D, et al. Diagnosing pulmonary embolism in outpatients with clinical assessment, D-dimer measurement, venous ultrasound, and helical computed tomography: a multi-center management study. Am J Med 2004;116(5):291 – 299

Remy-Jardin M, Mastora I, Remy J. Pulmonary embolus imaging with multislice CT. Radiol Clin North Am 2003;41(3):507 – 519

Remy-Jardin M, Remy J, Spiral CT. Spiral CT angiography of the pulmonary circulation. Radiology 1999;212(3):615 – 636

Remy-Jardin M, Tillie-Leblond I, Szapiro D, et al. CT angiography of pulmonary embolism in patients with underlying respiratory disease: impact of multislice CT on image quality and negative predictive value. Eur Radiol 2002;12(8):1971 – 1978

Simon M, Chiang EE, Boiselle PM. Paddle-wheel multislice helical CT display of pulmonary vessels and other lung structures. Radiol Clin North Am 2003;41(3):617 – 626

Wells PS, Anderson DR, Rodger M, et al. Derivation of a simple clinical model to categorize patients probability of pulmonary embolism: increasing the models utility with the SimpliRED D-dimer. Thromb Haemost 2000;83(3):416 – 420

Wells PS, Anderson DR, Rodger M, et al. Evaluation of D-dimer in the diagnosis of suspected deep-vein thrombosis. N Engl J Med 2003;349(13):1227 – 1235

Winer-Muram HT, Boone JM, Brown HL, Jennings SG, Mabie WC, Lombardo GT. Pulmonary embolism in pregnant patients: fetal radiation dose with helical CT. Radiology 2002;224(2):487 – 492

Imaging of Intensive Care Patients after Thoracic Surgery

Review Articles / Book Chapters

Bhalla M. Noncardiac thoracic surgical procedures. Definitions, indications, and postoperative radiology. Radiol Clin North Am 1996;34(1):137 – 155

Goodman LR. Imaging after Thoracotomy and Imaging after Cardiac Surgery. In: Goodman LR, Putman CE, eds. Critical Care Imaging. Philadelphia: Saunders; 1992

Goodman LR. Postoperative chest radiograph: II. Alterations after major intrathoracic surgery. AJR Am J Roentgenol 1980;134 (4):803 – 813

Sheehan RE, Sheppard MN, Hansell DM. Retained intrathoracic surgical swab: CT appearances. J Thorac Imaging 2000;15(1):61 – 64

Pneumonectomy and Lobectomy

Boiselle PM, Shepard JA, McLoud TC, Grillo HC, Wright CD. Postpneumonectomy syndrome: another twist. J Thorac Imaging 1997;12(3):209 – 211

Gruden JF, Campagna G, McGuinness G. The normal CT appearances of the second carina and bronchial stump after left upper lobectomy. J Thorac Imaging 2000;15(2):138 – 143

Kakeda S, Kamada K, Aoki T, Watanabe H, Nakata H. Postsurgical change in the tracheal bifurcation angle after upper lobectomy: radiographic evaluation. Acad Radiol 2003;10(6):644 – 649

Kim EA, Lee KS, Shim YM, et al. Radiographic and CT findings in complications following pulmonary resection. Radiographics 2002;22(1):67 – 86

Seo JB, Lee KS, Choo SW, Shim YM, Primack SL. Neofissure after lobectomy of the right lung: radiographic and CT findings. Radiology 1996;201(2):475 – 479

Shepard JA, Grillo HC, McLoud TC, Dedrick CG, Spizarny DL. Right-pneumonectomy syndrome: radiologic findings and CT correlation. Radiology 1986;161(3):661 – 664

Tsukada G, Stark P. Postpneumonectomy complications. AJR Am J Roentgenol 1997;169(5):1363 – 1370

Valji AM, Maziak DE, Shamji FM, Matzinger FR. Postpneumonectomy syndrome: recognition and management. Chest 1998;114 (6):1766 – 1769

Westcott JL, Volpe JP. Peripheral bronchopleural fistula: CT evaluation in 20 patients with pneumonia, empyema, or postoperative air leak. Radiology 1995;196(1):175 – 181

Lung Transplantation

Collins J. Imaging of the chest after lung transplantation. J Thorac Imaging 2002;17(2):102 – 112

Collins J, Kuhlman JE, Love RB. Acute, life-threatening complications of lung transplantation. Radiographics 1998;18(1):21 – 43, discussion 43 – 47

Collins J, Müller NL, Kazerooni EA, Paciocco G. CT findings of pneumonia after lung transplantation. AJR Am J Roentgenol 2000;175 (3):811 – 818

Diederich S, Scadeng M, Dennis C, Steward S, Flower CD. Radiological findings in lung transplantation. [Article in German] Rofo 1994;161(6):475 – 483

Engeler CE. Heart-lung and lung transplantation. Radiol Clin North Am 1995;33(3):559 – 580

Erasmus JJ, McAdams HP, Tapson VF, Murray JG, Davis RD. Radiologic issues in lung transplantation for end-stage pulmonary disease. AJR Am J Roentgenol 1997;169(1):69 – 78

Garg K, Zamora MR, Tuder R, Armstrong JD II, Lynch DA. Lung transplantation: indications, donor and recipient selection, and imaging of complications. Radiographics 1996;16(2):355 – 367

Gotway MB, Dawn SK, Sellami D, et al. Acute rejection following lung transplantation: limitations in accuracy of thin-section CT for diagnosis. Radiology 2001;221(1):207 – 212

Herman SJ. Radiologic assessment after lung transplantation. Radiol Clin North Am 1994;32(4):663 – 678

Ko JP, Shepard JA, Sproule MW, et al. CT manifestations of respiratory syncytial virus infection in lung transplant recipients. J Comput Assist Tomogr 2000;24(2):235 – 241

Ward S, Müller NL. Pulmonary complications following lung transplantation. Clin Radiol 2000;55(5):332 – 339

Cardiovascular Surgery

Apter S, Amir G, Taler M, et al. Unexpected subdiaphragmatic findings on CT of the chest in septic patients after cardiac surgery. Clin Radiol 2002;57(4):287 – 291

Gilkeson RC, Markowitz AH, Ciancibello L. Multisection CT evaluation of the reoperative cardiac surgery patient. Radiographics 2003;23 (Spec No):S 3 –S 17

Henry DA. Radiologic evaluation of the patient after cardiac surgery. Radiol Clin North Am 1996;34(1):119 – 135

Henry DA, Jolles H, Berberich JJ, Schmelzer V. The post-cardiac surgery chest radiograph: a clinically integrated approach. J Thorac Imaging 1989;4(3):20 – 41

Hornick PI, Harris P, Cousins C, Taylor KM, Keogh BE. Assessment of the value of the immediate postoperative chest radiograph after cardiac operation. Ann Thorac Surg 1995;59(5):1150 – 1153, discussion 1153 – 1154

Milot J, Perron J, Lacasse Y, Létourneau L, Cartier PC, Maltais F. Incidence and predictors of ARDS after cardiac surgery. Chest 2001;119(3):884 – 888

Mediastinitis / Sternal Dehiscence

Bitkover CY, Cederlund K, Aberg B, Vaage J. Computed tomography of the sternum and mediastinum after median sternotomy. Ann Thorac Surg 1999;68(3):858 – 863

Boiselle PM, Mansilla AV. A closer look at the midsternal stripe sign. AJR Am J Roentgenol 2002;178(4):945 – 948

Boiselle PM, Mansilla AV, Fisher MS, McLoud TC. Wandering wires: frequency of sternal wire abnormalities in patients with sternal dehiscence. AJR Am J Roentgenol 1999;173(3):777 – 780

Boiselle PM, Mansilla AV, White CS, Fisher MS. Sternal dehiscence in patients with and without mediastinitis. J Thorac Imaging 2001;16(2):106 – 110

Hayward RH, Knight WL, Reiter CG. Sternal dehiscence. Early detection by radiography. J Thorac Cardiovasc Surg 1994;108(4):616 – 619

Jolles H, Henry DA, Roberson JP, Cole TJ, Spratt JA. Mediastinitis following median sternotomy: CT findings. Radiology 1996;201 (2):463 – 466

Maddern IR, Goodman LR, Almassi GH, Haasler GB, McManus RP, Olinger GN. CT after reconstructive repair of the sternum and chest wall. Radiology 1993;186(3):665 – 670

Misawa Y, Fuse K, Hasegawa T. Infectious mediastinitis after cardiac operations: computed tomographic findings. Ann Thorac Surg 1998;65(3):622 – 624

Yamaguchi H, Yamauchi H, Yamada T, Ariyoshi T, Aikawa H, Kato Y. Diagnostic validity of computed tomography for mediastinitis after cardiac surgery. Ann Thorac Cardiovasc Surg 2001;7(2):94 – 98

Heart Transplantation

Austin JHM, Schulman LL, Mastrobattista JD. Pulmonary infection after cardiac transplantation: clinical and radiologic correlations. Radiology 1989;172(1):259 – 265

Janzen DL, Padley SPG, Adler BD, Müller NL. Acute pulmonary complications in immunocompromised non-AIDS patients: comparison of diagnostic accuracy of CT and chest radiography. Clin Radiol 1993;47(3):159 – 165

Kay HR, Goodman LR, Teplick SK, Mundth ED. Use of computed tomography to assess mediastinal complications after median sternotomy. Ann Thorac Surg 1983;36(6):706 – 714

Knisely BL, Mastey LA, Collins J, Kuhlman JE. Imaging of cardiac transplantation complications. Radiographics 1999;19(2):321 – 339, discussion 340 – 341

Knollmann FD, Hummel M, Hetzer R, Felix R. CT of heart transplant recipients: spectrum of disease. Radiographics 2000;20(6):1637 – 1648

Kuhlman JE. Thoracic imaging in heart transplantation. J Thorac Imaging 2002;17(2):113 – 121

Esophageal Surgery

Anbari MM, Levine MS, Cohen RB, Rubesin SE, Laufer I, Rosato EF. Delayed leaks and fistulas after esophagogastrectomy: radiologic evaluation. AJR Am J Roentgenol 1993;160(6):1217 – 1220

Gollub MJ, Bains MS. Barium sulfate: a new (old) contrast agent for diagnosis of postoperative esophageal leaks. Radiology 1997;202 (2):360 – 362

Levine MS, Fisher AR, Rubesin SE, Laufer I, Herlinger H, Rosato EF. Complications after total gastrectomy and esophagojejunostomy: radiologic evaluation. AJR Am J Roentgenol 1991;157(6):1189 – 1194

Swanson JO, Levine MS, Redfern RO, Rubesin SE. Usefulness of high-density barium for detection of leaks after esophagogastrectomy, total gastrectomy, and total laryngectomy. AJR Am J Roentgenol 2003;181(2):415 – 420

Acute Abdomen in Intensive Care Patients

Acute Pancreatitis

Clinical Aspects

Friedman LS. Liver, biliary tract, & pancreas. In: Tierney LM, McPhee SJ, Papadakis MA, ed. Current Medical Diagnosis and Treatment. 41st ed. New York: McGraw-Hill; 2002

Crass RA. Abdominal pain. In: Tierney LM, McPhee SJ, Papadakis MA, ed. Current Medical Diagnosis and Treatment. 41st ed. New York: McGraw-Hill; 2002

Review Articles

Memel DS, Balfe DM, Semelka RC. The biliary tract. In: Lee JKT, Stanley RJ, Heiken JP, eds. Computed Body Tomography with MRI Correlation. 3 rd ed. Philadelphia: Lippincott-Raven; 1998: 779 – 844

Sternbach GL, Barkin SZ. Acute abdominal pain. In: Rosen P, Doris PE, Barkin RM, Barkin SZ, Markovchick VJ, ed. Diagnostic Radiology in Emergency Medicine. St. Louis: Mosby; 1992: 359 – 378

Pancreatitis

Balthazar EJ, Freeny PC, vanSonnenberg E. Imaging and intervention in acute pancreatitis. Radiology 1994;193(2):297 – 306

Balthazar EJ, Robinson DL, Megibow AJ, Ranson JH. Acute pancreatitis: value of CT in establishing prognosis. Radiology 1990;174 (2):331 – 336

Balthazar EJ. Acute pancreatitis: assessment of severity with clinical and CT evaluation. Radiology 2002;223(3):603 – 613

Beger HG, Rau BM. Severe acute pancreatitis: clinical course and management. World J Gastroenterol 2007;13(38):5043 – 5051

Bradley EL III. A clinically based classification system for acute pancreatitis. Summary of the International Symposium on Acute Pancreatitis, Atlanta, Ga, September 11 through 13, 1992. Arch Surg 1993;128(5):586 – 590

Chen H, Li F, Sun JB, Jia JG. Abdominal compartment syndrome in patients with severe acute pancreatitis in early stage. World J Gastroenterol 2008;14(22):3541 – 3548

De Sanctis JT, Lee MJ, Gazelle GS, et al. Prognostic indicators in acute pancreatitis: CT vs APACHE II. Clin Radiol 1997;52(11):842 – 848

De Waele JJ, Delrue L, Hoste EA, De Vos M, Duyck P, Colardyn FA. Extrapancreatic inflammation on abdominal computed tomography as an early predictor of disease severity in acute pancreatitis: evaluation of a new scoring system. Pancreas 2007;34(2):185 – 190

Garcea G, Gouda M, Hebbes C, et al. Predictors of severity and survival in acute pancreatitis: validation of the efficacy of early warning scores. Pancreas 2008;37(3):e54 –e61

Jacobs JE, Birnbaum BA. Computed tomography evaluation of acute pancreatitis. Semin Roentgenol 2001;36(2):92 – 98

Jeffrey R. Acute abdominal pain. Rule out acute pancreatitis. In: Jeffrey R, Ralls P, Leung AN, Brant-Zawadzki M, ed. Emergency Imaging. Philadelphia: Lippincott Williams & Wilkins; 1999:149 – 154

Kim DH, Pickhardt PJ. Radiologic assessment of acute and chronic pancreatitis. Surg Clin North Am 2007;87(6):1341 – 1358, viii

Knoepfli AS, Kinkel K, Berney T, Morel P, Becker CD, Poletti PA. Prospective study of 310 patients: can early CT predict the severity of acute pancreatitis? Abdom Imaging 2007;32(1):111 – 115

Lecesne R, Taourel P, Bret PM, Atri M, Reinhold C. Acute pancreatitis: interobserver agreement and correlation of CT and MR cholangiopancreatography with outcome. Radiology 1999;211(3):727 – 735

Meek K, de Virgilio C, Murrell Z, et al. Correlation between admission laboratory values, early abdominal computed tomography, and severe complications of gallstone pancreatitis. Am J Surg 2000;180(6):556 – 560

Merkle EM, Görich J. Imaging of acute pancreatitis. Eur Radiol 2002;12(8):1979 – 1992

Pitchumoni CS, Patel NM, Shah P. Factors influencing mortality in acute pancreatitis: can we alter them? J Clin Gastroenterol 2005;39(9):798 – 814 [Review]

Ueda T, Takeyama Y, Yasuda T, et al. Simple scoring system for the prediction of the prognosis of severe acute pancreatitis. Surgery 2007;141(1):51 – 58

Yassa NA, Agostini JT, Ralls PW. Accuracy of CT in estimating extent of pancreatic necrosis. Clin Imaging 1997;21(6):407 – 410

Cholecystitis

Bloom RA, Libson E, Lebensart PD, et al. The ultrasound spectrum of emphysematous cholecystitis. J Clin Ultrasound 1989;17(4):251 – 256

Bouras G, Lunca S, Vix M, Marescaux J. A case of emphysematous cholecystitis managed by laparoscopic surgery. JSLS 2005;9 (4):478 – 480

Fidler J, Paulson EK, Layfield L. CT evaluation of acute cholecystitis: findings and usefulness in diagnosis. AJR Am J Roentgenol 1996;166(5):1085 – 1088

Hatzidakis AA, Prassopoulos P, Petinarakis I, et al. Acute cholecystitis in high-risk patients: percutaneous cholecystostomy vs conservative treatment. Eur Radiol 2002;12(7):1778 – 1784

Laurila J, Syrjälä H, Laurila PA, Saarnio J, Ala-Kokko TI. Acute acalculous cholecystitis in critically ill patients. Acta Anaesthesiol Scand 2004;48(8):986 – 991

Marchal GJ, Casaer M, Baert AL, Goddeeris PG, Kerremans R, Fevery J. Gallbladder wall sonolucency in acute cholecystitis. Radiology 1979;133(2):429 – 433

Mastoraki A, Mastoraki S, Kriaras I, Douka E, Geroulanos S. Complications involving gall bladder and biliary tract in cardiovascular surgery. Hepatogastroenterology 2008;55(85):1233 – 1237

Ott DJ. Acalculous gallbladder disease: a controversial entity and imaging dilemma revisited. Am J Gastroenterol 1998;93 (7):1181 – 1183

Pelinka LE, Schmidhammer R, Hamid L, Mauritz W, Redl H. Acute acalculous cholecystitis after trauma: a prospective study. J Trauma 2003;55(2):323 – 329

Ralls PW, Colletti PM, Lapin SA, et al. Real-time sonography in suspected acute cholecystitis. Prospective evaluation of primary and secondary signs. Radiology 1985;155(3):767 – 771

Ralls P. Right upper quadrant pain. Rule out acute cholecystitis. In: Jeffrey R, Ralls P, Leung AN, Brant-Zawadzki M, eds. Emergency Imaging. Philadelphia: Lippincott Williams & Wilkins; 1999:119 – 132

Simeone JF, Brink JA, Mueller PR, et al. The sonographic diagnosis of acute gangrenous cholecystitis: importance of the Murphy sign. AJR Am J Roentgenol 1989;152(2):289 – 290

Soyer P, Brouland JP, Boudiaf M, et al. Color velocity imaging and power Doppler sonography of the gallbladder wall: a new look at sonographic diagnosis of acute cholecystitis. AJR Am J Roentgenol 1998;171(1):183 – 188

Takada T, Yasuda H, Uchiyama K, Hasegawa H, Asagoe T, Shikata J. Pericholecystic abscess: classification of US findings to determine the proper therapy. Radiology 1989;172(3):693 – 697

Theodorou P, Maurer CA, Spanholtz TA, et al. Acalculous cholecystitis in severely burned patients: incidence and predisposing factors. Burns 2009;35(3):405 – 411

Uggowitzer M, Kugler C, Schramayer G, et al. Sonography of acute cholecystitis: comparison of color and power Doppler sonography in detecting a hypervascularized gallbladder wall. AJR Am J Roentgenol 1997;168(3):707 – 712

Cholangitis

Balthazar EJ, Birnbaum BA, Naidich M. Acute cholangitis: CT evaluation. J Comput Assist Tomogr 1993;17(2):283 – 289

Gelbmann CM, Rümmele P, Wimmer M, et al. Ischemic-like cholangiopathy with secondary sclerosing cholangitis in critically ill patients. Am J Gastroenterol 2007;102(6):1221 – 1229

Yoon KH, Ha HK, Lee JS, et al. Inflammatory pseudotumor of the liver in patients with recurrent pyogenic cholangitis: CT-histopathologic correlation. Radiology 1999;211(2):373 – 379

Hepatic Abscess

Barreda R, Ros PR. Diagnostic imaging of liver abscess. Crit Rev Diagn Imaging 1992;33(1-2):29 – 58

Mergo PJ, Ros PR. MR imaging of inflammatory disease of the liver. Magn Reson Imaging Clin N Am 1997;5(2):367 – 376

Rajak CL, Gupta S, Jain S, Chawla Y, Gulati M, Suri S. Percutaneous treatment of liver abscesses: needle aspiration versus catheter drainage. AJR Am J Roentgenol 1998;170(4):1035 – 1039

Terrier F, Becker CD, Triller JK. Morphologic aspects of hepatic abscesses at computed tomography and ultrasound. Acta Radiol Diagn (Stockh) 1983;24(2):129 – 137

Hepatitis and Liver failure

Chawla Y, Sreedharan A, Dhiman RK, Jain S, Suri S. Portal hemodynamics in fulminant hepatic failure as assessed by duplex Doppler ultrasonography. Dig Dis Sci 2001;46(3):504 – 508

Deasy NP, Wendon J, Meire HB, Sidhu PS. The value of serial Doppler ultrasound as a predictor of clinical outcome and the need for transplantation in fulminant and severe acute liver failure. Br J Radiol 1999;72(854):134 – 143

Valls C, Andía E, Roca Y, Cos M, Figueras J. CT in hepatic cirrhosis and chronic hepatitis. Semin Ultrasound CT MR 2002;23(1):37 – 61

Vascular Disorders of the Liver

Brancatelli G, Federle MP, Grazioli L, Golfieri R, Lencioni R. Large regenerative nodules in Budd-Chiari syndrome and other vascular disorders of the liver: CT and MR imaging findings with clinicopathologic correlation. AJR Am J Roentgenol 2002;178(4):877 – 883

Murphy FB, Steinberg HV, Shires GT III, Martin LG, Bernardino ME. The Budd–Chiari syndrome: a review. AJR Am J Roentgenol 1986;147(1):9 – 15

Complications and Interventions

Besselink MG, van Santvoort HC, Boermeester MA, et al; Dutch Acute Pancreatitis Study Group. Timing and impact of infections in acute pancreatitis. Br J Surg 2009;96(3):267 – 273

Bradley EL III, Howard TJ, van Sonnenberg E, Fotoohi M. Intervention in necrotizing pancreatitis: an evidence-based review of surgical and percutaneous alternatives. J Gastrointest Surg 2008;12 (4):634 – 639

Bruennler T, Langgartner J, Lang S, et al. Percutaneous necrosectomy in patients with acute, necrotizing pancreatitis. Eur Radiol 2008;18(8):1604 – 1610

Mortelé KJ, Girshman J, Szejnfeld D, et al. CT-guided percutaneous catheter drainage of acute necrotizing pancreatitis: clinical experience and observations in patients with sterile and infected necrosis. AJR Am J Roentgenol 2009;192(1):110 – 116

Rocha FG, Benoit E, Zinner MJ, et al. Impact of radiologic intervention on mortality in necrotizing pancreatitis: the role of organ failure. Arch Surg 2009;144(3):261 – 265

Segal D, Mortele KJ, Banks PA, Silverman SG. Acute necrotizing pancreatitis: role of CT-guided percutaneous catheter drainage. Abdom Imaging 2007;32(3):351 – 361

Werner J, Büchler MW. Infectious complications in necrotizing pancreatitis. [Article in German] Zentralbl Chir 2007;132(5):433 – 437

Wyncoll DL. The management of severe acute necrotising pancreatitis: an evidence-based review of the literature. Intensive Care Med 1999;25(2):146 – 156

Urosepsis / Acute Renal Failure

Book M, Lehmann LE, Schewe JC, Weber S, Stüber F. Urosepsis. Current therapy and diagnosis. Urologe A. 2005;44:413 – 422; Quiz 423 – 424

Calandra T, Cohen J; International Sepsis Forum Definition of Infection in the ICU Consensus Conference. The international sepsis forum consensus conference on definitions of infection in the intensive care unit. Crit Care Med 2005;33(7):1538 – 1548

Christoph F, Weikert S, Müller M, Miller K, Schrader M. How septic is urosepsis? Clinical course of infected hydronephrosis and therapeutic strategies. World J Urol 2005;23(4):243 – 247

Marx G, Reinhart K. Urosepsis: from the intensive care viewpoint. Int J Antimicrob Agents 2008;31(Suppl 1):S 79 –S 84

Shah K, Teng J, Shah H, Choe A, Darvish A, Newman D, Wiener D. Can bedside ultrasound assist in determining whether serum creatinine is elevated in cases of acute urinary retention? J Emerg Med 2009;[still E-pub]

Soulen MC, Fishman EK, Goldman SM, Gatewood OMB. Bacterial renal infection: role of CT. Radiology 1989;171(3):703 – 707

Wagenlehner FM, Pilatz A, Naber KG, Weidner W. Therapeutic challenges of urosepsis. Eur J Clin Invest 2008;38(Suppl 2):45 – 49

Acute Gastrointestinal Bleeding

Farrell JJ, Friedman LS. Review article: the management of lower gastrointestinal bleeding. Aliment Pharmacol Ther 2005;21(11):1281 – 1298

Nietsch H, Lotterer E, Fleig WE. Acute upper gastrointestinal hemorrhage. Diagnosis and management. [Article in German] Internist (Berl) 2003;44(5):519 – 528, 530 – 532

Zuckerman GR, Prakash C. Acute lower intestinal bleeding. Part II: etiology, therapy, and outcomes. Gastrointest Endosc 1999;49(2):228 – 238

CT Angiography

Anthony S, Milburn S, Uberoi R. Multi-detector CT: review of its use in acute GI haemorrhage. Clin Radiol 2007;62(10):938 – 949

Burke SJ, Golzarian J, Weldon D, Sun S. Nonvariceal upper gastrointestinal bleeding. Eur Radiol 2007;17(7):1714 – 1726

Duchesne J, Jacome T, Serou M, et al. CT-angiography for the detection of a lower gastrointestinal bleeding source. Am Surg 2005;71(5):392 – 397

Ernst O, Bulois P, Saint-Drenant S, Leroy C, Paris JC, Sergent G. Helical CT in acute lower gastrointestinal bleeding. Eur Radiol 2003;13(1):114 – 117

Ettorre GC, Francioso G, Garribba AP, Fracella MR, Greco A, Farchi G. Helical CT angiography in gastrointestinal bleeding of obscure origin. AJR Am J Roentgenol 1997;168(3):727 – 731

Filippone A, Cianci R, Milano A, Valeriano S, Di Mizio V, Storto ML. Obscure gastrointestinal bleeding and small bowel pathology: comparison between wireless capsule endoscopy and multidetector-row CT enteroclysis. Abdom Imaging 2008;33(4):398 – 406

Horton KM, Brooke Jeffrey R Jr, Federle MP, Fishman EK. Acute gastrointestinal bleeding: the potential role of 64 MDCT and 3 D imaging in the diagnosis. Emerg Radiol 2009

Laing CJ, Tobias T, Rosenblum DI, Banker WL, Tseng L, Tamarkin SW. Acute gastrointestinal bleeding: emerging role of multidetector

CT angiography and review of current imaging techniques. Radiographics 2007;27(4):1055 – 1070

Rajan R, Dhar P, Praseedom RK, Sudhindran S, Moorthy S. Role of contrast CT in acute lower gastrointestinal bleeding. Dig Surg 2004;21(4):293 – 296

Sabharwal R, Vladica P, Chou R, Law WP. Helical CT in the diagnosis of acute lower gastrointestinal haemorrhage. Eur J Radiol 2006;58(2):273 – 279

Angiography and Interventional Procedures

Gady JS, Reynolds H, Blum A. Selective arterial embolization for control of lower gastrointestinal bleeding: recommendations for a clinical management pathway. Curr Surg 2003;60(3):344 – 347

Karanicolas PJ, Colquhoun PH, Dahlke E, Guyatt GH. Mesenteric angiography for the localization and treatment of acute lower gastrointestinal bleeding. Can J Surg 2008;51(6):437 – 441

Koval G, Benner KG, Rösch J, Kozak BE. Aggressive angiographic diagnosis in acute lower gastrointestinal hemorrhage. Dig Dis Sci 1987;32(3):248 – 253

Padia SA, Geisinger MA, Newman JS, Pierce G, Obuchowski NA, Sands MJ. Effectiveness of coil embolization in angiographically detectable versus non-detectable sources of upper gastrointestinal hemorrhage. J Vasc Interv Radiol 2009;20(4):461 – 466

Pomoni M, Sissopoulos A, Condilis N, et al. Lower gastrointestinal bleeding treated with transcatheter arterial embolization. Case report and review of the literature. Ann Ital Chir 2008;79(4):281 – 286

Schürmann K, Bücker A, Jansen M, et al. Selective CT mesentericography in the diagnostics of obscure overt intestinal bleeding: preliminary results. [Article in German] Rofo 2002;174:444 – 451

Inflammatory Bowel Diseases

Pseudomembranous Enterocolitis

Ang CW, Heyes G, Morrison P, Carr B. The acquisition and outcome of ICU-acquired Clostridium difficile infection in a single centre in the UK. J Infect 2008;57(6):435 – 440

Bosseckert H. Antibiotic-associated diarrhea and pseudomembranous colitis. Treatment and prevention of recurrence. [Article in German] Med Monatsschr Pharm 2003;26(5):173 – 175

Garey KW, Dao-Tran TK, Jiang ZD, Price MP, Gentry LO, Dupont HL. A clinical risk index for Clostridium difficile infection in hospitalised patients receiving broad-spectrum antibiotics. J Hosp Infect 2008;70(2):142 – 147

Greenstein AJ, Byrn JC, Zhang LP, Swedish KA, Jahn AE, Divino CM. Risk factors for the development of fulminant Clostridium difficile colitis. Surgery 2008;143(5):623 – 629

Krämer S, Bischoff SC. Therapeutic possibilities of probiotics in antibiotic-related diarrhea. [Article in German] MMW Fortschr Med 2006;148(35-36):28 – 30

Lenzen-Grossimlinghaus R, Strohmeyer G. Antibiotic-associated diarrhea. [Article in German] Dtsch Med Wochenschr 2003;128(9):437 – 439

Graft versus Host Disease

Brodoefel H, Bethge W, Vogel M, et al. Early and late-onset acute GvHD following hematopoietic cell transplantation: CT features of gastrointestinal involvement with clinical and pathological correlation. Eur J Radiol 2010;73(3):594 – 600

Diverticulitis

Ambrosetti P, Becker C, Terrier F. Colonic diverticulitis: impact of imaging on surgical management—a prospective study of 542 patients. Eur Radiol 2002;12(5):1145 – 1149

Ambrosetti P. Acute diverticulitis of the left colon: value of the initial CT and timing of elective colectomy. J Gastrointest Surg 2008;12(8):1318 – 1320

Aschoff AJ. MDCT of the abdomen. Eur Radiol 2006;16(Suppl 7):M54 –M57

Chintapalli KN, Chopra S, Ghiatas AA, Esola CC, Fields SF, Dodd GD III. Diverticulitis versus colon cancer: differentiation with helical CT findings. Radiology 1999;210(2):429 – 435

Ferstl FJ, Obert R, Cordes M. CT of acute left-sided colonic diverticulitis and its differential diagnoses. [Article in German] Radiologe 2005;45(7):597 – 607

Floch MH, Bina I. The natural history of diverticulitis: fact and theory. J Clin Gastroenterol 2004; 38(5, Suppl 1)S 2 –S 7

Floch MH; NDSG. Symptom severity and disease activity indices for diverticulitis. J Clin Gastroenterol 2008;42(10):1135 – 1136

Horton KM, Corl FM, Fishman EK. CT evaluation of the colon: inflammatory disease. Radiographics 2000;20(2):399 – 418

Jang HJ, Lim HK, Lee SJ, Lee WJ, Kim EY, Kim SH. Acute diverticulitis of the cecum and ascending colon: the value of thin-section helical CT findings in excluding colonic carcinoma. AJR Am J Roentgenol 2000;174(5):1397 – 1402

Kaiser AM, Jiang JK, Lake JP, et al. The management of complicated diverticulitis and the role of computed tomography. Am J Gastroenterol 2005;100(4):910 – 917

Katz DS, Yam B, Hines JJ, Mazzie JP, Lane MJ, Abbas MA. Uncommon and unusual gastrointestinal causes of the acute abdomen: computed tomographic diagnosis. Semin Ultrasound CT MR 2008;29(5):386 – 398

Kirbaş I, Yildirim E, Harman A, Başaran O. Perforated ileal diverticulitis: CT findings. Diagn Interv Radiol 2007;13(4):188 – 189

Laméris W, van Randen A, Bipat S, Bossuyt PM, Boermeester MA, Stoker J. Graded compression ultrasonography and computed tomography in acute colonic diverticulitis: meta-analysis of test accuracy. Eur Radiol 2008;18(11):2498 – 2511

Lawrimore T, Rhea JT. Computed tomography evaluation of diverticulitis. J Intensive Care Med 2004;19(4):194 – 204

Lohrmann C, Ghanem N, Pache G, Makowiec F, Kotter E, Langer M. CT in acute perforated sigmoid diverticulitis. Eur J Radiol 2005;56(1):78 – 83

McCafferty MH, Roth L, Jorden J. Current management of diverticulitis. Am Surg 2008;74(11):1041 – 1049

Padidar AM, Jeffrey RB Jr, Mindelzun RE, Dolph JF. Differentiating sigmoid diverticulitis from carcinoma on CT scans: mesenteric inflammation suggests diverticulitis. AJR Am J Roentgenol 1994;163(1):81 – 83

Rotert H, Nöldge G, Encke J, Richter GM, Düx M. The value of CT for the diagnosis of acute diverticulitis. [Article in German] Radiologe 2003;43(1):51 – 58

Sarma D, Longo WE; NDSG. Diagnostic imaging for diverticulitis. J Clin Gastroenterol 2008;42(10):1139 – 1141

Sheth AA, Longo W, Floch MH. Diverticular disease and diverticulitis. Am J Gastroenterol 2008;103(6):1550 – 1556

Shyung LR, Lin SC, Shih SC, Kao CR, Chou SY. Decision making in right-sided diverticulitis. World J Gastroenterol 2003;9(3):606 – 608

Singh B, May K, Coltart I, Moore NR, Cunningham C. The long-term results of percutaneous drainage of diverticular abscess. Ann R Coll Surg Engl 2008;90(4):297 – 301

Urban BA, Fishman EK. Targeted helical CT of the acute abdomen: appendicitis, diverticulitis, and small bowel obstruction. Semin Ultrasound CT MR 2000;21(1):20 – 39

Zissin R, Hertz M, Osadchy A, Even-Sapir E, Gayer G. Abdominal CT findings in nontraumatic colorectal perforation. Eur J Radiol 2008;65(1):125 – 132

Acute Intestinal Ischemia

Berland T, Oldenburg WA. Acute mesenteric ischemia. Curr Gastroenterol Rep 2008;10(3):341 – 346

Betzler M. Surgical technical guidelines in intestinal ischemia. [Article in German] Chirurg 1998;69(1):1 – 7

Bradbury MS, Kavanagh PV, Bechtold RE, et al. Mesenteric venous thrombosis: diagnosis and noninvasive imaging. Radiographics 2002;22(3):527 – 541

Brophy CM. Gastrointestinal vascular and ischemic syndromes. Curr Opin Gen Surg 1993:225 – 231

Ernst S, Luther B, Zimmermann N, et al. Current diagnosis and therapy of non-occlusive mesenteric ischemia. [Article in German] Rofo 2003;175:515 – 523

Gore RM, Yaghmai V, Thakrar KH, et al. Imaging in intestinal ischemic disorders. Radiol Clin North Am 2008;46(5):845 – 875, v

Izbicki JR, Schneider CG, Kastl S. Partial ischemia. Occlusive and non-occlusive mesenteric ischemia, ischemic colitis, systemic lupus erythematosus. [Article in German] Chirurg 2003;74(5):413 – 418

Neri E, Sassi C, Massetti M, et al. Nonocclusive intestinal ischemia in patients with acute aortic dissection. J Vasc Surg 2002;36(4):738 – 745

Paterno F, Longo WE. The etiology and pathogenesis of vascular disorders of the intestine. Radiol Clin North Am 2008;46(5):877 – 885, v

Rha SE, Ha HK, Lee SH, et al. CT and MR imaging findings of bowel ischemia from various primary causes. Radiographics 2000;20(1):29 – 42

Schütz A, Eichinger W, Breuer M, Gansera B, Kemkes BM. Acute mesenteric ischemia after open heart surgery. Angiology 1998;49(4):267 – 273

Segatto E, Mortelé KJ, Ji H, Wiesner W, Ros PR. Acute small bowel ischemia: CT imaging findings. Semin Ultrasound CT MR 2003;24(5):364 – 376

Taourel P, Aufort S, Merigeaud S, Doyon FC, Hoquet MD, Delabrousse E. Imaging of ischemic colitis. Radiol Clin North Am 2008;46(5):909 – 924, vi

Wiesner W, Steinbrich W. Stellenwert der Computertomographie bei der Diagnostik der akuten Darmischämie. Radiologie up2date 2004;1:75 – 89

Yasuhara H. Acute mesenteric ischemia: the challenge of gastroenterology. Surg Today 2005;35(3):185 – 195

Imaging of Intensive Care Patients after Abdominal Surgery

Review Articles / Book Chapters

Gore RM, Levine MS, Laufer I, Eds. Textbook of Gastrointestinal Radiology. Philadelphia: Saunders; 1994

Halpert RD, Feczko PJ. The Requisites. Gastrointestinal Radiology: St. Louis: Mosby; 1999

Krestin GP, Choyke PL. Acute Abdomen. Stuttgart: Thieme; 1996

Abdominal Drainage

Benzer H, Buchardi H, Larsen R, Suter PM, Eds. Intensivmedizin. 7th ed. Berlin: Springer; 1994: 42

Benzer H, Buchardi H, Larsen R, Suter PM, Eds. Intensivmedizin. 7th ed. Berlin: Springer; 1994: 112

Durst J, Rohen JW. Chirurgische Operationslehre. Stuttgart: Schattauer; 1996: 353, 543

Felix R, Lüning M, eds. Komplexe bildgebende Diagnostik. Stuttgart: Thieme; 1989: 265

Vogel H. Postoperative Röntgenmorphologie. Landsberg: ecomed; 1986: 90

Postoperative Complications

Postoperative Bleeding

Miyamoto N, Kodama Y, Endo H, Shimizu T, Miyasaka K. Hepatic artery embolization for postoperative hemorrhage in upper abdominal surgery. Abdom Imaging 2003;28(3):347 – 353

Postoperative Sepsis

Barkhausen J, Stöblen F, Dominguez-Fernandez E, Henseke P, Müller RD. Impact of CT in patients with sepsis of unknown origin. Acta Radiol 1999;40(5):552 – 555

McDowell RK, Dawson SL. Evaluation of the abdomen in sepsis of unknown origin. Radiol Clin North Am 1996;34(1):177 – 190

Merrell RC. The abdomen as source of sepsis in critically ill patients. Crit Care Clin 1995;11(2):255 – 272

Velmahos GC, Kamel E, Berne TV, et al. Abdominal computed tomography for the diagnosis of intra-abdominal sepsis in critically injured patients: fishing in murky waters. Arch Surg 1999;134 (8):831 – 836, discussion 836 – 838

Peritonitis

Baker SR. Imaging of pneumoperitoneum. Abdom Imaging 1996;21 (5):413 – 414

Earls JP, Dachman AH, Colon E, Garrett MG, Molloy M. Prevalence and duration of postoperative pneumoperitoneum: sensitivity of CT vs. left lateral decubitus radiography. AJR Am J Roentgenol 1993;161(4):781 – 785

Gayer G, Jonas T, Apter S, Amitai M, Shabtai M, Hertz M. Postoperative pneumoperitoneum as detected by CT: prevalence, duration, and relevant factors affecting its possible significance. Abdom Imaging 2000;25(3):301 – 305

O'Connor AR, Coakley FV, Meng MV, Eberhardt SC. Imaging of retained surgical sponges in the abdomen and pelvis. AJR Am J Roentgenol 2003;180(2):481 – 489

Stapakis JC, Thickman D. Diagnosis of pneumoperitoneum: abdominal CT vs. upright chest film. J Comput Assist Tomogr 1992;16 (5):713 – 716

Abscess

Freed KS, Lo JY, Baker JA, et al. Predictive model for the diagnosis of intraabdominal abscess. Acad Radiol 1998;5(7):473 – 479

Gazelle GS, Mueller PR. Abdominal abscess. Imaging and intervention. Radiol Clin North Am 1994;32(5):913 – 932

Gervais DA, Ho CH, O'Neill MJ, et al. Recurrent abdominal and pelvic abscesses: incidence, results of repeated percutaneous drainage, and underlying causes in 956 drainages. AJR Am J Roentgenol 2004;182(2):463 – 466

Harisinghani MG, Gervais DA, Hahn PF, et al. CT-guided transgluteal drainage of deep pelvic abscesses: indications, technique, procedure-related complications, and clinical outcome. Radiographics 2002;22(6):1353 – 1367

Krumenacker JH, Panicek DM, Ginsberg MS, Bach AM, Hilton S, Schwartz LH. CT in searching for abscess after abdominal or pelvic surgery in patients with neoplasia: do abdomen and pelvis both need to be scanned? J Comput Assist Tomogr 1997;21 (4):652 – 655

Lal NR, Kazerooni EA, Bree RL. Development and implementation of an appropriateness guideline for use of CT in cases of suspected intraabdominal abscess. Acad Radiol 2000;7(9):711 – 716

Postoperative Bowel Obstruction

Frager DH, Baer JW, Rothpearl A, Bossart PA. Distinction between postoperative ileus and mechanical small-bowel obstruction: value of CT compared with clinical and other radiographic findings. AJR Am J Roentgenol 1995;164(4):891 – 894

Ha HK, Shin BS, Lee SI, et al. Usefulness of CT in patients with intestinal obstruction who have undergone abdominal surgery for malignancy. AJR Am J Roentgenol 1998;171(6):1587 – 1593

Kammen BF, Levine MS, Rubesin SE, Laufer I. Adynamic ileus after caesarean section mimicking intestinal obstruction: findings on abdominal radiographs. Br J Radiol 2000;73(873):951 – 955

Resnick J, Greenwald DA, Brandt LJ. Delayed gastric emptying and postoperative ileus after nongastric abdominal surgery: part I. Am J Gastroenterol 1997;92(5):751 – 762

Resnick J, Greenwald DA, Brandt LJ. Delayed gastric emptying and postoperative ileus after nongastric abdominal surgery: part II. Am J Gastroenterol 1997;92(6):934 – 940

Schuster TG, Montie JE. Postoperative ileus after abdominal surgery. Urology 2002;59(4):465 – 471

Small Bowel Obstruction

Bischof TP. Erbrechen. In: Krestin GP, ed. Akutes Abdomen. Stuttgart: Thieme; 1994:128 – 143

Bischof TP. Obstipation. In: Krestin GP, ed. Akutes Abdomen. Stuttgart: Thieme; 1994:144 – 155

DiSantis DJ, Ralls PW, Balfe DM, et al. The patient with suspected small bowel obstruction: imaging strategies. American College of Radiology. ACR Appropriateness Criteria. Radiology 2000;215 (Suppl):121 – 124

Herlinger H, Rubesin SE, Norris JB. Small bowel obstruction. In: Gore R, Levine MS, ed. Textbook of Gastrointestinal Radiology, Vol. 1. Philadelphia: Saunders; 2000: 815 – 837

Lappas JC, Reyes BL, Maglinte DD. Abdominal radiography findings in small-bowel obstruction: relevance to triage for additional diagnostic imaging. AJR Am J Roentgenol 2001;176(1):167 – 174

Maglinte DD, Kelvin FM, Rowe MG, Bender GN, Rouch DM. Small-bowel obstruction: optimizing radiologic investigation and nonsurgical management. Radiology 2001;218(1):39 – 46

Miller G, Boman J, Shrier I, Gordon PH. Etiology of small bowel obstruction. Am J Surg 2000;180(1):33 – 36

Small Bowel Feces Sign

Balthazar EJ. George W. Holmes Lecture. CT of small-bowel obstruction. AJR Am J Roentgenol 1994;162(2):255 – 261

Burkill G, Bell J, Healy J. Small bowel obstruction: the role of computed tomography in its diagnosis and management with reference to other imaging modalities. Eur Radiol 2001;11 (8):1405 – 1422

Maglinte DD, Reyes BL, Harmon BH, et al. Reliability and role of plain film radiography and CT in the diagnosis of small-bowel obstruction. AJR Am J Roentgenol 1996;167(6):1451 – 1455

Mayo-Smith WW, Wittenberg J, Bennett GL, Gervais DA, Gazelle GS, Mueller PR. The CT small bowel faeces sign: description and clinical significance. Clin Radiol 1995;50(11):765 – 767

Taourel PG, Fabre JM, Pradel JA, Seneterre EJ, Megibow AJ, Bruel JM. Value of CT in the diagnosis and management of patients with suspected acute small-bowel obstruction. AJR Am J Roentgenol 1995;165(5):1187 – 1192

Traub SJ, Hoffman RS, Nelson LS. Body packing—the internal concealment of illicit drugs. N Engl J Med 2003;349(26):2519 – 2526

Strangulated Bowel Obstruction

Balthazar EJ, Birnbaum BA, Megibow AJ, Gordon RB, Whelan CA, Hulnick DH. Closed-loop and strangulating intestinal obstruction: CT signs. Radiology 1992;185(3):769 – 775

Zalcman M, Van Gansbeke D, Lalmand B, Braudé P, Closset J, Struyven J. Delayed enhancement of the bowel wall: a new CT sign of small bowel strangulation. J Comput Assist Tomogr 1996;20(3):379 – 381

Ha HK, Kim JS, Lee MS, et al. Differentiation of simple and strangulated small-bowel obstructions: usefulness of known CT criteria. Radiology 1997;204(2):507 – 512

Furukawa A, Yamasaki M, Furuichi K, et al. Helical CT in the diagnosis of small bowel obstruction. Radiographics 2001;21(2):341 – 355

Complications of Specific Operations

After Gastric Surgery

Kim KW, Choi BI, Han JK, et al. Postoperative anatomic and pathologic findings at CT following gastrectomy. Radiographics 2002;22(2):323 – 336

Kim HC, Han JK, Kim KW, et al. Afferent loop obstruction after gastric cancer surgery: helical CT findings. Abdom Imaging 2003;28 (5):624 – 630

Pavone P, Laghi A, Catalano C, et al. CT of Nissen's fundoplication. Abdom Imaging 1997;22(5):457 – 460

Smith C, Deziel DJ, Kubicka RA. Evaluation of the postoperative stomach and duodenum. Radiographics 1994;14(1):67 – 86

After Pancreatic Surgery

Bluemke DA, Abrams RA, Yeo CJ, Cameron JL, Fishman EK. Recurrent pancreatic adenocarcinoma: spiral CT evaluation following the Whipple procedure. Radiographics 1997;17(2):303 – 313

Coombs RJ, Zeiss J, Howard JM, Thomford NR, Merrick HW. CT of the abdomen after the Whipple procedure: value in depicting postoperative anatomy, surgical complications, and tumor recurrence. AJR Am J Roentgenol 1990;154(5):1011 – 1014

Freed KS, Paulson EK, Frederick MG, Keogan MT, Pappas TN. Abdomen after a Puestow procedure: postoperative CT appearance, complications, and potential pitfalls. Radiology 1997;203 (3):790 – 794

Furukawa H, Kosuge T, Shimada K, Yamamoto J, Ushio K. Helical CT of the abdomen after pancreaticoduodenectomy: usefulness for detecting postoperative complications. Hepatogastroenterology 1997;44(15):849 – 855

Gervais DA, Fernandez-del Castillo C, O'Neill MJ, Hahn PF, Mueller PR. Complications after pancreatoduodenectomy: imaging and imaging-guided interventional procedures. Radiographics 2001;21 (3):673 – 690

Johnson PT, Curry CA, Urban BA, Fishman EK. Spiral CT following the Whipple procedure: distinguishing normal postoperative findings from complications. J Comput Assist Tomogr 2002;26(6):956 – 961

Mortelé KJ, Lemmerling M, de Hemptinne B, De Vos M, De Bock G, Kunnen M. Postoperative findings following the Whipple procedure: determination of prevalence and morphologic abdominal CT features. Eur Radiol 2000;10(1):123 – 128

Sohn TA, Yeo CJ, Cameron JL, et al. Pancreaticoduodenectomy: role of interventional radiologists in managing patients and complications. J Gastrointest Surg 2003;7(2):209 – 219

After Intestinal Surgery

Alfisher MM, Scholz FJ, Roberts PL, Counihan T. Radiology of ileal pouch-anal anastomosis: normal findings, examination pitfalls, and complications. Radiographics 1997;17(1):81 – 98, discussion 98 – 99

Blachar A, Federle MP. Gastrointestinal complications of laparoscopic roux-en-Y gastric bypass surgery in patients who are morbidly obese: findings on radiography and CT. AJR Am J Roentgenol 2002;179(6):1437 – 1442

Daly B, Sukumar SA, Krebs TL, Wong JJ, Flowers JL. Nonbiliary laparoscopic gastrointestinal surgery: role of CT in diagnosis and management of complication. AJR Am J Roentgenol 1996;167 (2):455 – 459

Seggerman RE, Chen MY, Waters GS, Ott DJ. Pictorial essay. Radiology of ileal pouch–anal anastomosis surgery. AJR Am J Roentgenol 2003;180(4):999 – 1002

After Liver Transplantation

Dinkel HP, Moll R, Gassel HJ, et al. Helical CT cholangiography for the detection and localization of bile duct leakage. AJR Am J Roentgenol 1999;173(3):613 – 617

Håkansson K, Leander P, Ekberg O, Håkansson HO. MR imaging of upper abdomen following cholecystectomy. Normal and abnormal findings. Acta Radiol 2001;42(2):181 – 186

Kapoor V, Baron RL, Peterson MS. Bile leaks after surgery. AJR Am J Roentgenol 2004;182(2):451 – 458

Letourneau JG, Steely JW, Crass JR, Goldberg ME, Grage T, Day DL. Upper abdomen: CT findings following partial hepatectomy. Radiology 1988;166(1 Pt 1):139 – 141

Millitz K, Moote DJ, Sparrow RK, Girotti MJ, Holliday RL, McLarty TD. Pneumoperitoneum after laparoscopic cholecystectomy: frequency and duration as seen on upright chest radiographs. AJR Am J Roentgenol 1994;163(4):837 – 839

Slanetz PJ, Boland GW, Mueller PR. Imaging and interventional radiology in laparoscopic injuries to the gallbladder and biliary system. Radiology 1996;201(3):595 – 603

Stockberger SM Jr, Johnson MS. Spiral CT cholangiography in complex bile duct injuries after laparoscopic cholecystectomy. J Vasc Interv Radiol 1997;8(2):249 – 252

Van Beers BE, Lacrosse M, Trigaux JP, de Cannière L, De Ronde T, Pringot J. Noninvasive imaging of the biliary tree before or after laparoscopic cholecystectomy: use of three-dimensional spiral CT cholangiography. AJR Am J Roentgenol 1994;162(6):1331 – 1335

vanSonnenberg E, D'Agostino HB, Easter DW, et al. Complications of laparoscopic cholecystectomy: coordinated radiologic and surgical management in 21 patients. Radiology 1993;188(2):399 – 404

Vazquez JL, Thorsen MK, Dodds WJ, et al. Evaluation and treatment of intraabdominal bilomas. AJR Am J Roentgenol 1985;144(5):933 – 938

Ward EM. Imaging after laparoscopic cholecystectomy. Gastroenterol Clin North Am 1995;24(2):239 – 257

Wright TB, Bertino RB, Bishop AF, et al. Complications of laparoscopic cholecystectomy and their interventional radiologic management. Radiographics 1993;13(1):119 – 128

Thoracic Imaging of the Pediatric Intensive Care Patient

Review Articles / Book Chapters

Cleveland RH. A radiologic update on medical diseases of the newborn chest. Pediatr Radiol 1995;25(8):631 – 637

Donnelly LF. Fundamentals of Pediatric Radiology. Philadelphia: Saunders; 2001

Gibson AT, Steiner GM. Imaging the neonatal chest. Clin Radiol 1997;52(3):172 – 186

Hedlund GL, Griscom NT, Cleveland RH, et al. Respiratory system. In: Kirks DR, Griscom NT, eds. Practical Pediatric Imaging. 3rd. ed. Philadelphia: Lippincott-Raven; 1998

Puig S, Hörmann M, Kuhle S, et al. Chest X-ray of the neonate. [Article in German] Radiologe 2000;40:43 – 51

Puig S, Hörmann M, Sandström S, et al. Acute, atraumatic changes of the lower respiratory tract in the child in thoracic roentgen imaging. Recognition and appreciation of radiological changes. [Article in German] Radiologe 2002;42:153 – 161

Swischuk LE. Emergency Imaging of the Acutely Ill or Injured Child. 3rd ed. Baltimore: Williams & Wilkins; 1994

Neuroradiology

Barkovich AJ, Hajnal BL, Vigneron D, et al. Prediction of neuromotor outcome in perinatal asphyxia: evaluation of MR scoring systems. AJNR Am J Neuroradiol 1998;19(1):143 – 149

Blankenberg FG, Loh NN, Bracci P, et al. Sonography, CT, and MR imaging: a prospective comparison of neonates with suspected intracranial ischemia and hemorrhage. AJNR Am J Neuroradiol 2000;21(1):213 – 218

Bydder GM, Rutherford MA, Cowan FM. Diffusion-weighted imaging in neonates. Childs Nerv Syst 2001;17(4-5):190 – 194

Roelants-van Rijn AM, Groenendaal F, Beek FJ, Eken P, van Haastert IC, de Vries LS. Parenchymal brain injury in the preterm infant: comparison of cranial ultrasound, MRI and neurodevelopmental outcome. Neuropediatrics 2001;32(2):80 – 89

Normal Thoracic Findings in Newborns

Frush DP, et al. Imaging evaluation of the thyms and thymic disorders in children. In: Strife JL, Lucaya J, eds. Pediatric Chest Imaging. Berlin: Springer; 2001

Infantile Respiratory Distress Syndrome (IRDS)

Donn SM, Dalton J. Surfactant replacement therapy in the neonate: beyond respiratory distress syndrome. Respir. Care 2009;54 (9):1203–1208

Swischuk LE, John SD. Immature lung problems: can our nomenclature be more specific? AJR Am J Roentgenol 1996;166(4):917 – 918

Meconium Aspiration Syndrome

Gregory GA, Gooding CA, Phibbs RH, Tooley WH. Meconium aspiration in infants—a prospective study. J Pediatr 1974;85(6):848 – 852

Complications during or after Mechanical Ventilation

Pulmonary Interstitial Emphysema

Donnelly LF, Frush DP. Localized radiolucent chest lesions in neonates. Causes and differentiation. AJR 1999;172(6):1651 – 1658

Congenital Lung Diseases with Respiratory Failure at Birth

Congenital Lobar Emphysema

Stigers KB, Woodring JH, Kanga JF. The clinical and imaging spectrum of findings in patients with congenital lobar emphysema. Pediatr Pulmonol 1992;14(3):160 – 170

Acute Obstruction of the Upper Airways

Donnelly LF, Frush DP, Bisset GS III. The multiple presentations of foreign bodies in children. AJR Am J Roentgenol 1998;170 (2):471 – 477

John SD, Swischuk LE. Stridor and upper airway obstruction in infants and children. Radiographics 1992;12(4):625 – 643, discussion 644

Kirse DJ, Roberson DW. Surgical management of retropharyngeal space infections in children. Laryngoscope 2001;111(8):1413 – 1422

Stone ME, Walner DL, Koch BL, Egelhoff JC, Myer CM. Correlation between computed tomography and surgical findings in retropharyngeal inflammatory processes in children. Int J Pediatr Otorhinolaryngol 1999;49(2):121 – 125

Asthma/Pneumomediastinum

Chalumeau M, Le Clainche L, Sayeg N, et al. Spontaneous pneumomediastinum in children. Pediatr Pulmonol 2001;31(1):67 – 75

Pneumonia

Donnelly LF, Klosterman LA. Pneumonia in children: decreased parenchymal contrast enhancement—CT sign of intense illness and impending cavitary necrosis. Radiology 1997;205(3):817 – 820

Donnelly LF, Klosterman LA. Cavitary necrosis complicating pneumonia in children: sequential findings on chest radiography. AJR Am J Roentgenol 1998;171(1):253 – 256

Donnelly LF. Maximizing the usefulness of imaging in children with community-acquired pneumonia. AJR Am J Roentgenol 1999;172 (2):505 – 512

Markowitz RI, Kramer SS. The spectrum of pulmonary infection in the immunocompromised child. Semin Roentgenol 2000;35(2):171 – 180

Acute Abdomen in the Pediatric Intensive Care Patient

Review Articles / Book Chapters

Barr LL. Sonography in the infant with acute abdominal symptoms. Semin Ultrasound CT MR 1994;15(4):275 – 289

Grier D. Radiology of gastrointestinal emergencies. In: Carty H, ed. Emergency Pediatric Radiology. Berlin: Springer; 1999: 117 – 181

Petit P, Pracros J. Role of ultrasound in children with emergency gastrointestinal diseases. [Article in German] J Radiol 2001;82(6 Pt 2):764 – 778, discussion 779 – 780

Meconium Ileus

Docherty JG, Zaki A, Coutts JAP, Evans TJ, Carachi R. Meconium ileus: a review 1972-1990. Br J Surg 1992;79(6):571 – 573

Necrotizing Enterocolitis

Hörmann M, Pumberger W, Puig S, Kreuzer S, Metz VM. Necrotizing enterocolitis (NEC) in the newborn. [Article in German] Radiologe 2000;40(1):58 – 62

Kreft B, Dalhoff K, Sack K. Necrotizing enterocolitis: a historical and current review. [Article in German] Med Klin (Munich) 2000;95 (8):435 – 441

Patton WL, Willmann JK, Lutz AM, Rencken IO, Gooding CA. Worsening enterocolitis in neonates: diagnosis by CT examination of urine after enteral administration of iohexol. Pediatr Radiol 1999;29(2):95 – 99

Malrotation and Volvulus

Ashley LM, Allen S, Teele RL. A normal sonogram does not exclude malrotation. Pediatr Radiol 2001;31(5):354 – 356

Bhat NA, Agarwala S, Mitra DK, Bhatnagar V. Duplications of the alimentary tract in children. Trop Gastroenterol 2001;22(1):33 – 35

Dilley AV, Pereira J, Shi EC, et al. The radiologist says malrotation: does the surgeon operate? Pediatr Surg Int 2000;16(1-2):45 – 49

Dufour D, Delaet MH, Dassonville M, Cadranel S, Perlmutter N. Midgut malrotation, the reliability of sonographic diagnosis. Pediatr Radiol 1992;22(1):21 – 23

Gastrointestinal Atresia and Stenosis

Lloyd-Still JD, Beno DW, Kimura RM. Cystic fibrosis colonopathy. Curr Gastroenterol Rep 1999;1(3):231 – 237

Sweeney B, Surana R, Puri P. Jejunoileal atresia and associated malformations: correlation with the timing of in utero insult. J Pediatr Surg 2001;36(5):774 – 776

Waldhausen JH, Sawin RS. Improved long-term outcome for patients with jejunoileal apple peel atresia. J Pediatr Surg 1997;32 (9):1307 – 1309

Congenital Megacolon (Hirschsprung Disease)

Lall A, Gupta DK, Bajpai M. Neonatal Hirschsprung's disease. Indian J Pediatr 2000;67(8):583 – 588

Martucciello G, Ceccherini I, Lerone M, Jasonni V. Pathogenesis of Hirschsprung's disease. J Pediatr Surg 2000;35(7):1017 – 1025

Hypertrophic Pyloric Stenosis

Cohen HL, Zinn HL, Haller JO, Homel PJ, Stoane JM. Ultrasonography of pylorospasm: findings may simulate hypertrophic pyloric stenosis. J Ultrasound Med 1998;17(11):705 – 711

Lowe LH, Banks WJ, Shyr Y. Pyloric ratio: efficacy in the diagnosis of hypertrophic pyloric stenosis. J Ultrasound Med 1999;18 (11):773 – 777

Sargent SK, Foote SL, Mooney DP, Shorter NA. The posterior approach to pyloric sonography. Pediatr Radiol 2000;30(4):256 – 257

Intussusception

DiFiore JW. Intussusception. Semin Pediatr Surg 1999;8(4):214 – 220

Rohrschneider W. Invagination. [Article in German] Radiologe 1997;37(6):446 – 453

Index

A

abdominal drainage 147–149
  anastomoses 148
  biliary 148–149
  bloody 148
  intra-abdominal abscess 162–163
  septic surgery 148
  urinary tract 149
abdominal drains 147–148
abdominal perforation, pediatric 209
abdominal surgery 147–182
  angiography 152–153
  biliary tract surgery 173
  bowel obstruction 163–166, 167, 168
  cholecystectomy 173–174
  colorectal surgery 174–176
  complications 151–168
    diagnostic strategy 151–153
  esophageal surgery 170, 171
  fluid collections 150
  gastric surgery 169–171
  hemorrhage 152–153, 152–154
  imaging 151–153
  intestinal atony 150
  intra-abdominal abscess 152, 157, 158–163
  liver transplantation 178–179, 180
  mesenteric hematoma 153–154, 155
  nephrectomy 176
  pancreatic surgery 171–173
  peristalsis resumption 150, 159
  peritonitis 156–158
  pneumoperitoneum 150–151
  postoperative bleeding 152–154
  postoperative findings complications 151–168
    normal 150–151
  renal transplantation 176–178
  sepsis 154–163
  septic 148
abdominal wall hematoma 154
abdominoperineal resection 175
abscess
  acute retropharyngeal 197–198
  cholecystectomy 174

colorectal surgery 175
  drainage of abdominal 148
  hepatic 122–123, 160, 161
  intra-abdominal 152, 157, 158–163
  intraparenchymal 160–161
  intraperitoneal 158
  pancreatic 115, 118, 172, 173
  pericholecystic 121
  pericolic 137, 138, 139
  pneumonia complication 205
  psoas 159
  renal 123, 124, 125–126
  renal transplantation 177
  subphrenic 162
accordion sign 136
N-acetylcysteine 162
acute abdomen 113–146
  acute cholecystitis 120–123
  acute gastrointestinal bleeding 129–130, 131, 132–135
  acute intestinal ischemia 140–143, 144, 145, 146
  acute pancreatitis 113–115, 116–117, 118, 119
  acute pyelonephritis 123–124, 125–126
  acute renal failure 127–128
  diverticulitis 135, 137, 138, 139
  graft-versus-host disease of bowel 136
  infectious enterocolitis 135–136
  inflammatory bowel diseases 135–137, 138, 139
  intussusception 166, 167, 215–218
  pediatric patients 207–218
    congenital megacolon 214
    examination technique 207–208
    gastrointestinal atresia/stenosis 213–214
    hypertrophic pyloric stenosis 215
    intussusception 215–218
    meconium ileus 208
    necrotizing enterocolitis 209–210, 211
  pseudomembranous enterocolitis 135, 136
  toxic megacolon 136–137
acute retropharyngeal abscess 197–198
acute tubular necrosis 177, 178
adult respiratory distress syndrome (ARDS) 37–49
  barotrauma 46, 47, 48, 49
  clinical parameters 37

complications 46, 47, 48–49
  CT 38, 40–42
  CT densitometry 41–42
  definitions 37
  diagnostic strategy 38
  differential diagnosis 44–46
  ECMO 43
  etiology 37
  fibrosis 49
  hydrostatic edema differential diagnosis 45, 46
  hyperinflated lung areas 42
  inhalation therapy 44
  liquid-assisted gas exchange 44
  Lung Injury Score 39
  multiorgan failure 49
  pathophysiology 37–38
  PEEP 40, 42–43
  phases 37–38, 38–39, 40–41
  pneumatocele 48
  pneumonia 48–49, 63, 70
    differential diagnosis 45–46
  pneumothorax 48
  positional changes 43–44
  pulmonary edema 36
  radiography 38–40
  scoring 39–40
  sepsis syndrome 49
  therapeutic measures effects on radiographic findings 42–44
  volutrauma 46, 47, 48
AIDS, pneumonia 66
air bronchograms, pulmonary edema 33
air-fluid level
  pleural empyema 96–97
  pneumonectomy 93, 94
allograft rejection
  heart transplantation 110
  lung transplantation 104, 105
alveolar edema 31–32
alveolar proteinosis 36
anal atresia 213
anastomotic leak
  biliary-enteric 173
  colorectal surgery 175, 176
  esophageal surgery 110, 111, 170, 171
  gastric surgery 171
  pancreatic surgery 172
  sleeve resection 103
anastomotic stricture 103
aneurysms
  gastrointestinal hemorrhage 130
  see also pseudoaneurysms

angel's wing sign 192
angiodysplasia 134, 135
angiography
  abdominal 152–153
  acute gastrointestinal bleeding 132–133, 134–135
  acute intestinal ischemia 145
antireflux operations 110
aortic aneurysm surgery/stenting 179–181
appendectomy, bleeding 176
apple-peel syndrome 214
arterial catheterization 21
arteriovenous fistula, renal transplantation 178
Aspergillus pneumonia 57
aspiration/aspiration pneumonia 56–61
asthma 200–201
atelectasis 70–74
  asthma 201
  bronchiolitis 201
  complete 71
  compression 71, 73
  esophageal surgery 111
  fibrotic 194
  foreign body aspiration 200
  imaging 71–73
  infantile respiratory distress syndrome 188, 190
  lobar 71, 72
  lobectomy 101, 102
  pathogenesis 70–71
  plate 70, 71
  pleural effusion differential diagnosis 73, 82, 84
  pneumonectomy 100
  pneumonia differential diagnosis 73–74
  postextubation 193
  postobstructive 72
  segmental 71
atrial arrhythmias 23

B

barotrauma
  ARDS 46, 47, 48, 49
  pneumomediastinum 192
  pneumothorax 76–77
  pulmonary interstitial emphysema 192
bile leaks 149, 174
bile peritonitis 149, 174
biliary drainage 148–149
biliary-enteric anastomosis 172
  leak 173, 174
biliary stents 148–149
biliary tract surgery 149, 173
bilioma 174

Billroth I and II operations
170–171
bladder catheterization 149
Bochdalek hernia *see* congenital
diaphragmatic hernia
bone marrow transplantation
64–65
bowel
adhesions 163, 164, 165
bird beak configuration 165,
213
graft-*versus*-host disease 136
malrotation 211–212, 213
rotation 211
thumbprinting 141, 212
see also colon; small bowel
bowel ischemia *see* intestinal
ischemia, acute
bowel obstruction
CT 164–165, 168
herniation 165, 166
imaging 164–165
incarceration 166, 168
intestinal ischemia 168
intussusception 166, *167*
mechanical 141, 163–164
dilatation of bowel 165
nephrectomy 176
toxic megacolon 137
transition zone 165
vesicular pneumatosis *146*
pneumatosis intestinalis *167*,
168
postoperative 163–166, *167*,
168
strangulated 165–166, *167*,
168
volvulus 165, 166, *167*
see also paralytic ileus
bowel wall thickening 165
bowel obstruction 168
hyperdense 143, *144*
bronchial cuffing in pulmonary
edema 33
bronchial dilatation 49
bronchiolitis 201–202
bronchiolitis obliterans 104,
201
bronchopleural fistula
pneumonia 68, 70
pneumothorax 97, *98*, *99*
bronchopulmonary dysplasia
193–194
bronchopulmonary fistula 26

C

cancer risk, radiation exposure
3, *5*
cardiac herniation 98
cardiac output monitoring 22
cardiac pacemakers 27–28
cardiac silhouette, enlarged 109
cardiac size 29

neonatal 185
cardiac surgery drains 28
cardiomegaly, pulmonary edema 33
cardiovascular surgery 106, *107*,
108–109
mediastinal hematoma 106,
107
mediastinitis 106, *108*
pseudoaneurysms 106, *107*
catheter jejunostomy 148
catheters for thoracic imaging
14–28
pediatric 185–186
celiac angiography, selective
132–133
central venous catheter
19–21, *22*
pediatric 186
chemical fibrinolysis, empyema
68, 70
chest radiography, portable
9–13
film–focus distance 10
grid effect 12
overexposure 12
poor image quality 11–12
projections 10
scatter-reduction grid 10
underexposure 12
undesired projections 11
chest tubes 24–26
complications 25–26
malposition 25, *26*
normal position 25
chest wall thickness 29–30
children *see* pediatric patients
cholangiography, T-tube 149
cholangitis 120–123
ascending bacterial 122
pathogenesis 120
cholascos 149
cholecystectomy 173–174, *175*
abscess 174
cholecystitis, acute 120–123
acalculous 120–121
emphysematous 121, *122*
gangrenous 121
choledochojejunostomy 171,
172
chylothorax 96, 111, 197
Clinical Pulmonary Infection
Score (CPIS) 62
Clostridium, emphysematous
cholecystitis 121
colitis, infectious/ischemic 137
colon
atresia 214
obstruction 164
wall thickening 142, *143*
colorectal surgery 174–176
colostomy 175
common bile duct drainage
148–149

communication, radiologists/
clinicians 13–14
computed radiography (CR) 2, 6
computed tomography (CT) 1
abdominal 151–152
ARDS 38, 40–42
atelectasis 72–73
catheter complications
15–16
chest radiography 15–16
dose reduction 5–6
dose–length product 6
with IV contrast for thrombosis 21
multislice spiral 15
pleural effusion 82, *85*
pneumonia 50–51, *54*,
55–56
pneumothorax 74, 75–77
pulmonary edema 34, *35*
pulmonary embolism 87, *88*,
89, *90*, *91*
radiation exposure in children 4–5
thoracic imaging 15–16
computed tomography (CT)
angiography 179
computed tomography (CT)
densitometry
abdominal 152
ARDS 41–42
computed tomography (CT)
Severity Index, acute pancreatitis *115*
congenital cystic adenomatoid
malformation 195, 196
congenital diaphragmatic hernia 196, *197*
congenital lobar emphysema
differential diagnosis 195
congenital heart disease, lobar
emphysema association 195
congenital lobar emphysema
195
congenital lung disease
194–197
congenital lymphangiectasia
197
congenital malformations,
radiation exposure 4
congenital megacolon 214
constrictive pericarditis, postpericardiotomy syndrome
109
contrast examination
acute renal failure 128
contraindication in toxic
megacolon 137
hypertrophic pyloric stenosis
215
lack of contrast in intestinal
ischemia 141, *142*
malrotation of gut 212
meconium ileus 208
pediatric acute abdomen 208

use in thoracic imaging
14–15
contrast extravasation, acute
gastrointestinal bleeding 133
conventional film-screen
radiography 2
creatinine 178
crescent-in-doughnut sign 216
Crohn disease 135
psoas abscess 159
toxic megacolon 136, 137
croup 200
crush kidney 127
cyclosporin A toxicity 177
cytomegalovirus (CMV)
heart transplantation 110
lung transplantation 104,
105
neonatal pneumonia 190

D

D-dimers, pulmonary embolism
86, *87*
defibrillators 27–28
devices, incomplete visualization 11
diagnostic imaging, problems in
ICU 1
digital radiography 2, 6
dose control 12–13
direct detector units 2
diverticulitis 135, 137, *138*, 139
perforated *138–139*
psoas abscess 159
toxic megacolon 137
diverticulosis 139
Doppler ultrasound, thrombosis
of subclavian vein/internal
jugular vein 21
dose indicators, digital radiography 13
dose–area product (DAP) 13
dose–length product (DLP) 6
double-target sign 123
duodenal atresia 213, 214
duodenal stenosis *212, 213*
duodenal stump leakage 171
duodenal tubes 26–27, 148
duodenal ulcer, bleeding/perfo-
rated *131*

E

echocardiography, pulmonary
embolism 87
embolization therapy 134
embryo, radiation exposure 3–4
emphysema
congenital lobar 195
mediastinal 199
pneumonia *58*

pulmonary interstitial 46, *47*, 191, *192*, 199
tracheostomy tube complications 17
empyema
  chemical fibrinolysis 68, 70
  hemithoracic opacity 205
  pediatric 205
  pneumonia 67–68, *69*
  sleeve resection 103
  thoracostomy 68
endobronchial intubation, endotracheal tube *16*, 17
endoleaks 179–180, *181*
endoscopic retrograde cholangiopancreatography (ERCP) 173
endotracheal tube 16–17, *18*
enterocolitis
  infectious 135–136
  pseudomembranous *135*, 136, 137
epiglottitis, acute 200
esophageal foreign body 200
esophageal intubation 17
esophageal myotomy, Heller technique 110
esophageal perforation 27
esophageal stricture *195*
esophageal surgery 110–111, 170, *171*
  anastomotic leak 110, *111*, 170, *171*
  tumor resection 170, *171*
esophageal varices, bleeding 129
esophagopleural fistula, pneumothorax 97–98, *99*
examinations, ordering 7
extra-corporeal membrane oxygenation (ECMO) 24, 28, 43
extracorporeal shock wave lithotripsy (ESWL) 176

F

feeding tubes 26–27, 148
fetal circulation, anatomy *185*
fetal lung fluid 183–184
fetus, radiation exposure 3–4
film–focus distance, portable chest radiography 10
fluorocarbon liquid-assisted gas exchange, ARDS 44
fluoroscopy
  portable machine 1
  thoracic imaging 15
football sign 209, *211*
foreign body aspiration 198–200
  empyema 205
fundoplication 170, *171*
fungal infections

G

gallbladder disorders 120–121
gallstone ileus 122
gastrectomy, partial/total 169–171
gastric surgery 169–171
gastric tubes 26–27
  pediatric 186
gastroduodenal artery aneurysm *130*
gastroduodenectomy, total 170
gastrointestinal bleeding, acute 129–130, *131*, 132–135
  angiography 132–133, 134–135
  causes 133, *134*
  contrast extravasation 133
  CT 129–130, *131*, 132, *133–134*
  diagnostic strategy 129–130, *131*, 132–133
  embolization therapy 134
  endoscopy 129
  extravasated blood 133
  imaging 129–130, *131*, 132, 133–135
  intramural bleeding 133–134
  pathogenesis 129
  provocation of bleeding 133
  pseudoaneurysms 130, 135
  vasopressin infusion 134
gastrointestinal tract
  arterial occlusion 140, 141, *142*
  atresia 213–214
  blood supply *140*
  hyperdense thickening of bowel wall 143, *144*
  malrotation 211–212, 213
  stenosis 213–214
  thumbprinting 141, 212
  venous occlusion 140, 141, *142*
gastrojejunostomy 171, *172*
Goodpasture syndrome *36*, 45
graft-*versus*-host disease, bowel 136
grid effect, portable chest radiography 12

H

halo sign 141, 168
heart transplantation 109–110

heart transplantation 110
lung transplantation 105
pneumonia 51, *57*

heart valve surgery 109
Heller technique of modified esophageal myotomy 110
hemidiaphragm, midclavicular line 11, *12*
hemithorax, opaque 200, 205
hemopericardium, pacemaker complication 28
hemothorax *21*, 95
hepatic abscess 160, *161*
  acute pancreatitis 122–123
hepatic artery thrombosis *180*
hepaticojejunostomy 173
Hirschsprung disease 214
HIV infection 66, *146*
hyaline membrane disease *see* infantile respiratory distress syndrome
hydrocarbon liquid ingestion 199–200
hydronephrosis 127–128
  decompression 149
  urinary tract obstruction 178
hydrothorax, lobectomy 101
hypertrophic pyloric stenosis (HPS) 215

I

ileal atresia 213, 214
ileal conduit construction 176
immunodeficiency
  infections in children 203, *204*
  pneumonia 64–66
  recurrent lung infections 203
immunosuppression, pneumonia 64–66
Impella device 24, *25*
implantable cardioverter defibrillators (ICDs) 27
incarceration, bowel obstruction 166, 168
infantile respiratory distress syndrome 188, *189*, 190
  neonatal pneumonia differential diagnosis 191
  transient tachypnea of the newborn differential diagnosis 187
infections
  acute pancreatitis 116, *117*, 118
  aortic aneurysm surgery/ stenting 180
  bronchiolitis 201, 202
  cholecystectomy 174
  emphysematous cholecystitis 121, *122*
  heart transplantation 110
  lobectomy 101, *102*
  lung transplantation 104, 105, 109
  recurrent lung 203

staphylococcal hematogenous spread 123
  see also abscess; pyelonephritis, acute
infectious colitis, toxic megacolon 137
infectious enterocolitis 135–136
inflammatory bowel disease 135–137, *138*, 139
inhalation therapy, ARDS 44
inspiration, inadequate depth 11, *12*
internal jugular vein thrombosis 21
International Commission on Radiological Protection (1991), risk coefficients 3
intestinal ischemia, acute 140–143, *144*, 145, *146*
  angiography 145
  bowel obstruction 168
  diagnostic strategy 140
  pathogenesis 140
  pneumatosis intestinalis 141, 143, *145*, *146*
intra-abdominal abscess 152, 157, 158–163
  catheters for drainage 162–163
  clinical aspects 159
  density 160, *161*
  differential diagnosis 161–162
  drainage 162–163
  gas collections 160, *161*
  intraparenchymal 160–161
  N-acetylcysteine treatment 162
  pathogenesis 158–159
  pyogenic 160, *161*
  rim enhancement 159–160
  site of occurrence 158, *159*
  urokinase treatment 162, *163*
intra-aortic balloon pump 23–24
intraparenchymal abscess 160–161
intraparenchymal hematoma 154, *155*
intraperitoneal abscess 158
intrapulmonary hemorrhage 193
intrapulmonary vessels 29
intussusception 215–218
  bowel obstruction 166, *167*
  recurrence 218
  reduction methods 217–218

J

jejunal atresia *213*, 214
jejunal tubes 26–27
jejunostomy tube 148

L

Ladd bands *212*, 213
laryngotracheobronchitis 200
lead aprons, equivalency 5
lead screens 5
left superior vena cava, persistent 20–21
leukemia, latent period 3
liquid-assisted gas exchange, ARDS 44
listeriosis, transplacental 190
lithiasis, gallbladder 120
liver transplantation 178–179, *180*
lobar torsion 101, *102*
lobectomy 101, *102*
lung(s)
  cavitation in pneumonia 67
  hyperinflation 42
    asthma 200
    bronchiolitis 200, 202
    foreign body aspiration 198, *199*
    lobectomy 101
    meconium aspiration *189*
    neonatal pneumonia 191
  incomplete visualization 11
  volume in pulmonary edema 33
lung disease
  congenital 194–197
  drug-induced/immunologic 45
  HIV infection *66*
  see also named conditions
lung fluid, fetal 183–184
Lung Injury Score (LIS) 39
lung resection
  segmental 102
  sleeve 103
  see also pneumonectomy
lung transplantation 103–105
  airway complications 104, *105*
  anastomotic leak 104, *105*
  imaging 103–104
  infections 104, 105, 109
  initial dysfunction 104
  osteomyelitis 108–109
  postoperative findings 103–105
  postpericardiotomy syndrome 109
  rejection 104, *105*
  sternal dehiscence 106, 108–109
  valvular surgery complications 109
lymphocele 177

M

magnetic resonance cholangio-pancreatography (MRCP) 174
malrotation of gut 211–212, 213
mechanical ventilation 191
  infantile respiratory distress syndrome *189*
  pediatric complications 185, *189*, 191–194
  pneumonia 61–63
meconium aspiration/meconium aspiration syndrome *189*, 190
meconium ileus 208
mediastinal emphysema 199
mediastinal hematoma
  cardiovascular surgery 106, *107*
  central venous catheter complication *21*
mediastinal lipomatosis 110
mediastinal shift
  pleural empyema 96
  pneumonectomy 93, *94*, 95
mediastinitis, cardiovascular surgery 106, *108*
Mendelson syndrome 56, 59–61
mesenteric insufficiency, non-occlusive 140
middle lobe syndrome 101, *102*
monitoring devices, thoracic imaging 14–28
multiorgan dysfunction syndrome (MODS) 156
multiorgan failure, ARDS 49
Murphy sign 121
myocardial perforation 28

N

N-acetylcysteine, intra-abdominal abscess treatment 162
necrotizing enterocolitis 209–210, *211*
neonates
  cardiac size 185
  intrapulmonary hemorrhage 193
  lung fluid 183–184
  mechanical ventilation 185
  normal thoracic findings 183–185
  pleural effusion 197, 204–205
  pneumothorax 192
  postextubation atelectasis 193
  preterm 190, 193
  thymus 184–185
  transient tachypnea of the newborn 187
  see also congenital *conditions*
nephrectomy 176
nephritis
  focal bacterial 124, *125*
  see also pyelonephritis, acute
neutropenia, pneumonia-associated 64, 65
Nissen fundoplication 170, *171*
nitric oxide inhalation 44

O

organ transplantation
  bone marrow 64–65
  cardiac 109–110
  pneumonia in immunodeficient/immunosuppressed patients 64
  renal 176–178
  see also lung transplantation
osteomyelitis, lung transplantation 108–109

P

pancreas, annular 213
pancreatic abscess 115, 118, 172, *173*
pancreatic surgery 171–173
pancreaticoenteric anastomosis 172
pancreaticojejunostomy 171, *172*
pancreatitis, acute 113–115, *116–117*, 118, *119*
  bacterial contamination 114
  classification 114–115
  complications 115, *117*, 118, *119*
  CT Severity Index 115
  gallstone ileus 122
  hemorrhage 118, *119*
  hemorrhagic necrotizing form 114, *116–117*
  hepatic abscess 122–123
  infections 116, *117*, 118
  necrotizing 114, *116–117*, 118, *119*
  pseudoaneurysms 118, *119*
  pseudocysts *115*, 118
  serous exudative form 114, *116*
  suppurative form 115, *117*
  vascular complications 118, *119*
paralytic ileus 141, 154, 163
pediatric patients

radiation dose reduction 5
radiation exposure 4–5
  see also acute abdomen, pediatric patients; thoracic imaging, pediatric patients
percutaneous endoscopic gastrostomy (PEG) tube 148
percutaneous nephrostomy 149
pericardial drainage 28
pericardial effusion 110
pericardial tamponade 28, 109
pericardiocentesis 28
pericholecystic abscess 121
pericolic abscess 137, *138*, 139
peristalsis resumption after surgery 150, 159
peritoneal compartments 157, *158*
peritonitis 156–158
  biliary 149, 174
  with septic shock 137, *138–139*
plain abdominal radiography 151
  pediatric patients 207–208
pleural effusion *69*, 80–82, *83–85*
  atelectasis differential diagnosis 73, 82, *84*
  lung transplantation 103
  mediastinitis association 106
  neonates 191, 197
  pediatric 204–205
  pneumonia
    differential diagnosis 82, *85*
    neonatal 191
pleural empyema 96–97
pleural fluid, draining 25
pneumatocele 48, 67
  pediatric 205
pneumatosis intestinalis 141, 143, *145*, 146
  bowel obstruction *167*, 168
  pediatric patients 209
Pneumocystis jirovecii infection *53*, *58*, 66
pneumomediastinum 191–192, 201
  foreign body aspiration 199
pneumonectomy 93, *94*, 95–98, *99*, 100, 102
  air-fluid level 93, *94*
  air leaks 102
  anastomotic leak 98
  atelectasis 100
  chylothorax 96
  edema 95
  fluid collection 102
  hemothorax 95
  mediastinal shift 93, *94*, 95
  pneumonia 100
  pneumothorax 102
  pseudotumor 102
  segmental 102

sleeve 103
pneumonectomy syndrome 98,
100
pneumonia 49–70
abscess complication 205
alveolar edema differential
diagnosis 32
ARDS 48–49, 63, 70
differential diagnosis
45–46
aspiration 56–61
atelectasis differential diagnosis 73–74
atypical infections 51, *55, 56*
bilateral lobar 54
bone marrow transplantation
64–65
bronchopleural fistula 68, 70
causative organisms 50–51,
53
children 203–205
classification 49–50
complications 67–70
pediatric 204–205
congenital cystic adenomatoid malformation differ-
ential diagnosis 196
consolidation *59*
CT 50–51, 51–52, *54, 55–56*
differential diagnosis 52, 56
emphysema *58*
empyema 67–68, *69*
esophageal surgery 111
feeding tube complication 27
foreign body aspiration 199
fungal infections 51, *57*
heart transplantation 110
HIV infection 66
imaging 51–52
immunodeficient/immuno-
suppressed patients 64–66
infantile respiratory distress
syndrome differential
diagnosis 190
lung cavitation 67
mechanical ventilation
61–63
necrotizing 67, 100
neonatal 190–191
nosocomial infections 49, 50
opacification patterns 51, *52*
opportunistic infections 49
organ transplantation 64
pathogen classification
50–51
pathogenesis 50
pleural effusion differential
diagnosis 82, *85*
pneumatocele 67
pneumonectomy 100
pulmonary abscess 67
pulmonary edema 36
radiography 51–52
recurrent 201
round 203

septic *54,* 63
transient tachypnea of the
newborn differential diagnosis 187
tree-in-bud sign 51, *54*
ventilator-associated 61–63
viral infections 51, *56*
pneumonitis, chemical 190, 200
pneumoperitoneum
after abdominal surgery
150–151, 157
necrotizing enterocolitis 209,
210
peritonitis 157
pneumothorax 74–77, *78, 79*
ARDS 48
barotrauma 76–77
bronchopleural fistula 97, *98,
99*
cardiac herniation 98
central venous catheter complications 21
congenital lobar emphysema
differential diagnosis 195
differential diagnosis 77, *78,
79*
esophagopleural fistula
97–98, *99*
evacuation 25
feeding tube complication 27
foreign body aspiration 199
lobectomy 101
meconium aspiration syn-
drome *189,* 190
neonates 192
pacemaker complication 28
pleural empyema 96–97
pneumonectomy 102
pulmonary interstitial emphysema as precursor 191
tracheostomy tube complications 17, 19
volume estimation 75–76
see also tension pneumothorax
positive end-expiratory pressure (PEEP)
ARDS 40, 42–43
radiolucency changes 61
postpericardiotomy syndrome
109
postpneumonectomy edema 95
pregnancy, radiation exposure
3–4
preterm infants 190, 193
proctectomy 174–175
prostacyclin inhalation 44
prostaglandin inhalation 44
pseudoaneurysms
acute pancreatitis 118, *119*
cardiovascular surgery 106,
107
gastrointestinal hemorrhage
130, 135
renal transplantation 178

pseudocavitation 205
pseudocysts, acute pancreatitis
115, 118
pseudomembranous entero-
colitis *135,* 136, 137
Pseudomonas 104, 105, 110
psoas abscess 159
pulmonary abscess 67
pulmonary artery aneurysm/
rupture 23
pulmonary artery catheter
22–23
pulmonary capillary wedge
pressure 22
pulmonary edema 30–36
alveolar 31–32
crazy paving pattern 34, 36
evaluation 30–34, *35,* 36
foreign body aspiration 199
gravity-dependent 36
hydrostatic 30, 33, 44–45, 46
infiltrative spread *35*
interstitial 30, *31,* 32
neurogenic *33, 34*
noncardiogenic 33, 103
permeability 30, 32, 33, *34*
postobstructive *33, 34*
re-expansion *33, 35*
reactive 199
pulmonary embolism 86–89,
90–91
D-dimers 86, *87*
differential diagnosis 86, 87
mosaic perfusion 87, *89*
pretest probability 86
pulmonary infarction 87, *88*
pulsation/respiratory artifacts *90*
segmental 89, *90*
pulmonary fibrosis, ARDS 49
pulmonary hemodynamics
29–30
pulmonary hemorrhage 36, 45
pulmonary infarction 23, 87, *88*
pulmonary interstitial emphysema (PIE) 46, *47,* 191, *192*
pulmonary vascular redistribution to upper zones 33
pyelonephritis, acute 123–124,
125–126
emphysematous 123, 124,
126
renal abscess 123, 124,
125–126
pyeloplasty 176
pyloric stenosis, hypertrophic
215
pylorospasm 215
pylorus-preserving pancreaticoduodenectomy 171, *172*
pyonephrosis 123, 124, *125, 126*
pyoserothorax 96

R

radiation, scattered 5
radiation dose reduction 5
radiation exposure 3–5
radiation safety 3–6
radiographic equipment 1
radiographic techniques 1–2
radiological examination 4
radiology findings 7
radiology services, ordering 13
radionuclide imaging 153
recurrent laryngeal nerve palsy
111
renal abscess 123, 124,
125–126
renal artery stenosis 178
renal cortical necrosis 127, 128
renal failure, acute 127–128
renal surgery 176–178
renal transplantation
176–178
renal vein thrombosis 178
reperfusion edema 103
respiratory failure in esophageal surgery 111
retroperitoneal hematoma 154,
155
retropharyngeal abscess
197–198
right-heart overload 87, 89
Rigler sign 209, *211*
ring sign 159, *160*
Roux-en-Y reconstruction 170,
171

S

scatter-reduction grid 10
Schoenlein–Henoch purpura
130
scintigraphy, abdominal surgery 153
selective celiac angiography
132–133
sepsis, abdominal surgery
154–163
sepsis syndrome, ARDS 49
septal lines, pulmonary edema
33
shock bowel 143, *145*
sigmoid volvulus 212–213
bowel obstruction 165, 166,
167
skin folds, pneumothorax
differential diagnosis 77, *78*
small bowel
adhesions 163, *164*
contrast series 164
faeces sign 165
graft-*versus*-host disease 136
hyperdense thickening 143,
144
infarction 142–143, *144*

intramural bleeding 129, 133–134
ischemia 129, 143, *144*
mechanical obstruction 176
wall thickening 142
spinnaker sail sign 192
splenic artery aneurysms 118, *119*
sternal dehiscence, lung transplantation 106, 108–109
stomach tube 148
subclavian vein thrombosis 21
subphrenic abscess *162*
surfactant administration
ARDS 44
infantile respiratory distress syndrome 190
surfactant deficiency disease
see infantile respiratory distress syndrome
Swan–Ganz catheter 22, *23*
Swyer–James syndrome 201

T

target sign 168
tension pneumothorax 48, 78, 80
meconium aspiration syndrome *189*, 190
sleeve resection 103
thoracic imaging 9–92
after surgery 93–112
ARDS 37–49
atelectasis 70–74
cardiovascular surgery 106, *107*, 108–109
catheters 14–28
computed tomography 15–16
contrast use 14–15
device localization 14
diagnostic strategy 14–15
emergency orders 13, 14
esophageal surgery 110–111
fluoroscopy 15

heart transplantation 109–110
lobectomy 101, *102*
lung transplantation 103–105
monitoring devices 14–28
pediatric patients 183–206
acute obstruction of upper airways 197–200
asthma 200–201
bronchiolitis 201–202
bronchopulmonary dysplasia 193–194
catheter position 185–186
congenital lung disease 194–197
foreign body aspiration 198–200
infantile respiratory distress syndrome 188, *189*, 190
intrapulmonary hemorrhage 193
mechanical ventilation complications 191–194
neonatal pneumonia 190–191
normal findings in newborns 183–185
pneumomediastinum 191–192
pneumonia 203–205
pneumothorax 192
postextubation atelectasis 193
pulmonary interstitial emphysema 191, *192*
tracheoesophageal fistula 194–195
transient tachypnea of the newborn 187
pleural effusion 80–82, *83–85*
pneumonectomy 93, *94*, 95–98, *99*, 100
pneumonia 49–70
pneumothorax 74–77, *78, 79*
portable chest radiography 9–13

pulmonary embolism 86–89, *90–91*
radiology service ordering 13
reporting 14
routine orders 13, 14
segmental lung resection 102
sleeve resection 103
tension pneumothorax 78, 80
thoracic veins 20–21
thoracostomy 68
thoracostomy tubes 24–26
thrombosis, intravenous with central venous catheter 21
thymus
neonatal 184–185
pneumomediastinum/pneumothorax 192
tonsillitis 200
toxic megacolon 136–137
trachea
iatrogenic rupture 17, *18*
necrosis after esophageal surgery 111
tracheitis, exudative 200
tracheoesophageal fistula 194–195
tracheostomy tube 17, *18*, 19
transient tachypnea of the newborn 187
transurethral resection of the prostate (TUR) 127
Treitz ligament 212, 213
triangle sign 209, *211*
TUR syndrome 127

U

ulcerative colitis 135
subtotal colectomy 175–176
toxic megacolon 136, 137
ultrasonography
abdominal 151, 152
pediatric patients 207
pleural effusion 80, 81, *83*
pneumothorax 74, 77
thoracic imaging 15
umbilical artery catheter 185–186

umbilical vein catheter 186
upper airways, acute obstruction 197–200
ureteral outflow obstruction 177
ureteral reconstruction 176
ureteral stenosis 175
ureteral stenting 149
ureteroneocystostomy 176
urinary tract drainage 149
urinary tract obstruction, renal transplantation 178
urinoma 177
urokinase 162, *163*
urosepsis 123–124, *125–126*

V

vascular pedicle 29, 33
vascular prostheses 180–181
vasopressin 134
ventilator-associated pneumonia (VAP) 61–63
ventilator-induced lung injury 46, *47*, 48
ventricular arrhythmias 23
viral infections
pneumonia 51, *56*
see also cytomegalovirus (CMV)
volume CT dose index (CTDI$_{vol}$) 5–6
volvulus 212–213
bowel obstruction 165, 166, *167*

W

wet lung 187
Whipple operation 171–173
whirlpool sign 212

X

x-ray fluoroscopy 15